Chronic Care Nursing

A Framework for Practice

Second edition

Chronic conditions have a substantial and increasing global impact on life and health care. Health systems need to adapt to address these shifting health priorities, while nurses require specialised skills to implement changes and create better client outcomes. *Chronic Care Nursing: A Framework for Practice* provides a comprehensive and accessible overview of the role of the nurse in managing chronic conditions across a variety of settings in Australia and New Zealand.

The first part of the book outlines two essential approaches to chronic care management – the Chronic Care Model and the World Health Organization's Innovative Care for Chronic Conditions Framework – while the second part covers key conditions within chronic care nursing. The second edition has been fully updated to include the latest research, and features new chapters covering self-management and empowerment; living with mental health issues; chronic bowel conditions; and eye, ear and dental health.

Written by an expert author team of practising nurses and academics, *Chronic Care Nursing* continues to provide students and practising nurses with the essential skills required to be effective in evolving health systems.

Linda Deravin is a lecturer in the School of Nursing, Midwifery and Indigenous Health at Charles Sturt University.

Judith Anderson is an adjunct senior lecturer in the School of Nursing, Midwifery and Indigenous Health at Charles Sturt University and General Manager at Opal Specialist Aged Care, Bathurst, New South Wales.

Second edition

Chronic Care Nursing

A Framework for Practice

Edited by
Linda Deravin and
Judith Anderson

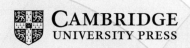

CAMBRIDGE
UNIVERSITY PRESS

University Printing House, Cambridge CB2 8BS, United Kingdom

One Liberty Plaza, 20th Floor, New York, NY 10006, USA

477 Williamstown Road, Port Melbourne, VIC 3207, Australia

314–321, 3rd Floor, Plot 3, Splendor Forum, Jasola District Centre, New Delhi – 110025, India

79 Anson Road, #06–04/06, Singapore 079906

Cambridge University Press is part of the University of Cambridge.

It furthers the University's mission by disseminating knowledge in the
pursuit of education, learning and research at the highest international
levels of excellence.

www.cambridge.org
Information on this title: www.cambridge.org/9781108701020

© Cambridge University Press 2016, 2019

First published 2016
Second edition 2019

Cover designed by Fiona Byrne
Typeset by SPi Global
Printed in Singapore by Markono Print Media Pte Ltd, March 2019

A catalogue record for this publication is available from the British Library

A catalogue record for this book is available from the National Library of Australia

ISBN 978-1-108-70102-0 Paperback

Additional resources for this publication at www.cambridge.edu.au/academic/chronic

....

The editors would like to dedicate this
text to nurses of the future.

Linda Deravin and Judith Anderson

Contents

Preface

Impact of chronic conditions in Australia and New Zealand, and worldwide

This is the second edition of *Chronic Care Nursing: A Framework for Practice*, which we believe will be a useful resource for this area of clinical nursing practice. This book has been developed for undergraduate nurses and registered nurses who wish to develop their knowledge about the care of people living with chronic conditions in our communities.

The structure of this book is based on the Innovative Care for Chronic Conditions Framework (ICCCF), which is an internationally recognised framework for the delivery of chronic care. The ICCCF extends the Chronic Care Model (CCM) that was developed by Wagner (Wagner et al., 1999). The CCM is well recognised to provide a systematic approach to chronic care management. It incorporates six components: health system (organisation of health care), self-management support, decision support, delivery-system design, clinical information systems, and community resources and policies (Stellefson, Dipnarine & Stopka, 2013). The model provides a multidimensional solution to the complex problem of the provision of chronic care (Bodenheimer, Wagner & Grumbach, 2002).

The CCM has been expanded and internationalised by the World Health Organization (WHO) to be developed into the ICCCF. Nurses need to lead the redesign of the health care system in order to improve health outcomes through the implementation of the CCM. The ICCCF extends the CCM by adding micro, meso and macro levels and incorporates six guiding principles: evidence-based decision making, population health approach, focus on prevention, quality focus, integration, and flexibility and adaptability (WHO, 2002; 2018). These levels extend the involvement of community, and describe policies and financing as the drivers at the macro level (Epping-Jordan et al., 2004). An important aspect of the implementation of this model and framework is how well it is integrated into undergraduate nursing education so that an informed and well-prepared nursing workforce is established in Australia and New Zealand (Anderson & Malone, 2015). For this reason, the following competencies table outlines how each chapter aligns to the standards of practice for registered nurses in Australia and New Zealand.

The first section of this textbook focuses on the ICCCF to support the learning of undergraduate student nurses about the complexity of chronic conditions and how it is best implemented to improve patient outcomes at both a national and international level. An additional chapter has been included in the second edition that focuses on self-management of the person with chronic conditions. The second section supports the ICCCF and includes a chapter on each of the Australian National Health Priority Areas of asthma, cancer, diabetes, cardiovascular disease, injury prevention and control, arthritis and musculoskeletal conditions, mental health, obesity, and dementia. There are also chapters about other chronic conditions such as chronic kidney disease, disability, end of life care, and Parkinson's disease and multiple sclerosis. Additional chapters have been added to address chronic bowel conditions; and chronic eye, ear and dental health. This is provided within the Australian and New Zealand context.

Linda Deravin and Judith Anderson

REFERENCES

Anderson, J. & Malone, L. (2015). Chronic care undergraduate nursing education in Australia. *Nurse Education Today*, 35(12), 1135–8. doi: http://10.1016/j.nedt.2015.08.008

Bodenheimer, T., Wagner, E. H. & Grumbach, K. (2002). Improving primary care for patients with chronic illness. *Journal of the American Medical Association*, 288(15), 1909–14.

Epping-Jordan, J. E., Pruitt, S. D., Bengoa, R. & Wagner, E. H. (2004). Improving the quality of health care for chronic conditions. *Quality and Safety in Health Care*, 13(4), 299–305. doi: http://10.1136/qshc.2004.010744

Stellefson, M., Dipnarine, K. & Stopka, C. (2013). The Chronic Care Model and diabetes management in US primary care settings: A systematic review. *Preventing Chronic Disease*, 10, E26. doi: http://10.5888/pcd10.120180

Wagner, E. H., Davis, C., Schaefer, J., Von Korff, M. & Austin, B. T. (1999). A survey of leading chronic disease management programs: Are they consistent with the literature? *Managed Care Quarterly*, 7, 56–66.

World Health Organization (WHO) (2002). *Innovative Care for Chronic Conditions: Building Blocks for Action Global Report.* Geneva: WHO.

—— (2018). *Global Action Plan for the Prevention and Control of Noncommunicable Diseases (NCDs): 2013–2020.* Geneva: WHO. Retrieved from www.who.int/nmh/events/ncd_action_plan/en/

Contributors

Judith Anderson (RN, PhD, MHSM, MN, BN, FACN) is an adjunct senior lecturer in the School of Nursing, Midwifery and Indigenous Health at Charles Sturt University and General Manager at Opal Specialist Aged Care, Bathurst, New South Wales. She has been a registered nurse for more than 20 years, working in a variety of clinical, education, research and managerial positions. Judith has worked in a variety of settings, including chronic care, acute care, rural health, aged care and community health in the public and private sectors. Judith develops nursing curricula and supervises higher degree students and is a fellow of the Australian College of Nursing.

Kathryn Anderson (RN, BN) is a registered nurse with a keen interest in chronic care areas of health.

Melissa Arnold-Chamney is a lecturer in the Nursing School at the University of Adelaide. She has worked in the renal care setting for over 20 years, first in the clinical setting and since 2001 in the higher education sector. Melissa is the Chief Editor of the *Renal Society of Australasia Journal*.

Kylie Ash (RN) is a registered nurse with over 20 years' experience in clinical and education roles in oncology and haematology practice settings. She completed a Master of Nursing (Cancer Nursing) from Queensland University of Technology in 2008. Kylie has been involved in a number of large national workforce development projects to improve the intersection of health education and evidence-based practice with health policy. She is the National Manager for the Palliative Care Curriculum for Undergraduates project (PCC4U). Kylie is also the Vice President of the Cancer Nurses Society of Australia.

Michelle Baird (RN, CTC Certificate, BA Liberal Studies, MN – Nurse Practitioner) is a chronic and complex care nurse practitioner who has worked in chronic care in rural Western New South Wales for the past 20 years. Michelle is interested in chronic heart failure, chronic obstructive pulmonary disease (COPD), smoking cessation and self-management. She has recently completed research in COPD self-management. Michelle is the Chair of the COPD Nurse Committee for the Lung Foundation Australia.

Marguerite Bramble is Associate Professor in the School of Nursing, Midwifery and Indigenous Health at Charles Sturt University. As a senior nurse academic, Marguerite's extensive clinical, education and research expertise is chronic care nursing, with a focus on neurological conditions affecting the older population such as dementia and Parkinson's disease. She has national recognition for her expertise in managing and implementing innovative, evidence-based models and clinical trial interventions.

Sally Bristow (RN, BN MN, RM Grad Dip Mid, PhD candidate) is a registered nurse, registered midwife and lecturer at the School of Health in Nursing, University of New England. Sally researches and teaches in the area of chronic health conditions. Her research mainly lies in the fields of carer experience. Sally joined the School of Health in 2013. She was previously a clinical nurse consultant in Aboriginal chronic care, the Director of Nursing and Midwifery and, prior to this, an area nurse manger in renal service. Before working in senior nursing and executive positions, Sally worked as a registered nurse and midwife in remote, rural and metropolitan hospitals across Australia.

Rhonda Brown (RN) is a senior lecturer at Deakin University. She is an experienced clinician and educator, with a background in community and mental health nursing, counselling and family therapy, and community and tertiary education.

Kate Cameron is a senior lecturer in the Adelaide Nursing School at the University of Adelaide, and the Nursing Service Director for the Michael Rice Centre for Haematology and Oncology at the Women's and Children's Hospital in South Australia. Kate's professional experience over the past 25 years encompasses clinical, management, leadership and academic roles in cancer nursing. Her areas of interest include the impact of rurality on people with cancer, effective and sustainable consumer engagement in cancer care and policy development, clinical governance, and tertiary education for specialist clinicians.

Ysanne Chapman (RN, PhD, MSc (Hons), BEd (Nsg), GDE, DNE) has retired from academic life and is now an independent scholar. She is a former Dean of Nursing and Midwifery at CQU in Mackay, Queensland. Ysanne's professional research interests have included dying and death, curriculum issues, caring, and diabetes. She now consults on matters of curriculum, advanced nursing practice and international community care. She also edits and marks PhD dissertations and masters' theses, and is an adjunct professor at James Cook University. Ysanne has instructed undergraduate and postgraduate nursing students in many aspects of nursing practice. She has published several books, chapters and journal articles in all areas of nursing.

Lyn Croxon (RN, MEd, Grad Dip Geront) is a lecturer at Charles Stuart University, and has worked in clinical and academic roles for more than 40 years. Lyn has taught across a range of subjects and coordinated the Bachelor of Nursing course across five campuses. Her research interests include care of older person, the impact of delirium, palliative care education, and models of clinical placement supervision.

Maria Davies works as a chronic care clinical nurse consultant for Dubbo Health Service. Maria coordinates the cardiopulmonary rehabilitation programs and works closely with the Dubbo respiratory teams. As part of her role, Maria conducts ward reviews of patients, coordinates exercise and self-management classes, and provides patient education on chronic disease risk factor modification and behavioural change. Maria also coordinates the long-term and short-term Home Oxygen Programs at Dubbo, and the patient enable-based CPAP loan program. Prior to this, Maria worked for over 10 years in intensive care.

Linda Deravin (RN, BN, MHM, Grad Cert in L&T in Higher Ed, Grad Cert Anaes & Rec Room Nurs, Grad Dip Gerontology, Grad Cert E Health, FCHSM) is a lecturer in nursing at Charles Sturt University. Throughout her 30-year nursing career, she has worked as a clinician, an educator, a senior nurse and a health manager. She has a keen interest in Indigenous health, nursing workforce and chronic care issues that influence and impact on health systems and the delivery of nursing care.

Alison Devitt (RN, MN, Grad Cert Teaching and Learning in Higher Education, Grad Dip Divinity, Cert Health Coaching) is a lecturer in nursing at Charles Sturt University. She is known for her passion exploring the use of educational technologies for online learning. Alison's interest in technology stems from her past role as a telemonitoring nurse. She continues to provide consultancy and contributes to research in this innovative area of chronic disease management.

Tracey Doherty is the Nursing Director of the Centre for Health Innovation at Gold Coast Health and a PhD candidate at Griffith University. Her strategic and research interests include development and implementation of innovative nursing and midwifery models of care to better meet the needs of the community. With a nursing and health leadership career spanning over 30 years, Tracey remains committed to partnering with consumers and clinicians to deliver person-centred, integrated care that is safe, effective and sustainable. She completed a Master of Nursing (Nurse Practitioner) in 2004 and was Australia's first endorsed Oncology Nurse Practitioner in 2005.

Marion Eckert is the Chair of the Cancer Care Research Group, University of South Australia, and the inaugural Professor of Cancer Nursing in South Australia. She is also the inaugural Director at the Rosemary Bryant AO Research Centre at the School of Nursing and Midwifery, University of South Australia, which was established as a partnership with the Australian Nursing and Midwifery Federation (South Australia branch). Marion brings more than 25 years' experience in the health care industry and has a strong clinical academic background. She completed her professional doctorate from University of Adelaide in 2004. Marion has won peer-reviewed excellence awards for her clinical leadership, and was awarded the 2015 Winston Churchill Fellowship for her dedication and passion for cancer survivorship research.

Karen Francis (RN, PhD, MEd, MHlth Sc PHC, Grad Cert Uni Teach/Learn, B Hlth Sc Nsg, Dip Hlth Sc Nsg, FRCNA, FJBI) holds the position of Professor and Head of the Nursing Discipline at the University of Tasmania. Her research interests include nursing and midwifery workforce, rural nursing and midwifery, primary health care, and rural health.

Michelle Francis is a senior therapist in drug treatment and has a master's degree in addictive behaviours. She has been working in health and human services for over 10 years as a clinician, in leadership and in research. Michelle's practice domains have included homelessness, complex care, mental health, and emergency and drug treatment. Her research focus has been long-term homelessness and access to drug treatment, stigma and dual diagnosis.

Julia Gilbert is a lecturer in the School of Nursing and Healthcare Professions at Federation University in Ballarat, Victoria. She has over 30 years' experience in a variety of clinical and academic settings with an interest in dementia care. Julia also completed a Bachelor of Laws and a Graduate Diploma of Legal Practice and was admitted to the Supreme Court of Queensland as a legal practitioner in 2008.

Amali Hohol is a lecturer in nursing at Charles Sturt University. Amali is a registered nurse with extensive experience and knowledge in critical care nursing, and she continues to practise clinically.

Melissa Johnston (RN, BN, Grad Cert N (Critical Care), Grad Dip N(Cardiovascular)) is a clinical nurse educator in the Coronary Care Department of Orange Health Service. Melissa has worked in critical care throughout her career with extensive experience and knowledge in cardiovascular and intensive care nursing.

Kathryn Kent was the Family and Carer Mental Health Support Worker/Education Officer with CentaCare Wilcannia-Forbes in the Family and Carer Mental Health Program, funded by NSW Health. Her involvement in supporting the education of nursing students in chronic and complex care of mental health issues began in 2011, with the introduction of carers and those living with mental health issues presenting their lived experience of mental health problems to nursing and paramedic students at Charles Sturt University.

Mooreen Macleay is the Clinical Nurse Consultant for Cancer Care Coordination in the Western NSW Local Health District (Bathurst Region). Mooreen has extensive clinical experience in palliative care as well as primary, secondary and tertiary nursing in the public and private sectors.

Jennifer Manning (RN, BA, Grad Dip OH&S, Grad Dip Education, MN, MACN) is an associate lecturer in nursing at Charles Sturt University. Jennifer has spent over 30 years working in many different care environments including cardiothoracic, spinal and emergency nursing, occupational health and rehabilitation, and education. Jennifer's passion is education and facilitating undergraduate nursing students in their passage to becoming registered.

Denise McGarry is a Credentialed Mental Health Nurse with life-long experience in mental health nursing as an academic in tertiary education and in the clinical environment. She has taught undergraduate paramedic and nursing programs, and post-graduate mental health nursing programs. She has also had roles in staff training and education in the clinical arena, as well as a variety of management positions. Denise is a fellow of the Australian College of Mental Health Nurses.

Maureen Miles is the Coordinator of Midwifery Programs at Deakin University. She has worked in hospitals and the community as a nurse, midwife, and maternal and child health nurse.

Amanda Moses (BN, Grad Dip Onc Nursing, MN (NP)) has over 30 years' nursing experience – covering metropolitan, rural and remote locations – and in many diverse settings including ICU, coronary care, paediatrics, community health, surgical and acute medical care. Amanda's interest in primary and community health led her to a focus in this field, specifically within rural and remote areas; her specialisation has included oncological nursing. Her passion for improving the quality of life for people with chronic and complex conditions led Amanda to qualify as an endorsed nurse practitioner, with a scope of practice for chronic disease management. Amanda now lectures at Charles Sturt University, teaching undergraduate primary health care and chronic disease management, and postgraduate chronic disease management and clinical education.

Patience Moyo (RN, GradCertAcutMed/SurgNurs, MA (AdvNursPract)) is a lecturer in nursing at Charles Sturt University. She qualified as a nurse in Zimbabwe and has gained experience in the fields of medical-surgical nursing, paediatric nursing, critical care nursing, emergency care nursing, midwifery, nursing education, and surgical and post-anaesthetic care nursing.

Maryanne Podham is a lecturer in nursing at Charles Sturt University, with a passion for student-centred education and improving clinical practice. She has over 20 years' experience in clinical nursing in rural New South Wales.

Amanda Stott is a lecturer in nursing at Charles Sturt University, where she teaches health law and clinical skills to undergraduate students. Amanda has worked as a generalist nurse in metropolitan and regional locations, as well as in the United Kingdom.

Louise Wells (RN, MN, Grad Cert Periop, Grad Cert Crit Care) is a lecturer in nursing at Charles Sturt University and has extensive experience teaching medical-surgical nursing subjects. Her clinical background is predominantly in critical care nursing and education.

Sally-Anne Wherry is a lecturer of nursing at the University of Canberra. She has eight years of clinical experience in her field, specialising in Parkinson's disease and movement disorders.

Acknowledgements

The editors wish to acknowledge the work and contribution of nursing clinicians, health professionals and academics who contributed to the development of this book. We would also like to thank Bronwen Ashcroft, Jessica Biles, Simone Brown, Elizabeth Forbes, Donna Hodgson, Sharon Hooge, Jody Hook, Catherine Hungerford, Heather Latham and Amy Vaccaro for their contribution to the first edition; and in this edition, Lee Hunt for her personal cancer journey, featured in Chapter 7. Your enthusiasm and willingness to contribute demonstrates your commitment to this area of nursing practice. We would also like to acknowledge the publishing team for their ongoing support and great work which allowed this book to be published.

The authors and Cambridge University Press would like to thank the following for permission to reproduce material in this book.

Figure 3.2 and **8.1**: © Getty Images/wetcake; **3.3**: Reprinted from *The Ottawa Charter for Health Promotion*, World Health Organization, Geneva, © 1986. Retrieved from www.who.int/healthpromotion/conferences/previous/ottawa/en/index.html; **7.2**: Reproduced with permission from Cancer Australia; **12.1**: © Emma Hammett, First Aid for Life (FirstAidforLife.org.uk) and onlinefirstaid.com, 2014, reproduced with permission; **12.2**: © Getty Images/normaals; **12.3**: © Getty Images/Mario Tama; **13.1**: © Getty Images/TefiM; **13.2**: Wikimedia Commons/James Heilman, MD, Osteoarthritis left knee, https://commons.wikimedia.org/wiki/File:Osteoarthritis_left_knee.jpg, licensed under CC BY-SA 3.0, https://creativecommons.org/licenses/by-sa/3.0/deed.en; **13.3**: © Getty Images/colematt; **13.4**: © Getty Images/JodiJacobson; **13.5**: © Getty Images/Stocktrek Images; **16.1**: © Getty Images/PIXOLOGICSTUDIO/SCIENCE PHOTO LIBRARY; **19.1**: © Getty Images/RUSSELLTATE-dotCOM; **19.2**: © Getty Images/Alan Gesek/Stocktrek Images; **21.2**: Wong-Baker FACES Foundation (2016). Retrieved 28 November 2017with permission from http://www.wongbakerFACES.org. Originally published in *Whaley & Wong's Nursing Care of Infants and Children*. © Elsevier.

Every effort has been made to trace and acknowledge copyright. The publisher apologises for any accidental infringement and welcomes information that would redress this situation.

Competencies

	1	2	3	4	5	6	7	8	9	10	11	12	13	14	15	16	17	18	19	20	21
Registered Nurse Standards for Practice (Australia, 2016)																					
Standard 1: Thinks critically and analyses nursing practice						×	×	×	×	×	×	×	×	×	×	×	×	×	×	×	×
Standard 2: Engages in therapeutic and professional relationships	×	×	×	×	×	×	×	×	×	×	×	×	×	×	×	×	×	×	×	×	×
Standard 3: Maintains the capability for practice				×		×	×	×	×	×	×	×	×	×	×	×	×	×	×	×	×
Standard 4: Comprehensively conducts assessments			×	×	×	×	×	×	×	×	×	×	×	×	×	×	×	×	×	×	×
Standard 5: Develops a plan for nursing practice				×	×	×	×	×	×	×	×	×	×	×	×	×	×	×	×	×	×
Standard 6: Provides safe, appropriate and responsive quality nursing practice	×	×	×	×	×	×	×	×	×	×	×	×	×	×	×	×	×	×	×	×	×
Standard 7: Evaluates outcomes to inform nursing practice	×		×			×	×	×	×	×	×	×	×	×	×	×	×	×	×	×	×
Competencies for Registered Nurses (New Zealand, 2016)																					
Domain 1: Professional responsibility	×	×	×	×	×	×	×	×	×	×	×	×	×	×	×	×	×	×	×	×	×
Domain 2: Management of nursing care	×		×	×		×	×	×	×	×	×	×	×	×	×	×	×	×	×	×	×
Domain 3: Interpersonal relationships			×	×		×	×	×	×	×	×	×	×	×	×	×	×	×	×	×	×
Domain 4: Interprofessional healthcare and quality improvement	×	×	×	×	×	×	×	×	×	×	×	×	×	×	×	×	×	×	×	×	×

An 'x' indicates that this standard or competency for practice is being addressed in this chapter

Nursing and Midwifery Board of Australia (2016). *Registered Nurse Standards for Practice*. Melbourne: Nursing & Midwifery Board of Australia. Retrieved from http://www.nursingmidwiferyboard.gov.au/Codes-Guidelines-Statements/Professional-standards.aspx

Nursing Council of New Zealand ([2007] 2016). *Competencies for Registered Nurses*. Wellington: Nursing Council of New Zealand. Retrieved from http://www.nursingcouncil.org.nz/Nurses.

PART 1

Frameworks for chronic care management

Frameworks for chronic care management

Judith Anderson, Linda Deravin
and Karen Francis

LEARNING OBJECTIVES

After studying this chapter, you should be able to:

1. understand the impact of chronic disease burden on communities in Australia and New Zealand
2. describe what a model of care is and how this applies to chronic care management
3. outline the Chronic Care Model (CCM) developed by Wagner and colleagues
4. describe the Innovative Care for Chronic Conditions Framework (ICCCF)
5. explain the value of evidence-based practice (EBP) to patient outcomes and the nursing profession in relation to chronic conditions.

Introduction

Chronic conditions are prolonged and unable to be cured. They frequently have multiple causes, take a long time to develop and can lead to complications (Australian Institute of Health and Welfare (AIHW), 2012; 2017). In 2018, chronic conditions accounted for 63 per cent of deaths in the world (World Health Organization (WHO), 2018). The burden of **chronic conditions** is estimated to account for approximately 80 per cent of **disability adjusted life years (DALYs)** and continues to increase, according to the Australian National Chronic Disease Strategy (National Health Priority Action Council, 2006). In 2014, chronic conditions accounted for 90 per cent of deaths in Australia and New Zealand (WHO, 2017).

These figures indicate the substantial impact that chronic conditions have on life worldwide, and this will also impact on health systems (Nuño et al., 2012). Nurses, who are the majority of workers within those systems, can have a significant impact on dealing with the issues that are arising from the increase in chronic conditions. Health systems will need to reorganise from a focus on acute health care to a focus on addressing and preventing chronic conditions. A focus on prevention, self-management, organisational change and political change is required to create better client outcomes; this will require specialised skills from nurses if they are to be an effective part of the workforce to make these changes (Nuño et al., 2012). As indicated by the International Council of Nurses (2010), there is a growing global need for nurses to engage with communities and other sectors to intervene at the earliest stages to prevent chronic conditions. In order for nurses to do this effectively, they need to implement EBPs that have demonstrated positive outcomes. Not only does this apply to the practices related to direct patient/client care, but also to the models of care that organisations use to guide care for people with chronic conditions (Nuño et al., 2012).

This chapter provides an overview of the CCM, how it was developed, the evidence base behind the model and how it has been implemented. The necessity for the evolution of the CCM into the ICCCF to address issues at an international level is discussed, together with an overview of the ICCCF. The importance of EBP is also described.

Chronic conditions – persistent illnesses or disabilities lasting for more than six months, which cannot be cured.

Disability adjusted life years (DALYs) – a statistical term that measures the numbers of years lost due to illness or disability.

Models of care

A model of care is a framework that articulates how health care services are delivered to meet the needs of people, population groups and/or patient cohorts. It aims to ensure that these groups obtain the right care by the right service at the right time as they progress through the stages of their condition (Agency for Clincial Innovation, 2013). Broadly speaking, a model of care describes concepts or aspects of health care and how they interrelate with each other. Models of care can vary to identify different levels of relationships, such as the ICCCF, which describes three levels of care (the micro, meso and macro levels) (Frogner, Waters & Anderson, 2011). Models of care indicate to staff what their roles are, who they may interact with and what pressures they may face as they undertake their tasks. A good model of care will identify aspects of health care that may otherwise be overlooked. For this reason, a model of care is especially useful for new practitioners to assist them in providing appropriate care for people (Agency for Clinical Innovation, 2013).

At higher levels, identifying how patients/clients move through a model of care can assist in identifying gaps in the care being provided or a duplication of services that could be altered. This level of a model of care is useful for managers and organisations (Agency for Clinical Innovation, 2013). Models of care should also cover situations that are unusual or unlikely and be adaptable to change in order to maintain their currency.

Research into successful models of providing chronic care has been undertaken over many years. Due to the overarching nature of many proposed models of care for people with chronic conditions, sometimes parts of the models, rather than the entire model, are evaluated or researched (Nuño et al., 2012). Although some specific models to implement chronic care exist in Australia, such as those developed for Indigenous peoples, this text will focus on a model developed for the international market as it is important for nurses to be aware of what is happening globally and to have a framework that can be implemented in any environment. The ICCCF, which has evolved from the earlier work of the CCM, guides this text and will be described in greater detail.

The Chronic Care Model

Effective management of chronic conditions requires a coordinated, system-wide approach. Wagner and colleagues (1999) developed the CCM (CCM; see Figure 1.1) to provide a systematic approach to chronic care management that bridges the gap between knowledge and practice, and supports patients (Kadu & Stolee, 2015).The CCM has been identified as being effective in a wide variety of settings and environments (Coleman et al., 2009; Nuño et al., 2012) and of particular significance in the Australian environment for Indigenous peoples (Si et al., 2008). The CCM focuses on involving the individual with a chronic condition in their care, as well as on the responsibility of organisations to provide a system-wide approach to managing chronic disease burden (Wagner et al., 1999; Wagner et al., 2001).

The CCM incorporates six components: health system (organisation of health care); self-management support; decision support; delivery system design; clinical information systems; and community resources and policies (Stellefson, Dipnarine & Stopka, 2013). The CCM outlines a multidimensional solution to the provision of chronic care (Bodenheimer, Wagner & Grumbach, 2002), acknowledging that effective chronic care management requires an organised approach where health systems support both the **activated patient** alongside a prepared and adequately resourced health provider team (Wagner et al., 1999). Self-management is valued within the CCM as being of significant benefit to the patient/client.

Activated patient – a person who is informed and engages in the decision-making process related to their own health care needs.

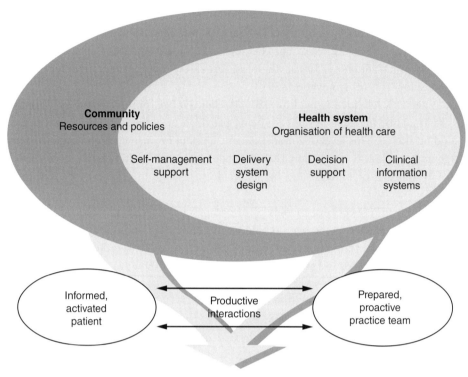

Figure 1.1   The Chronic Care Model
Source: Wagner (1998)

Health system (organisation of health care)

The CCM recognises that the management of chronic conditions will have a limited effect unless the system changes in the way services are coordinated and delivered. Pivotal to this system change occurring are health service leaders who are instrumental in obtaining resources to support programs. Conversely, these health service leaders are also crucial in removing barriers that may potentially inhibit the implementation of system-wide change. Reducing duplication through realigning and integrating services is required to achieve efficiencies. Ensuring that organisations include chronic care improvement targets and goals as part of their strategic and business plans encourages senior leaders to take responsibility for and support chronic care programs (Wagner et al., 2001).

Another strategy to support system-wide change is in the provision of financial and non-financial incentives that may be offered to encourage providers to take on case management roles to coordinate care. In Australia, general practitioners are encouraged to claim levies through Medicare for case-management roles. Where health services have met targets or key performance indicators, additional funding also provides an incentive for leaders to support changes to the way care is organised (Bodenheimer et al., 2002).

Self-management support

Reducing the symptoms and complications that result from many chronic conditions often requires a change in lifestyle. Models of care where health providers set goals for the patient, with minimal involvement from the patient, have been shown to be less effective than self-care management strategies. Enabling patients (and their family/carers) to care better for themselves and make decisions about their own care is a fundamental principle in self-care management (Epping-Jordan et al., 2004). A collaborative approach between patients and health providers, which includes defining the issues or problems, setting realistic goals and creating mutually agreed treatment plans that can be modified if problems arise, is a key feature of successful management programs. Evidence demonstrates that when patients are provided with information about their chronic condition, and have the support and encouragement to make their own decisions about their care, including control over their own lives, outcomes are significantly improved (Wagner et al., 2001). The focus in health care has, therefore, moved towards individual and group interventions that promote empowerment and the gaining of skills that assist in the management of chronic conditions.

SKILLS IN PRACTICE

Coordinating care

Mary is a 44-year-old woman with diabetes and renal failure. She has missed several appointments with her family doctor, the diabetes clinical nurse consultant and the podiatrist.

QUESTION

As the visiting community nurse who sees Mary on a weekly basis, what do you do to help improve the coordination of care for Mary and her chronic conditions?

Decision support

To provide quality care for the person with a chronic condition, health providers need access to professionals with clinical expertise and experience that supports the delivery of that care. Evidence-based guidelines or protocols should be available to health providers where decisions about ongoing treatment and management of chronic conditions are required. Access to reminders and standing orders that support decisions in the delivery of care to the person with a chronic condition should be available. Health teams, including doctors, nurses and allied health professionals, require access to ongoing professional development and education to support adherence to best practice and to adapt to changing models of care. Through education, the ability to make informed decisions is enhanced (Wagner et al., 2001).

Delivery system design

Historically, health care systems have been developed to manage acute care conditions. People with chronic conditions do not fit in to this model easily. Single transactions of care, which focus on assessment, treatment and discharge, generally do not recognise the complexity of chronic conditions and the need for ongoing care. Wagner and colleagues (2001) emphasise that **productive interactions** between the patient and practice team are more likely to occur with planning for future interactions and visits. People with complex conditions need access to a wide range of health providers. Multidisciplinary health care teams and outreach services can provide follow up to ensure adherence to the ongoing management of chronic conditions. Therefore, for there to be an improved management of people with chronic conditions, the ways in which health systems are designed must change (Wagner et al., 2001).

Productive interactions – individualised care where health care teams optimise patient outcomes through a series of exchanges.

Clinical information systems

Coordinated care is reliant on timely access to data and information. Chronic care patients may engage multiple health providers over long periods of time. This presents challenges in the care and treatment of people with chronic conditions. Clinical information systems, such as databases and registries that have the ability to flag follow ups and client recalls, are tools that can be used in the coordination of care (Wagner et al., 2001). Computerised information systems should have the ability to share information across various platforms so that information is readily accessible to a variety of health providers. This is not without its own set of issues and is one of the many challenges in supporting coordinated and integrated care for people with chronic conditions.

Community resources and policies

People with chronic conditions are multiple users of a variety of health services. Not all services can provide everything that a person with a chronic condition may need. For this reason, it is important that access to a wide range of services, expertise and resources is promoted. Increasing access to community programs, where multiple health agencies have agreed to share resources, can lead to improved cost efficiencies in the delivery of health care. For this to occur, health policy that is supported by senior leaders who are in a position to modify or change policy is required (Wagner et al., 2001).

REFLECTION

Models of care are commonly modified to improve health care for patients. What model of care is used in your area of practice? Is this model effective in addressing the needs of chronic care patients/clients?

Evolution of the Innovative Care for Chronic Conditions Framework

The ICCCF extends the CCM by adding micro, meso and macro levels to it (see Figure 1.2). This framework incorporates six guiding principles: evidence-based decision making, population health approach, focus on prevention, quality focus, integration, and flexibility and adaptability (WHO, 2002). These levels extend the involvement of community, and describe policies and financing as the drivers for implementation of the framework at the macro level (Epping-Jordan et al., 2004). The CCM, although useful, was found to be based on the US health care system, and thereby on evidence from high-income countries. The ICCCF, however, is more suitable for low- to middle-income countries as it emphasises policy development, the role of the community and integration between services (Nuño et al., 2012).

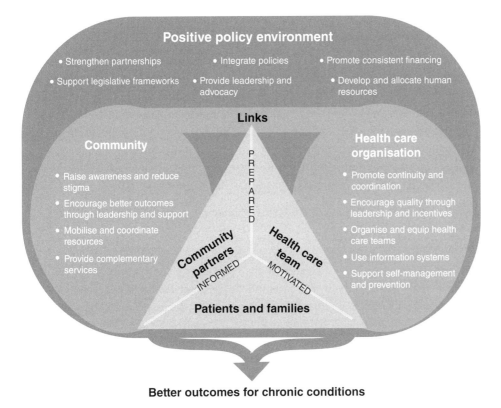

Figure 1.2 Innovative Care for Chronic Conditions Framework
Source: WHO (2002)

The three levels (macro, meso and micro) of the ICCCF will be the focus of further chapters where they will be discussed in greater detail. At this stage, the six guiding principles will be discussed to provide an overview of the ICCCF and how it should be implemented within health care services. Nursing staff, who make up the majority of the health workforce, should be educated in the use of the ICCCF (Anderson & Malone, 2015). All six guiding principles complement each other and are designed to be followed at all levels of the ICCCF.

Evidence-based decision making

Evidence (in the form of research) should be the basis for all decision making in health care (Wagner et al., 2005). For nurses, this involves finding the latest research that is available and using it to inform clients so that their decisions can be based on evidence. This is especially the case in the management of chronic conditions if nurses are to reduce the impact of those conditions on their clients. Evidence should inform not only clinical care, but also policy-making and service-delivery decisions (WHO, 2002). Evidence-based practice will be discussed in greater detail later in this chapter.

Population health approach

A focus on the entire population is the most efficient way to utilise health service resources. It allows for the development of long-term, proactive strategies to organise often limited resources to provide good-quality services to many people (WHO, 2002). Entire populations are at risk of contracting chronic conditions. Patterns of behaviour regarding nutrition and physical activity are often found within communities, and individuals can find it difficult to change these behaviours when acting alone. Promoting healthy lifestyles among groups can provide the support that individuals need to make effective lifestyle changes. Such support to populations benefits individuals (Nuño et al., 2012); for example, the Australian National Heart Foundation campaign 'Move More, Sit Less' targets the whole population through national and state media campaigns that impact on individuals who are exposed to repeated messages about increasing exercise as a preventative strategy to reduce cardiovascular disease, which is a national health priority (AIHW, 2015; Heart Foundation, 2015).

Focus on prevention

The ICCCF is based on a recognition that preventing chronic conditions is more effective than treating them and attempts to reorient health services to focus on prevention (Gardner et al., 2011). Prevention should focus on both the population and the individual levels to be most effective. There is sufficient evidence regarding risk factors: to allow intervention to take place before chronic conditions and their complications become apparent, to delay their onset and to limit their progression once they have begun (Nuño et al., 2012). It is also known that risk factors often exist in combination. People who smoke, for example, are more likely to drink than those who do not smoke (AIHW, 2012). Increasing the incidence of risk-reducing behaviours, which is the current focus of prevention activities (AIHW, 2014), can dramatically reduce the incidence of chronic conditions in the future, but requires commitment at all levels of the ICCCF (WHO, 2002).

Emphasis on quality of care and systematic quality

It has been demonstrated that continuous quality improvement can lead to positive changes in health service systems, safety, delivery and outcomes for clients (Hickey &

Brosnan, 2012). Although there are some variations, most quality improvement programs follow a cyclical process of 'plan, do, study, act', which leads to incremental improvement that is contextualised to address the needs of individual services (Gardner et al., 2011). Quality can increase accountability for the health provider and is most effective when applied at all levels of the ICCCF (WHO, 2002).

Integration

The need to build an integrated health system is one of the reasons that the ICCCF comprises micro, meso and macro levels. It is recognised that all of these levels need to work together to inform a single health system and to be integrated to produce the best possible outcomes for clients (Nuño et al., 2012). A good integration would see the blurring of levels to provide seamless, effective and efficient client care, including primary health care, in-patient care and chronic care (Humphries & Wenzel, 2015). Literature indicates that the majority of research in this area focused on the meso level and the need to integrate and communicate effectively across health services. However, the need for an integrated service at the micro level is also obvious as this is where actual contact with the clients occurs. The overarching aspect of the macro level and how it impacts on service provision and funding for clients is also essential if outcomes are to be maximised (Nuño et al., 2012).

Flexibility and adaptability

Flexibility and adaptability are required if the ICCCF is to meet the diverse needs of the populations it is designed to service. As an international model, the ICCCF needs to be adaptable to an extensive variety of settings. If it is to be applicable over time, then it needs to be able to adapt to changes in government and economic conditions. Adaptability and quality improvement are designed to lead to a framework that can change to meet the needs of the clients that it is serving (WHO, 2002). In Australia and New Zealand, the complexities of the geographic environment (among other issues) have led to the development of 'fly in, fly out' models of care (Gardner et al., 2011). These are particularly designed to address rural and remote settings where services and expertise are often lacking. The flexibility and adaptability aspects of the ICCCF encourage this type of adaptation to meet the needs of communities that are unable to be addressed otherwise.

REFLECTION

What type of health prevention, risk reduction and promotion programs are available in your community? Are they driven by the needs of people with chronic conditions or by health service needs?

Evidence-based practice

Evidence-based practice (EBP) refers to the use of current best evidence to inform clinical decision making and the delivery of health services (Gillespie et al., 2012; Nagy et al., 2010). Prior to the EBP epoch, health professionals relied on tradition, guesswork or logic when determining clinical actions (Nagy et al., 2010). This approach was criticised as it resulted in wide variations in care and unpredictable health outcomes (Stevens, 2013). Evidence generated from systematic approaches to inquiry that are subjected to critique and extensive evaluation, and subsequently incorporated into clinical practice guidelines, have realised the standardisation of health care in Australia and New Zealand and greatly improved health outcomes (Stevens, 2013). An example of a standardisation of health care that has improved the quality of life of individuals and health outcomes nationally is Australia's National Guidelines for Asthma Management (National Asthma Council Australia, 2015). Asthma is a debilitating airways disease affecting over two million Australians and approximately 334 million people globally (Global Asthma Network, 2014). Evidence-based practice is the mechanism for quality care improvement at global, national and local levels and, therefore, is the means by which preventable morbidity and mortality are addressed (Stevens, 2013).

Hoffman, Bennett and Del Mar (2010) assert that EBP promotes attitudes of inquiry among health professionals that support clinician accountability, enhance the transparency of the decision-making process, and promote fiscal efficiencies and the achievement of positive health outcomes. Health professionals' engagement with people who have a chronic condition is a fundamental aspect of the CCM and the ICCCF. Open, ongoing communication that accommodates the centrality of the patient/client is encouraged and accepted as necessary to support the individual's self-management of their chronic condition (Australian Health Ministers' Advisory Council, 2017; Wagner et al., 2005). As the body of evidence is ever evolving, health professionals must constantly update their knowledge and practice to keep abreast of new research and the implications for their practice.

The Joanna Briggs Institute, for example, has designed a model of evidence-based health care that provides a detailed overview of the methods by which health care providers make clinical decisions. The model suggests that discourse, talking with others, experience and research are techniques by which information is garnered, processed and utilised to inform practice (Pearson et al., 2005). The model highlights the process by which research is generated, understood, verified and incorporated into the body of evidence, and ultimately shared and translated into practice by health care providers globally (see Figure 1.3).

The evidence base for the CCM (and the ICCCF that is derived from it) is strong. Several authors have published reviews of the literature supporting this (for example, see Coleman et al., 2009, and Nuño et al., 2012). However, as the CCM and ICCCF are complex and would require implementation by many agencies and organisations to be researched effectively, much of the existing research has been limited to specific aspects that are more easily implemented. Self-care management, for example, has been demonstrated to have significant health benefits for people with chronic conditions (Hibbard, 2012; Wagner et al., 2001).

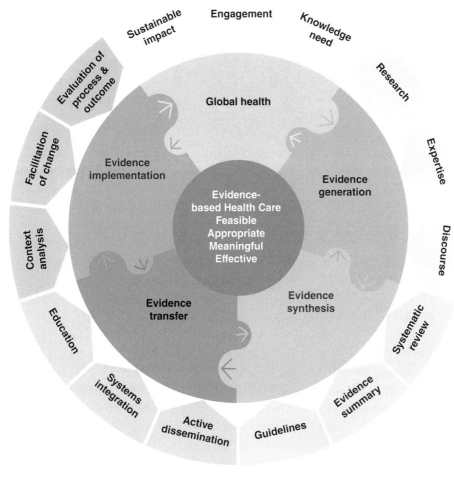

Figure 1.3   Conceptual model of evidence-based health care
Source: Jordan et al. (2016), p. 4

Evidence-based practice and professional accountability

Regulated health professionals, such as nurses, are required as part of their registration to maintain currency in their knowledge and practice by participating in professional development activities and incorporating contemporary scientific evidence into their practice, thus ensuring public safety (Hoffman et al., 2010; Nursing and Midwifery Board of Australia, 2016). Employing scientific evidence to underpin practice is referred to as **evidence utilisation** (Pearson et al., 2005) or **knowledge transfer** (Bannigan, 2009) (see Figure 1.4). Evidence alone, however, is not the only factor that health professionals utilise when making clinical decisions. The Duke University Medical Center (2015) asserts that EBP should reflect 'the integration of clinical expertise, patient values, and the best research evidence into the decision making process for patient care.'

Evidence utilisation – denotes the use of evidence to inform clinical decision making and practice.

Knowledge transfer – the transmission of knowledge generated from research, expert opinion and discourse to stakeholders to inform policy, education, service development and delivery, and practice.

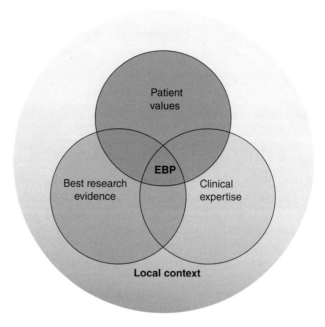

Figure 1.4   Model of evidence-based practice
Source: Strauss et al., 2018

Clinical expertise relates to the knowledge and skills of individual clinicians that has been developed through experience, education and practice (Bobay, Gentile, & Hagle, 2009; Melnyk & Fineout-Overolt, 2005). Patient values and beliefs must be a central consideration of health care professionals when making any clinical decisions, including therapeutic health interventions (Cochrane Community (beta), 2015; Duke University Medical Center, 2015; Joanna Briggs Institute, 2015). Pearson and colleagues (2005) highlight that the local context is a significant consideration in this decision-making process. The local context covers the health care system, the practice environment, available resources (fiscal, physical environment, equipment and access to medicines (see University of South Australia, 2015)), organisational policies, staffing levels and mix, health provider preferences, geographic location and patient preferences (Pearson et al., 2005). The resources that are available can facilitate or impede the implementation of EBP. Adapting best practice evidence to accommodate these contextual factors is often necessary.

Best practice guidelines

Best practice guidelines – evidence-informed recommendations that support clinical practice and guide practitioner and patient decisions regarding appropriate health care in specific clinical practice settings and circumstance (Australian Nursing and Midwifery Federation (SA Branch), 2015).

Organisations such as the Joanna Briggs Institute (2015) and the Cochrane Collaboration produce **best practice guidelines** that are widely accessible (Cochrane Community (beta), 2015) to facilitate the translation of research to practice (McDonnell, 2004).

These guidelines are updated regularly to ensure that the most current evidence is accessible and incorporated in the practice guidelines of health services. Individual health services often develop their own clinical guidelines to meet local needs. The currency of the evidence informing such guidelines has been identified as a potential limitation that all health professionals need to be mindful of (McDonnell, 2004).

SKILLS IN PRACTICE

Falls risk in the community

You are a health professional employed at the local community health centre, and you live and work in a small rural town that is renowned for its historical significance. You know that the streets are very old and to access footpaths from the road requires people to step up approximately 30 cm. Several older clients/patients, who have sought assistance from you at the community health centre, have commented on how difficult it is for them to do their shopping as they find it hard to step up to the footpaths from the road when they park their cars. You are concerned that people, particularly older people, are at risk of falling. You feel it is your duty to bring this concern to the attention of the local council.

QUESTION

In preparing a submission for the local council, what evidence would you gather to support your concerns and what recommendations would you suggest? Identify three chronic conditions people might have that would make access issues such as this relevant.

REFLECTION

How do nurses access evidence? How do they accommodate new knowledge into their practice?

SUMMARY

Learning objective 1: Understand the impact of chronic disease burden on communities in Australia and New Zealand.

The burden of chronic conditions is estimated to account for approximately 80 per cent of disability adjusted life years and is continuing to increase rapidly. In Australia and New Zealand, chronic conditions accounted for 90 per cent of deaths in 2014. This places a significant burden on health care provision in both countries.

Learning objective 2: Describe what a model of care is and how this applies to chronic care management.

A model of care is a framework that articulates how health care services are delivered and managed to meet the needs of people with chronic conditions. Models of care describe concepts or aspects of health care and how they interrelate with each other. An example of a model of care is the ICCCF.

Learning objective 3: Outline the CCM developed by Wagner and colleagues.

The CCM provides an evidence-based framework that bridges the gap between knowledge and practice, and supports the delivery of patient-centred care (Kadu & Stolee, 2015). The CCM includes the involvement of the individual with a chronic illness as well as the responsibility of organisations to provide a system-wide approach to managing chronic illness (Wagner et al., 1999; Wagner et al., 2001).

Learning objective 4: Describe the ICCCF.

The ICCCF is based on the CCM and adds micro, meso and macro levels to it. The micro level describes interaction between the patient, community and the health care provider. The meso level describes the health care organisation and the overarching community. The macro level describes the environment in which the framework is situated, with its policies and legislative requirements. The ICCCF incorporates six guiding principles: evidence-based decision making; population health approach; focus on prevention; quality focus; integration; and flexibility and adaptability (WHO, 2002).

Learning objective 5: Explain the value of EBP to patient outcomes and the nursing profession in relation to chronic conditions.

Evidence-based practice supports the care of the person with a chronic condition as it incorporates patient expectations, definitive diagnoses, therapeutic interventions, quality of nursing care and quality of life.

REVIEW QUESTIONS

1. List the six components of the CCM.
2. Outline the differences between the ICCCF and the CCM.
3. Identify potential issues in sharing information among health care providers to improve care for people with chronic conditions.
4. Discuss the relationship of research evidence to clinical decision making by health care providers.
5. Identify potential barriers to implementation of EBP and outline methods for limiting the impact of these on evidence utilisation in practice.

RESEARCH TOPIC

Identify a chronic condition that you may be interested in; for example, diabetes or asthma. What type of services are available to people with chronic conditions in your local community? Is there more than one provider of the same service? How do people access these services if they have a chronic condition?

FURTHER READING

Hoffman, T., Bennett, S. & Del Mar, C. (2010). Introduction to evidence-based practice. In T. Hoffman, S. Bennett & C. Del Mar (eds), *Evidence-Based Practice Across the Health Professions* (pp. 1–15). Sydney: Churchill Livingstone, Elsevier.

Nuño, R., Coleman, K., Bengoa, R. & Sauto, R. (2012). Integrated care for chronic conditions: The contribution of the ICCC Framework. *Health Policy*, 105(1), 55–64. doi: http://dx.doi.org/10.1016/j.healthpol.2011.10.006

Wagner, E. H., Austin, B. T., Davis, C., Hindmarsh, M., Schaefer, J. & Bonomi, A. (2001). Improving chronic illness care: Translating evidence into action. *Health Affairs*, 20(6), 64–78. doi: http://10.1377/hlthaff.20.6.64

Wagner, E. H., Bennett, S. M., Austin, B. T., Greene, S. M., Schaefer, J. K. & Vonkorff, M. (2005). Finding common ground: Patient-centeredness and evidence-based chronic illness care. *Journal of Alternative & Complementary Medicine*, 11(Suppl. 1), 7–15.

World Health Organization (WHO). (2002). *Innovative Care for Chronic Conditions: Building Blocks for Action: Global Report.* Geneva: WHO.

REFERENCES

Agency for Clinical Innovation. (2013). *Understanding the Process to Develop a Model of Care: An ACI Framework.* Chatswood, NSW: Agency for Clinical Innovation. Retrieved from www.aci.health.nsw.gov.au/__data/assets/pdf_file/0009/181935/HS13-034_Framework-DevelopMoC_D7.pdf

Anderson, J. & Malone, L. (2015). Chronic care undergraduate nursing education in Australia. *Nurse Education Today.* doi: http://10.1016/j.nedt.2015.08.008

Australian Health Ministers' Advisory Council. (2017). *National Strategic Framework for Chronic Conditions.* Canberra: Australian Government.

Australian Institute of Health and Welfare (AIHW). (2012). *Risk Factors Contributing to Chronic Disease.* Canberra: AIHW. Retrieved from www.aihw.gov.au/chronic-disease/risk-factors/

—— (2014). *Australia's Health 2014. Australia's Health Series No. 14.* Cat. no. AUS 178. Canberra: AIHW.

—— (2015). National health priority areas. Retrieved from www.aihw.gov.au/national-health-priority-areas

—— (2017). Evidence for chronic disease risk factors. Retrieved from www.aihw.gov.au/reports/chronic-disease/evidence-for-chronic-disease-risk-factors/summary

Australian Nursing and Midwifery Federation (SA Branch). (2015). Best practice guidelines. Retrieved from www.anmfsa.org.au

Bannigan, K. (2009). Evidenced-based practice is an evolving concept. *International Journal of Disability, Development & Education*, 56(3), 301–5.

Bobay, K., Gentile, D. L. & Hagle, M. E. (2009). The relationship of nurses' professional characteristics to levels of clinical nursing expertise. *Applied Nursing Research*, 22(1), 48–53. doi: http://10.1016/j.apnr.2007.03.005

Bodenheimer, T., Wagner, E. H. & Grumbach, K. (2002). Improving primary care for patients with chronic illness. *Journal of the American Medical Association*, 288(15), 1909–14.

Cochrane Community (beta). (2015). Evidence-based health care and systematic reviews. Retrieved from http://community.cochrane.org/about-us/evidence-based-health-care

Coleman, K., Austin, B. T., Brach, C. & Wagner, E. H. (2009). Evidence on the Chronic Care Model in the new millennium. *Health Affairs*, 28(1), 75–85.

Duke University Medical Center. (2015). Introduction to evidenced-based practice. Retrieved from http://guides.mclibrary.duke.edu/c.php?g=158201&p=1036002

Epping-Jordan, J. E., Pruitt, S. D., Bengoa, R. & Wagner, E. H. (2004). Improving the quality of health care for chronic conditions. *Quality and Safety in Health Care*, 13(4), 299–305. doi: http://10.1136/qhc.13.4.299

Frogner, B. K., Waters, H. R. & Anderson, G. F. (2011). Comparative health systems. In A. R. Kovner & J. R. Knickman (eds), *Jonas and Kovner's Health Care Delivery in the United States* (10th edn, pp. 67–84). New York: Springer.

Gardner, K., Bailie, R., Si, D., O'Donoghue, L., Kennedy, C., Liddle, H., ... & Beaver, C. (2011). Reorienting primary health care for addressing chronic conditions in remote Australia and the South Pacific: Review of evidence and lessons from an innovative quality improvement process. *Australian Journal of Rural Health*, 19(3), 111–17. doi: http://10.1111/j.1440-1584.2010.01181.x

Gillespie, L. D., Robertson, M., Gillespie, W. J., Sherrington, C., Gates, S., Clemson, L. M. & Lamb, S. E. (2012). Interventions for preventing falls in older people living in the community. Retrieved from www.cochrane.org/CD007146/MUSKINJ_interventions-for-preventing-falls-in-older-people-living-in-the-community

Global Asthma Network. (2014). *The Global Asthma Report 2014*. Auckland: Global Asthma Network. Retrieved from www.globalasthmareport.org/index.php

Heart Foundation. (2015). Move more, sit less. Retrieved from www.heartfoundation.org.au/active-living/sit-less

Hibbard, J. (2012). Forging a tool to guide patients in self-care management. *Health Affairs*, 31(3), 569.

Hickey, J. V. & Brosnan, C. A. (2012). Evaluation in advanced practice nursing. In J. V. Hickey (ed.), *Evaluation of Health Care Quality in Advanced Practice Nursing* (pp. 1–24). New York: Springer.

Hoffman, T., Bennett, S. & Del Mar, C. (2010). Introduction to evidenced-based practice. In T. Hoffman, S. Bennett & C. Del Mar (eds), *Evidenced-Based Practice Across the Health Professions* (pp. 1–15). Sydney: Churchill Livingstone, Elsevier.

Humphries, R. & Wenzel, L. (2015). *Options for Integrated Commissioning: Beyond Barker*. London: The King's Fund.

International Council of Nurses. (2010). *Delivering Quality, Serving Communities: Nurses Leading Chronic Care.* Geneva: International Council of Nurses.

Joanna Briggs Institute. (2015). The JBI Approach. Retrieved from http://joannabriggs.org/jbi-approach.html#tabbed-nav=JBI-approach

Jordan, Z., Lockwood, C., Aromataris, E. & Munn, Z. (2016). *The JBI Model of Evidence-based Healthcare: A Model Reconsidered.* Adelaide: The Joanna Briggs Institute. Retrieved from http://joannabriggs.org/assets/docs/approach/The_JBI_Model_of_Evidence_-_Healthcare-A_Model_Reconsidered.pdf

Kadu, M. K. & Stolee, P. (2015). Facilitators and barriers of implementing the chronic care model in primary care: a systematic review. *BMC Family Practice*, 16(1), 1–14. doi: http://10.1186/s12875-014-0219-0

McDonnell, A. (2004). Factors which may inhibit the application of research findings in practice and some solutions. In P. A. Crooks & S. Davies (eds), *Research into Practice, Essential Skills for Reading and Applying Research in Nursing and Health Care* (pp. 185–198). Sydney: Ballière Tindall.

Melnyk, B. M. & Fineout-Overolt, E. (2005). *Evidenced-Based Practice in Nursing and Healthcare: A Guide to Best Practice.* Philadelphia, PA: Lippincott, Williams & Wilkins.

Nagy, S., Mills, J., Waters, D. & Birks, M. (2010). *Using Research in Healthcare Practice.* Sydney: Wolters Kluwer, Lippincott, Williams & Wilkins.

National Asthma Council Australia. (2015). *Australian Asthma Handbook – Quick Reference Guide, Version 1.1.* Melbourne: National Asthma Council Australia.

National Health Priority Action Council. (2006). *National Chronic Disease Strategy.* Canberra: Australian Government Department of Health and Ageing.

Nuño, R., Coleman, K., Bengoa, R. & Sauto, R. (2012). Integrated care for chronic conditions: The contribution of the ICCC Framework. *Health Policy*, 105(1), 55–64. doi: http://dx.doi.org/10.1016/j.healthpol.2011.10.006

Nursing and Midwifery Board of Australia. (2016). *Registered Nurse Standards for Practice.* Melbourne: Nursing and Midwifery Board of Australia.

Pearson, A., Weichula, R., Court, A. & Lockwood, C. (2005). The JBI model of evidence-based healthcare. *International Journal of Evidenced Based Healthcare*, 3, 207–15.

Si, D., Bailie, R., Cunningham, J., Robinson, G., Dowden, M., Stewart, A., ... & Weeramanthri, T. (2008). Describing and analysing primary health care system support for chronic illness care in Indigenous communities in Australia's Northern Territory: Use of the Chronic Care Model. *BMC Health Services Research*, 8, 1–14. doi: http://10.1186/1472-6963-8-112

Stellefson, M., Dipnarine, K. & Stopka, C. (2013). The Chronic Care Model and diabetes management in US primary care settings: A systematic review. *Preventing Chronic Disease*, 10, E26. doi: http://10.5888/pcd10.120180

Stevens, K. R. (2013). The impact of evidence-based practice in nursing and the next big ideas. *Online Journal of Issues in Nursing*, 18(2). doi: http://10.3912/OJIN. Vol18 No02Man04

Strauss, S., Glasziou, P., Richardson, P. W. & Haynes, R. B. (2018). *Evidence-Based Medicine: How to Practice and Teach EBM* (5th edn). New York: Elsevier.

University of South Australia. (2015). Evidence based practice in the Philippines. Retrieved from www.unisa.edu.au/Research/Sansom-Institute-for-Health-Research/Research-at-the-Sansom/Research-Concentrations/Allied-Health-Evidence/Quality-Care/EBPPhil

Wagner, E. (1998) Chronic disease management: What will it take to improve care for chronic illness? *Effective Clinical Practice,* 1(1), 2–4. Retrieved from https://ecp.acponline.org/augsep98/cdm.pdf

Wagner, E. H., Austin, B. T., Davis, C., Hindmarsh, M., Schaefer, J. & Bonomi, A. (2001). Improving chronic illness care: Translating evidence into action. *Health Affairs,* 20(6), 64–78. doi: http://10.1377/hlthaff.20.6.64

Wagner, E. H., Bennett, S. M., Austin, B. T., Greene, S. M., Schaefer, J. K. & Vonkorff, M. (2005). Finding common ground: Patient-centeredness and evidence-based chronic illness care. *Journal of Alternative & Complementary Medicine,* 11(Suppl. 1), 7–15.

Wagner, E. H., Davis, C., Schaefer, J., Von Korff, M. & Austin, B. T. (1999). A survey of leading chronic disease management programs: Are they consistent with the literature? *Managed Care Quarterly,* 7, 56–66.

World Health Organization (WHO). (2002). *Innovative Care for Chronic Conditions: Building Blocks for Action: Global Report.* Geneva: WHO.

—— (2017). *Noncommunicable Diseases Progress Monitor 2017.* Geneva: WHO. Retrieved from http://apps.who.int/iris/bitstream/handle/10665/258940/9789241513029-eng.pdf?sequence=1

—— (2018). *Global Action Plan for the Prevention and Control of Noncommunicable Diseases 2013–2020.* Geneva: WHO. Retrieved from www.who.int/nmh/events/ncd_action_plan/en/

Implementing the macro level of the Innovative Care for Chronic Conditions Framework

Linda Deravin, Karen Francis
and Judith Anderson

LEARNING OBJECTIVES

After studying this chapter, you should be able to:

1. explain how the macro level of the Innovative Care for Chronic Conditions Framework (ICCCF) addresses care for the person with a chronic condition
2. understand the importance of national health policy and strategic initiatives to improve primary care services
3. describe quality and monitoring systems within a chronic care nursing context
4. understand the importance of education for the nurse and other health professionals in the specialty of chronic care.

Introduction

The macro level of the ICCCF reviews policy development and resource allocation. This level also considers the legislative framework and the ability of policy makers to adapt policies to meet changes in health care requirements and create effective intersectoral links. The fragmentation of **financial incentives** and its impact on health outcomes and services are considered. Maintaining **quality** health care and monitoring systems are included, together with continuing education for registered nurses.

A positive **policy environment** is the macro level that is required to support the micro and meso levels of the ICCCF. It is this level that provides the leadership, regulation and financial support for the health organisation, community and patient interaction (Epping-Jordan et al., 2004).

Chronic conditions can be viewed as being on a continuum, spanning those with the condition to those without the condition, as these conditions develop over time — beginning with risk, developing into diagnosis and then moving into complications. An awareness of this continuum is required to understand the need to invest at all points in the development of chronic conditions to manage them effectively. This is why the ICCCF requires three levels to manage chronic conditions (Epping-Jordan et al., 2004).

Describing the macro level

The macro level of the ICCCF describes the positive policy environment that supports the care provided for people with chronic conditions (see Figure 2.1). It includes legislation, leadership, policy, partnerships, financial support and human resource allocation (Davey & Burridge, 2009; Epping-Jordan et al., 2004). An appropriate legislative structure is essential to protect human rights and to delineate the roles of private and public health service provision (World Health Organization (WHO), 2002).

Policy naturally develops in a political environment so, at the macro level of the ICCCF, politics needs to be considered. Aligning policies at this level, so that they complement each other, will produce the best possible outcomes for people with chronic conditions. It is important that, with the increasing rates of chronic conditions, health care policies focus on the people with these conditions, rather than being limited to acute, episodic provision of health care, as has previously been the case. This focus would include not only health policies, but also labour policies, agricultural regulations, education and other legislative areas that have a significant impact on population health (WHO, 2002). Best practice guidelines, such as those produced by the Joanna Briggs Institute (2017) and the Cochrane Community (2017), should also inform the development of local policies and procedures and support evidence-based practice. Such guidelines and evidence-based practice are discussed in Chapter 1. From an international perspective, it is at the macro level that most differences exist in the support provided to people with chronic conditions. Poorer, underdeveloped countries, in particular, have significant issues at this level and those

Financial incentives – monetary benefit offered to health providers to motivate actions that might not occur without this enticement.

Quality – a measure of how well a service meets the established standards or satisfies clients.

Policy environment – supports the care provided for people with chronic conditions and includes legislation, leadership, policy, partnerships, financial support and human resource allocation.

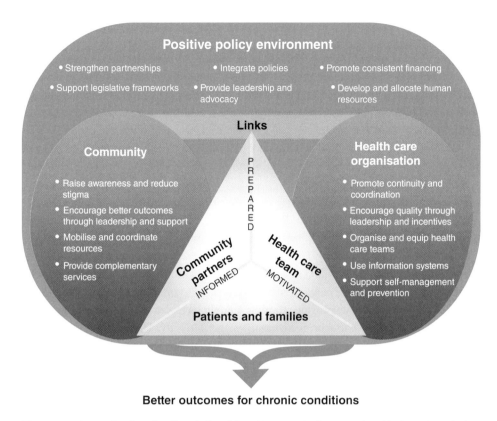

Figure 2.1   Innovative Care for Chronic Conditions Framework: the macro level (coloured section)
Source: WHO (2002)

that are unstable politically are particularly lacking in their ability to support people (Davey & Burridge, 2009).

Chronic conditions are not equally distributed among the population. This unequal distribution indicates areas where macro level policies can have an impact; for example, additional support for Indigenous populations, people with low socio-economic status or the elderly (Australian Institute Health and Welfare (AIHW), 2016; New Zealand Ministry of Health (NZMOH), 2017). The WHO (2018) has issued a worldwide call to take action to prevent and control chronic conditions in its publication *Global Action Plan for the Prevention and Control of Noncommunicable Diseases 2013–2020*. The action plan provides targets for member organisations to report against in order to measure outcomes and allows comparisons between countries to guide further learning about how best to implement such actions (WHO, 2018).

REFLECTION

Identify and describe two features of the macro level that directly impact on your practice as a registered nurse in caring for people with chronic conditions.

National health policy and strategic initiatives

Both the Chronic Care Model (CCM) (Wagner et al., 1999) and the ICCCF (Nuño et al., 2012) recognise that implementing sustainable change requires the support of government and global entities such as the WHO. For this to occur, key components at the macro level of the ICCCF include the integration of health policy, supportive legislative frameworks, and leadership that is able to make decisions and influence change.

Currently in Australia there are a number of health policy documents that are relevant to chronic care. These include the *National Health Reform Agreement* (Council of Australian Governments, 2011), the *National Disability Agreement* (Council of Australian Governments, 2012), the *National Primary Health Care Strategic Framework* (Standing Council on Health, 2013) and the *National Strategic Framework for Chronic Conditions* (Australian Health Ministers' Advisory Council, 2017). Similar frameworks exist in New Zealand, including *The Primary Health Care Strategy* (NZOMH, 2001), the *Meeting the Needs of People with Chronic Conditions* (National Health Committee, 2007) policy document and the *New Zealand Health Strategy: Future Direction* (NZMOH, 2016). All these documents provide strategic guidelines for how to improve the coordination of care for people with chronic conditions and disability. These strategic guidelines give health providers direction, with the expectation that they will implement these health policies at the level appropriate for their health services. A brief description of each of these major health policies is provided in Table 2.1. This list may change and grow as different political parties influence the way health budgets are distributed.

As can be seen from Table 2.1, the priorities of these policies are similar. For these priorities to be achieved, adequate resources need to be made available to support them.

Strategic guidelines – integrate planning and quality concepts and techniques to improve practice.

Table 2.1 Health policy documents relevant to chronic care in Australia and New Zealand

Health policy	Priorities related to chronic condition management
Australia	
National Health Reform Agreement, 2011	Commonwealth and state governments work in partnership to improve access and hospital efficiencies, improve quality and safety for all health consumers, develop an integrated primary health care system and further define the funding responsibility for aged and disability client groups.
National Disability Agreement, 2012	People with disability and their carers have an enhanced quality of life where choice, wellbeing and the opportunity to live independently is supported; and that people with disability are socially included within their community and that services are available to assist families and carers within the caring role.
National Primary Health Care Strategic Framework, 2013	Strategic outcomes include developing an integrated primary health care system which meets the needs of the consumer; to improve access and reduce health inequity; to focus on health promotion and prevention, screening and early intervention; and to improve the quality, safety, performance and accountability of health services that are provided.
National Strategic Framework for Chronic Conditions, 2017	A healthier future for the community requires improvement in prevention, detection and management of chronic disease. By preventing or delaying the onset of chronic illness, the impetus is to reduce avoidable hospital admissions, maximise the quality of life of individuals and invest in the health workforce to meet the demand for chronic disease prevention and care.

Health policy	Priorities related to chronic condition management
New Zealand	
The Primary Health Care Strategy, 2001	Primary health care services in New Zealand will work towards reducing health inequalities; providing access to health services that are designed to improve, restore and maintain people's health; coordinating care across multiple services; and develop the primary health workforce to deliver the care.
Meeting the Needs of People with Chronic Conditions, 2007	Primary objectives are to provide effective chronic care management and coordination of services, to develop the health workforce to meet the needs of this population group, to integrate structures and services that deliver health care, and to involve communities in the planning of this realignment of services.
New Zealand Health Strategy: Future Direction, 2017	After an extensive review of health services New Zealand developed a framework to guide health care for the people of New Zealand. It incorporates five themes including: value and high performance, people powered, close to home, smarter systems and one team to help improve the health of population by maintaining wellness, the prevention of illness and providing support with services across the lifespan

REFLECTION

From the policy documents outlining changes to health care services (see Table 2.1), identify the following.

- Which policy will have the most impact on chronic condition management?
- What level of government is responsible for the funding of chronic care?
- What might be some of the issues between who holds the funding and who provides the service?
- Are there any similarities in what they are trying to achieve?

Legislation

In Australia and New Zealand, laws protect the rights of people to have access to health care, to work and live in safe environments, and to participate in many other aspects of daily living. A number of legislative acts are in place to protect people with chronic conditions from being treated unfairly (**discrimination**) within the community. Some examples in Australia are:

- *Age Discrimination Act 2004*
- *Australian Human Rights Commission Act 1986*
- *Disability Discrimination Act 1992*
- *Mental Health Act 2014.*

Some examples in New Zealand are:

- *Human Rights Act 1993*
- *New Zealand Bill of Rights Act 1990.*

Discrimination – the act of treating people or individuals unfairly or differently from others.

In each country, these laws work together to protect the rights of individuals and are supported by additional legislation which, even if not directly related to people with chronic conditions, provides protection for all people and may be relevant depending on the context.

SKILLS IN PRACTICE

Putting legislation into practice

Mrs Jane Smith is 65 years old and has type 1 diabetes mellitus. She recently retired from a senior executive position. Mrs Smith qualified as a physiotherapist in her early 20s and practised as a physiotherapist in private practice for 10 years while completing higher degrees at university. In her mid-30s, she accepted a position at a university and advanced her career within this setting. A telephone call was made to the police by a shopping centre security guard, who had been alerted by a shop assistant and some other shoppers to Mrs Smith's strange behaviour. The guard told the police that Mrs Smith appeared to be either drunk or 'high on drugs', was walking into things, appeared glassy-eyed and when asked if she needed help, didn't respond. When the police arrived, Mrs Smith was disoriented and vague, and appeared pale and clammy. She could not respond to questions and directions, and appeared to be very drowsy. The police called an ambulance as they believed that Mrs Smith required medical intervention.

QUESTIONS
1. What do you think might have been happening to Mrs Smith?
2. What do you think the people who reported Mrs Smith were thinking?
3. How do you think Mrs Smith would feel when she realised what had happened?
4. What legislation protects a person's reputation against libellous accusations and other people's preconceived assumptions and biases?

Financial incentives and support

Primary health care – the first level of contact with individuals, families and the community within the health care system.

The 2011 *National Health Reform Agreement* (Council of Australian Governments, 2011) was designed to align the Australian federal and state governments in the provision of health care. The federal government was seen to take the lead on this policy document, with the state governments agreeing to the reallocation of resources and being responsible for implementing the changes. In Australia, funding for **primary health care** comes from the Commonwealth government. Two of the major changes within the *National Health Reform Agreement* were that the Commonwealth government would establish Medicare locales as a way to promote the coordination of primary health care services delivery, and to work with each level of state government to develop policy and planning for primary care services (Council of Australian Governments, 2011). These changes have had a significant effect on the way chronic disease is managed. However, policy alone cannot bring about all the changes that are required. For these other changes to occur, realignment of health services and investment in both physical and human resources is necessary.

Similarly, in New Zealand, a national health reform process occurred in 2002 with the introduction of district health boards and primary health organisations. The reform process recognised that the existing health system would be ineffectual in dealing with an ageing and disabled population if changes were not made. The changes included a focus on prevention and early intervention to decrease acute hospital presentations and improve the quality of life for the New Zealand population (NZMOH, 2001; WHO, 2014). More detail is provided on the health systems of Australia and New Zealand in Chapter 5.

In Australia, Medicare, the national health insurance scheme, provides rebates for medical services that are provided by general practitioners outside of the acute care hospital system (Connelly & Butler, 2012). As many people with chronic conditions are managed within the community, and health policy encourages this to occur to reduce the pressure on acute care services, one of the ways to encourage private medical providers is to look at alternative funding models that might support this approach (Standing Council on Health, 2013). General practitioners provide a pivotal role in the coordination of care to people with chronic conditions. The use of financial incentives to medical practitioners, in the form of increased medical rebates through the health insurance scheme, has been suggested as a way to improve chronic care management. There has been some debate about whether this is an effective strategy (Mayor, 2011; Scott & Harris, 2012). It is suggested, for example, that financial incentives should not be the sole driver of change for improved chronic care management, and that investment in staff training and education through **cross-discipline collaboration** for all health providers is a pre-ferred long-term strategy (Anderson & Malone, 2015; Bonney & Farmer, 2010; Dolor & Schulman, 2013). Australia and New Zealand both provide financial support for people with chronic conditions who are unable to work and therefore support themselves. Debate continues about the allocation and level of funding provided in this manner, as it is frequently considered to be minimal and perpetu-ates the disadvantage felt by vulnerable members of the population (Davey & Burridge, 2009; Epping-Jordan et al., 2004).

Cross-discipline collaboration – working in partnership with more than two health professions; for example, nurses and medical staff.

SKILLS IN PRACTICE

Caring for people with cancer

Care for people with cancer receives a great deal of publicity and financial incentives and support.

QUESTION

Identify three sources of such support and how they can be accessed to assist patients.

Human resource allocation

Fundamental to supporting any changes in health system delivery and health policy is to have an educated and adequately resourced health workforce. Legislation to protect the health and safety of communities in both Australia and New Zealand includes the regulation of health workers. Funding for the health workforce is provided at national, state or regional and community levels. The effects of an ageing population continue to place additional pressure on available funding, which has consequences for human resource allocations. This frequently leads to the use of unqualified staff (Malone & Anderson, 2014) and a growing burden on unpaid carers who provide support to people with chronic conditions. When considering the provision of holistic care to people with chronic conditions, its ICCCF, particularly at the micro level, incorporates family and carers as part of its triad. The macro level, with its focus on human resource allocation, provides some support to these people in the form of carer pensions; however, the criteria to qualify for a pension results in these pensions going to those with greatest need. This means that people who are somewhere in between qualifying to receive a pension and being financially independent have the potential to fall through the cracks and may not be serviced adequately by the system (Kidd, Watts & Saltman, 2008).

Quality and monitoring systems

The logic behind the CCM, when it was developed, was to build a system that encouraged collaboration between members of the health care team, organisations and communities, and government and regulatory bodies. This was based on the belief that working smarter, not harder, would improve the quality of care provided to clients; it has been demonstrated to be effective in improving overall client outcomes (Wagner et al., 2001).

PDSA – Plan, Do, Study, Act is a cyclical approach to incremental quality improvement.

Quality is a measure of how well a service meets the established standards or satisfies clients (Ross, 2013). Many authors (Anderson et al., 2008; Gardner et al., 2011; Moule, Evans & Pollard, 2013) recommend a **PDSA** (Plan, Do, Study, Act) cyclical approach to continuous quality improvement. PDSA involves planning for change, doing or implementing the change, studying or observing the results of the change, and acting on what has been learned from implementing the change. The model is considered to be cyclical, focusing on the introduction of continuous, incremental change, as one cycle follows another (Anderson et al., 2008; Gardner et al., 2011; Moule et al., 2013).

Although a good evidence base exists in relation to preventative interventions, many clients do not receive them. Quality improvement strategies that target health systems (for example, use of multidisciplinary teams), health professionals (for example, reminders) or clients (for example, provision of equipment) can be useful in improving the management of chronic conditions. Identifying desired outcomes or key performance indicators can assist with monitoring how well best practice is being implemented (Tricco et al., 2012). Key performance indicators frequently include assessment of effectiveness, efficiency, accessibility, timeliness and safety (Nurullah, Northcott & Harvey, 2014). Quality in health care is now more closely aligned with clinical guidelines and quality measures than ever before (Nigam, 2012).

At the macro level of the ICCCF, several organisations exist to assist and guide quality improvement in health services, including the Australian Commission on Safety and Quality in Health Care (Australian Council on Healthcare Standards International, 2015) and the Health Quality and Safety Commission New Zealand (Health Quality and Safety Commission New Zealand, 2015). Other organisations can accredit health services to be of good quality, such as the Australian Council on Healthcare Standards International (see Australian Council on Healthcare Standards International, 2015) and HealthCERT within New Zealand (NZMOH, 2014).

REFLECTION

Nurses participate in and lead quality improvement activities. Why is this important for your own nursing practice, for the health system and for the person with a chronic condition?

Continuing education for nurses
Learning: a lifelong activity

Learning occurs continuously throughout a person's lifetime (Pool et al., 2015). Pool and colleagues (2015) suggest that people are inherently lifelong learners, being consciously and unconsciously exposed to, and processing and assimilating, information that informs who they are and how they interact with the world around them.

Accelerated learning occurs when an individual is motivated to acquire specific knowledge and skills (Pool et al., 2015). For example, a nurse who is interested in specialising in addiction studies may participate in relevant online training programs, undertake a pertinent postgraduate qualification and/or complete an accredited professional development program that leads to specialist credentialing (Drug and Alcohol Nurses of Australasia, 2015). Pool and colleagues (2015) proffer that to be employed today does not guarantee lifetime employment. To ensure employability, they assert that people must constantly update their knowledge and skills.

Mandatory continuing professional development

Nurses in Australia (Nursing and Midwifery Board of Australia, 2016), New Zealand (Nursing Council of New Zealand, 2018) and many other countries have mandatory requirements for hours of continuing professional development (CPD) that must be met annually to qualify for renewal of practice licences (Ross, Barr & Stevens, 2013). Nursing regulatory authorities, such as the Nursing and Midwifery Board of Australia (2016) and the Nursing Council of New Zealand (2018), assert that mandating continuing education is a recognised method for promoting currency of practice, thus protecting the public from outdated treatment and care that is not based on validated evidence (Ross et al., 2013). Protection of the public is enhanced if nurses are competent, confident and current in their practice (Ross et al., 2013; Wenghofer et al., 2015).

Nurses can make choices about the CPD activities they undertake. Their choices will be informed by an array of motivators, such as personal preferences, access to educational opportunities, type of program (academic award or no award program), modality of delivery (face-to-face, online, self-directed), cost, time available, career aspirations and the requirements of the regulatory authorities (National Health Committee, 2010; Nursing and Midwifery Board of Australia, 2016; Nursing Council of New Zealand, 2018; Polifko, 2010; Pool et al., 2015; Ross et al., 2013). Furthermore, nurses are often required to complete training and education programs mandated by their employers. Typically, work-based obligatory training includes cardiopulmonary resuscitation, hand hygiene and medication calculations. Such training programs are employer-mandated as risk-reduction measures to improve patient safety and health outcomes. Continuing professional development activities should be accompanied by a self-reflective process that enables individual nurses to consider what they have learned, how that knowledge can be used and what additional learning is required (Nursing and Midwifery Board of Australia, 2016; Nursing Council of New Zealand, 2018). Such CPD activities often form the basis of credentialing for advanced nursing practice, which is discussed further in relation to specific conditions in subsequent chapters.

SUMMARY

Learning objective 1: Explain how the macro level of the ICCCF addresses care for the person with a chronic condition.

The macro level within the ICCCF is where leadership, regulation and financial support for the health organisation, community and patient interaction occurs. This level supports health policy that affects the management of chronic conditions at a strategic level, setting the direction for the delivery of health care.

Learning objective 2: Understand the importance of national health policy and strategic initiatives to improve primary care services.

Through policy and strategic initiatives, implementing sustainable change requires the support of government and global entities to work in partnership to improve access, equity, safety, quality and the efficient use of resources in the management of chronic conditions.

Learning objective 3: Describe quality and monitoring systems within a chronic care nursing context.

Most quality improvement systems use a PDSA cyclical approach to produce incremental change that is contextualised to the setting. Monitoring quality is frequently supported by key performance indicators that consider effectiveness, efficiency, accessibility, timeliness and safety.

Learning objective 4: Understand the importance of education for the nurse and other health professionals in the specialty of chronic care.

The burden of chronic disease is expanding. Nurses and other health professionals will need to develop their knowledge and skills in this area to address future health needs within their communities. Nurses are required to maintain their professional knowledge through further education. This now also forms part of required mandatory education standards to maintain professional registration.

REVIEW QUESTIONS

1. How does health policy influence the management of resources in health care?
2. For a coordinated approach to health care, what needs to change in the way health care services are delivered?
3. What is CPD?
4. Why do nurses need to engage in CPD?
5. What is meant by the term 'discrimination'? Provide an example relevant to people with chronic conditions.

RESEARCH TOPIC

Identify a chronic condition you are interested in and locate some best practice guidelines that suggest how this condition should be managed. Next, locate the national government policies that address this condition and comment on how well aligned the two are.

FURTHER READING

Australian Health Ministers' Advisory Council. (2017). *National Strategic Framework for Chronic Conditions*. Canberra: Australian Government.

Cochrane Community. (2017). The need for systematic reviews. Retrieved from http://community.cochrane.org/handbook-sri/chapter-1-introduction/11-cochrane/12-systematic-reviews/121-need-systematic-reviews

Council of Australian Governments. (2011). *National Health Reform Agreement*. Canberra: Council of Australian Governments. Retrieved from http://www.federalfinancialrelations.gov.au/content/npa/health/_archive/national-agreement.pdf

New Zealand Ministry of Health (NZMOH). (2016). *New Zealand Health Strategy: Future Direction*. Wellington: Ministry of Health. Retrieved from www.health.govt.nz/new-zealand-health-system/new-zealand-health-strategy-future-direction

World Health Organization (WHO). (2018). *Global Action Plan for the Prevention and Control of Noncommunicable Diseases 2013–2020*. Geneva: WHO. Retrieved from www.who.int/nmh/events/ncd_action_plan/en/

REFERENCES

Anderson, J. K. & Malone, L. (2015). Chronic care undergraduate nursing education in Australia. *Nurse Education Today*, 35(12), 135–8. doi: http://10.1016/j.nedt.2015.08.008

Anderson, J. K., Rae, J. B., Grenade, L. E. & Boldy, D. P. (2008). Residents' satisfaction with multi-purpose services. *Australian Health Review*, 32(2), 349–55. doi: http://10.1071/ AH080349

Australian Council on Healthcare Standards International. (2015). Evaluation and Quality Improvement Program (EQuIP) overview. Retrieved from www.achs.org.au/achs-international/products-and-services/evaluation-and-quality-improvement-program-(equip)

Australian Health Ministers' Advisory Council. (2017). *National Strategic Framework for Chronic Conditions*. Canberra: Australian Government.

Australian Institute of Health and Welfare (AIHW). (2016). *Australia's Health 2016*. *Australia's Health Series No. 15*. Cat. no. AUS 199. Canberra: AIHW.

Bonney, A. & Farmer, E. A. (2010). Health care reform: Can we maintain personal continuity? *Australian Family Physician*, 39(7), 455–6.

Cochrane Community. (2017). The need for systematic reviews. Retrieved from http://community.cochrane.org/handbook-sri/chapter-1-introduction/11-cochrane/12-systematic-reviews/121-need-systematic-reviews

Connelly, L. B. & Butler, J. R. G. (2012). Insurance rebates, incentives and primary care in Australia. *Geneva Papers on Risk and Insurance – Issues and Practice*, 37(4), 745–62. doi: http://10.1057/gpp.2012.40

Council of Australian Governments. (2011). *National Health Reform Agreement*. Canberra: Council of Australian Governments.

—— (2012). *National Disability Agreement*. Canberra: Council of Australian Governments.

Davey, G. & Burridge, E. (2009). Community-based control of a neglected tropical disease: The mossy foot treatment and prevention association. *PLOS Neglected Tropical Diseases*, 3(5), e424. doi: http://10.1371/journal.pntd.0000424

Dolor, R. J. & Schulman, K. A. (2013). Financial incentives in primary care practice: The struggle to achieve population health goals. *Journal of the American Medical Association*, 310(10), 1031–2.

Drug and Alcohol Nurses of Australasia. (2015). Pathways to credentialling program, journey to excellence! Retrieved from www.danaonline.org/wp-content/uploads/2013/02/Credentialling-Brochure-AUS.pdf

Epping-Jordan, J. E., Pruitt, S. D., Bengoa, R. & Wagner, E. H. (2004). Improving the quality of health care for chronic conditions. *Quality and Safety in Health Care*, 13(4), 299–305. doi: http://10.1136/qhc.13.4.299

Gardner, K., Bailie, R., Si, D., O'Donoghue, L., Kennedy, C., Liddle, H., ... & Beaver, C. (2011). Reorienting primary health care for addressing chronic conditions in remote Australia and the South Pacific: Review of evidence and lessons from an innovative quality improvement process. *Australian Journal of Rural Health*, 19(3), 111–17. doi: http://10.1111/j.1440-1584.2010.01181.x

Health Quality and Safety Commission New Zealand. (2015). About us. Retrieved from www.hqsc.govt.nz/about-the-commission

Joanna Briggs Institute. (2017). JBI about us. Retrieved from http://joannabriggs.org/about.html

Kidd, M. R., Watts, I. T. & Saltman, D. C. (2008). Primary health care reform: Equity is the key. *Medical Journal of Australia*, 189(4), 221–2.

Malone, L. M. & Anderson, J. K. (2014). The right staffing mix for inpatient care in rural multi-purpose service health facilities. *Rural Remote Health*, 14(4), 2881.

Mayor, S. (2011). Evidence is poor that financial incentives in primary care improve patients' wellbeing. Cochrane review finds. *British Medical Journal*, 343, d5682. doi: http://10.1136/bmj.d5682

Moule, P., Evans, D. & Pollard, K. (2013). Using the plan-do-study-act model: Pacesetters' experiences. *International Journal of Health Care Quality Assurance*, 26(7), 593–600.

National Health Committee. (2007). *Meeting the Needs of People with Chronic Conditions – Häpai te whänau mo ake ake tonu*. Wellington: National Advisory Committee on Health and Disability.

—— (2010). *Rural Health, Challenges of Distance, Opportunities for Innovation*. Retrieved from www.rgpn.org.nz/Network/media/documents/pdfs/rural-health-challenges-opportunities.pdf

New Zealand Ministry of Health (NZMOH). (2001). *The Primary Health Care Strategy*. Wellington: Ministry of Health.

—— (2014). Certification of health care services. Retrieved from www.health.govt.nz/our-work/regulation-health-and-disability-system/certification-health-care-services

—— (2016). *New Zealand Health Strategy: Future Direction*. Wellington: Ministry of Health. Retrieved from www.health.govt.nz/new-zealand-health-system/new-zealand-health-strategy-future-direction

—— (2017). *Annual Update of Key Results 2016/17: New Zealand Health Survey*. Wellington: Ministry of Health. Retrieved from www.health.govt.nz/publication/annual-update-key-results-2016-17-new-zealand-health-survey

Nigam, A. (2012). Changing health care quality paradigms: The rise of clinical guidelines and quality measures in American medicine. *Social Science & Medicine*, 75(11), 1933–7. doi: http://10.1016/j.socscimed.2012.07.038

Nuño, R., Coleman, K., Bengoa, R. & Sauto, R. (2012). Integrated care for chronic conditions: The contribution of the ICCC Framework. *Health Policy*, 105(1), 55–64. doi: http://10.1016/j.healthpol.2011.10.006

Nursing Council of New Zealand. (2018). Continuing competence. Retrieved from www.nursingcouncil.org.nz/Nurses/Continuing-competence

Nursing and Midwifery Board of Australia. (2016). Registration standard: Continuing professional development. Retrieved from www.nursingmidwiferyboard.gov.au/registration-standards/continuing-professional-development.aspx

Nurullah, A., Northcott, H. & Harvey, M. (2014). Public assessment of key performance indicators of healthcare in a Canadian province: The effect of age and chronic health problems. *SpringerPlus*, 3(1), 28.

Polifko, K. A. (ed.). (2010). *The Practice Environment of Nursing, Issues and Trends*. Clifton Park, NY: Delmar Cengage Learning.

Pool, I. A., Poell, R. F., Berings, M. G. M. C. & ten Cate, O. (2015). Strategies for continuing professional development among younger, middle-aged, and older nurses: A biographical approach. *International Journal of Nursing Studies*, 52(5), 939–50. doi: http://10.1016/j.ijnurstu.2015.02.004

Ross, K., Barr, J. & Stevens, J. (2013). Mandatory continuing professional development requirements: What does this mean for Australian nurses? *BMC Nursing*, 12, 9. doi: http://10.1186/1472-6955-12-9

Ross, T. K. (2013). Health care quality management: Tools and applications. Retrieved from http://CSUAU.eblib.com/patron/FullRecord.aspx?p=1580438

Scott, A. & Harris, M. F. (2012). Designing payments for GPs to improve the quality of diabetes care. *Medical Journal of Australia*, 196(1), 24–6.

Standing Council on Health. (2013). *National Primary Health Care Strategic Framework*. Canberra: Commonwealth of Australia.

Tricco, A. C., Ivers, N. M., Grimshaw, J. M., Moher, D., Turner, L., Galipeau, J., ... & Shojania, K. (2012). Effectiveness of quality improvement strategies on the management of diabetes: A systematic review and meta-analysis. *The Lancet*, 379(9833), 2252–61. doi: http://10.1016/S0140-6736(12)60480-2

Wagner, E. H., Austin, B. T., Davis, C., Hindmarsh, M., Schaefer, J. & Bonomi, A. (2001). Improving chronic illness care: Translating evidence into action. *Health Affairs*, 20(6), 64–78. doi: http://10.1377/hlthaff.20.6.64

Wagner, E. H., Davis, C., Schaefer, J., Von Korff, M. & Austin, B. T. (1999). A survey of leading chronic disease management programs: Are they consistent with the literature? *Managed Care Quarterly*, 7, 56–66.

Wenghofer, E. F., Campbell, C., Marlow, B., Kam, S. M., Carter, L. & McCauley, W. (2015). The effect of continuing professional development on public complaints: A case-control study. *Medical Education*, 49(3), 264–75. doi: http://10.1111/medu.12633

World Health Organization (WHO). (2002). *Innovative Care for Chronic Conditions: Building Blocks for Action: Global Report*. Geneva: WHO.

—— (2014). *New Zealand Health System Review. Health Systems in Transition*, 4(2). Wellington: WHO.

—— (2018). *Global Action Plan for the Prevention and Control of Noncommunicable Diseases 2013–2020*. Geneva: WHO. Retrieved from www.who.int/nmh/events/ncd_action_plan/en/

Implementing the meso level of the Innovative Care for Chronic Conditions Framework

Karen Francis, Judith Anderson
and Linda Deravin

LEARNING OBJECTIVES

After studying this chapter, you should be able to:

1. explain how the meso level of the Innovative Care for Chronic Conditions Framework (ICCCF) addresses care for the person with a chronic condition
2. understand how to build a supportive environment with the person with a chronic condition and other health partners
3. explore aspects of health promotion and education within chronic care nursing
4. consider the available resources within the community that support the care of the person with a chronic condition and identify methods to develop future resources within health care organisations
5. describe the impact of stigma in relation to chronic illness.

Introduction

This chapter describes the meso level of the ICCCF, which focuses on the health care environment and how care is organised. Tools and expertise that are required by nurses to provide evidence-based care within health care organisations, and the need to provide health education and promotion are discussed. This level of the ICCCF, with its focus on the entire organisation, is where other members of the team are valued for their involvement and support of the client. The benefits of information systems and community resources to provide comprehensive chronic care are also addressed.

Combining large health care organisations and community groups to provide health care can lead to very effective interventions, but may require assistance to coordinate and support clients who may have difficulty understanding the roles of such a variety of groups and people. Nurses are in a unique position to coordinate such care and to advise clients (Anderson & Malone, 2015) about what is available both within their own organisations and in the community, and thereby ensure the best possible outcomes.

The meso level of the ICCCF is the link between the interaction of the client and the health care team (the micro level) and the overall environment in which care is provided (the macro level). In this way, the meso level supports the interaction with clients by providing the space and services where the interaction takes place, while the macro level provides the regulation and funding to ensure the safety and functioning of the meso-level organisations and community.

Describing the meso level

The meso level of the ICCCF is the level at which health care organisations and communities exist (see Figure 3.1). Organisations need to coordinate workers, resources and expertise to provide suitable care to meet the needs of people with chronic conditions. These factors are commonly associated with risk factors that are often related to the **social determinants of health**. Communities have important resources that can support people with chronic conditions when they need them. Support groups, advocates and agencies are all valuable resources that can be found within communities. The links between the levels of the ICCCF are important. The organisation, for example, needs to focus on the person rather than the condition, which could be interpreted to be a function of the micro level of the framework (World Health Organization (WHO), 2002).

Chronic conditions follow known and predictable progressions, so an organisation can work towards preventing and delaying onset and complications in a proactive and organised manner. The organisation should be instigating contact with the client (that is, follow up, which is described in Chapter 4) rather than waiting for the client to experience symptoms or complications that leads them to making contact with the organisation. To effectively predict the progression of a chronic condition or how to best manage it, organisations need systems that allow them to access and implement evidence-based practice and information systems that support this kind of work through reminders and monitoring. This type of follow up allows continuity of care and should exist at an organisational level to overcome staffing issues that may arise. If this was to be implemented at the micro

Social determinants of health – refers to the conditions in which people are born, grow, work, live and age, and the wider sets of forces and systems shaping the conditions.

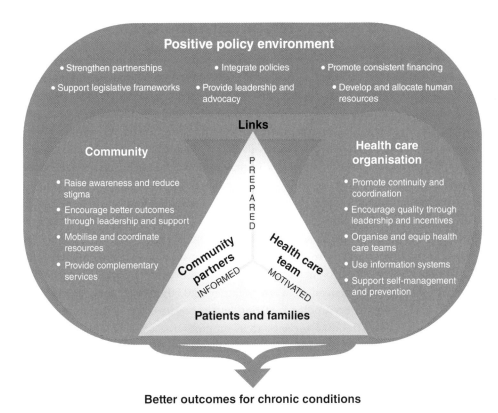

Figure 3.1 Innovative Care for Chronic Conditions Framework: the meso level (coloured section)
Source: WHO (2002)

level of the ICCCF then it would rely solely on individuals and may not occur, such as, for example, when staff take leave (WHO, 2002).

Coordination of services is more effective, then, when it occurs at the meso level of the ICCCF. Coordination of multiple health care workers enhances the collection of information about clients, and combines their knowledge and skills. Sometimes this coordination is enhanced with the employment of a care coordinator to ensure the integration and coordination of care when there is a variety of staff (WHO, 2002).

Integrating the health care organisation within the community that it serves has significant benefits. Communities can provide a broad range of resources that may have great potential to assist people with chronic conditions, especially when their own resources are stretched, which often occurs due to the impact that chronic conditions have on their ability to work and earn an income (WHO, 2002).

REFLECTION

Promoting continuity and coordination of services is a key component of the meso level. Identify four key health professional roles and describe how they might support this coordination of care.

Supportive health care environments

At the meso level of the ICCCF, the integration and coordination of care is one of the core principles to effectively deliver health care to patients with chronic conditions (Department of Health and Human Services, Victoria, 2018; Nuño et al., 2012). Health care services have been traditionally set up to focus on acute episodes of care where assessment, treatment and cure are the priorities. These traditional models do not work effectively in the management of chronic conditions (Wagner et al., 2001). People who experience chronic illness may need to engage multiple providers to achieve effective health outcomes. It has been shown that coordinated and integrated care improves health outcomes, as opposed to disjointed and singular episodes of care without follow up (Australian Bureau of Statistics, 2015; Nuño et al., 2012). For this reason, the ICCCF suggests that changing the model of care to account for the long-term management of chronic conditions is essential. This means that health care providers and different levels of health care provision need to work together and, therefore, the way services are delivered needs to be modified. Strong and innovative leadership is required to help build bridges across services that supports the sharing of information and ways of working towards a coordinated approach to chronic disease management.

Primary health reform

With the introduction of the *National Health Reform Agreement* in Australia (Council of Australian Governments, 2011; see also Chapter 2), the impetus for better coordination of services has been articulated. In Australia, the focus on primary health services with the development of primary health networks, incentives for general practitioners to better manage chronic care patients, and a commitment to the reduction of duplicated services has seen much turmoil over the past 10 years. Essentially, these changes were undertaken so that resources would be better utilised (Council of Australian Governments, 2011).

In New Zealand a similar approach has been adopted with the integration of primary and secondary health care provision, and a new focus on the patient rather than the institution. District health boards, primary health organisations and general practices have been urged to work together in the provision of primary care with the aim to provide care closer to patients' homes to reduce health inequalities in New Zealand (New Zealand Ministry of Health (NZMOH), 2014; 2016).

With the restructure of health services and the reallocation of resources to support changes in the way primary care services are delivered and to improve chronic care management, another supporting feature is the investment in staff. This requires the development of staff through education at the undergraduate (Anderson & Malone, 2015) and postgraduate levels, and that staff have the resources to effectively perform their roles (Nuño et al., 2012).

Information systems

People with chronic conditions have far greater access to **health information** than in previous years through the use of information technology and the Internet, and have the ability to become more informed about their condition (Kim & Xie, 2017). Health providers also require timely access to data and information so that care can be coordinated. People with chronic conditions may need to engage with multiple health providers to receive the care that they need. The use of databases and client registries to flag follow ups and client recalls can facilitate coordination of care (Wagner et al., 2001). Many health care organisations are now transitioning towards electronic health care records, which allow improved accessibility to information that supports coordination of care for the person with a chronic condition (Andrews, Gajanayake & Sahama, 2014).

Health information – can include information about the health or disability of an individual, the services provided by a health entity and the personal information about an individual that is used in their care and treatment.

Organising health care teams

The skills, knowledge and resources of a variety of health care professionals need to be managed effectively at the meso level by the health care organisation (WHO, 2002). Frequently, the managers at this level of the organisation are nurses who not only need to manage interactions with clients but also to ensure that there are no gaps in the care provided to clients by other services or health professionals. This type of care coordination role is now common for nurses and has been demonstrated to improve client outcomes (Zangerle, 2017).

The nature of chronic conditions, in that they are managed rather than cured, means that people will often live with these conditions for long periods of time. Also, having one condition or problem often predisposes a person to other conditions. This means that people who are managing chronic conditions often present to health services with multiple, complex issues that a single health professional may not be able to treat. Collaboration with other health professionals to form a multidisciplinary team is essential to provide the most suitable treatment options for such clients (Zangerle, 2017). Multidisciplinary teams are groups of professionals with diverse professional backgrounds (for example, nurses, doctors, physiotherapists, occupational therapists, speech pathologists, social workers, Indigenous health workers and pastoral carers) who work autonomously and in collaboration to plan and provide health care. Care coordination involves the organisation of health care activities provided by a minimum of two health care providers to facilitate the effective delivery of services and the best possible health outcomes for the client (Zangerle, 2017). A study by Harris and colleagues (2011) discovered that Australian clients with team care arrangements (funded under Medicare) self-assessed their quality of care as being higher than people without such arrangements, and they were associated with improved health outcomes. The study also found that people living in rural areas were less likely to receive care from a multidisciplinary team than people living in metropolitan areas. Although this may not always be rectifiable, due to limited availability of staff in these areas, technology can assist in ensuring that people in rural or remote areas are not disadvantaged (Malone & Anderson, 2014).

Services within the community

Syd has had a stroke, which has resulted in a left-sided hemiparesis. He is now ready for discharge from the rehabilitation unit back to his home, where he lives with his wife, Shirley. As a nurse who has to offer information to Syd, who requires ongoing services within his community, answer the following questions.

QUESTIONS

Identify three services within the community to which you may be able to refer Syd.

1. What kind of service do they provide?
2. Who do they provide services to and are there any restrictions?
3. How do these services network or share information with other health providers?
4. How long are people allowed to stay within these services or do they offer care for an unlimited time?
5. What type of health professionals work within these organisations?

Health promotion and education

Health promotion is defined as 'the process of enabling people to increase their control over, and to improve, their health' (Francis et al., 2013). Health is a personal resource that encapsulates social, economic and political determinants (Francis et al., 2013). The equitable distribution of available resources (wealth, education, political stability) that support health and wellbeing continue to be recognised as key drivers of health promotion policy and practice (Talbot & Verrinder, 2014). In 1978, member nations of the WHO met at Alma-Ata in Russia and advocated urgent action by all governments to protect and promote the health and wellbeing of all of the people of the world (Moodie, 2008; Standing Council on Health, 2013). This call to action was adopted as an outcome of deliberations on why global health had not improved significantly in the aftermath of World War II. Member nations were concerned about growing disparities in the health status of peoples in developing countries compared with those in developed nations, and within developed nations where there were marked differences within populations, such as Indigenous peoples compared to non-Indigenous peoples (WHO, 2015). The **Declaration of Alma-Ata** identified 'health for all people by 2000' as a goal. The WHO asserted that this goal was achievable if basic needs were met (Francis et al., 2013). As **Maslow's hierarchy of needs** indicates, access to biological and physiological needs such as air, food, clean water, clothing and shelter are essential for sustaining life (see Figure 3.2). Next come safety needs, such as being free of threats to life from war, natural disasters, domestic violence, abuse and economic insecurity. The third level of needs encapsulates interpersonal relationships: belongingness and being loved. Esteem is the fourth level. Having self-esteem and self-respect, being valued and respected by others, impacts on an individual's sense of self-worth, and

Declaration of Alma-Ata – 1978 outcome of a World Health Organization conference that identified primary health care as the key to achieving 'health for all'.

Maslow's hierarchy of needs – a theory of human motivation. Maslow argued that the most basic needs of humans must be met before individuals will aspire to achieve higher-order motivators.

overall health and wellbeing. The last level of need Maslow termed 'self-actualisation'. This concept refers to the achievement of a person's full potential; that is, being what they aspire to be (Kozier et al., 2015).

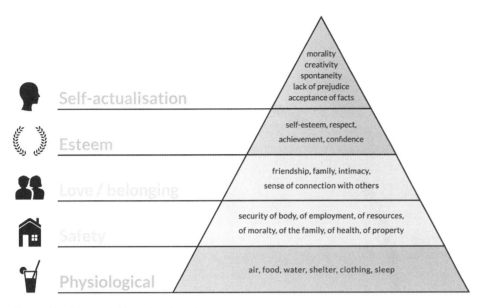

Figure 3.2   Maslow's hierarchy of needs

The Ottawa Charter for Health Promotion: primary health care

Maslow's hierarchy of needs established basic needs for human existence and postulated that unless they are met, individuals are not motivated or able to aspire to achieve higher-order motivators. For individuals who need assistance to meet these needs, interventions that support their health may be required. Primary health care, with its focus on preventing ill health, is particularly suitable to provide such support. Primary health care is a strategy that was identified by the WHO in 1986 and enshrined in the **Ottawa Charter for Health Promotion** (see Figure 3.3), which provided a blueprint for achieving 'health for all' (Francis et al., 2013; Kozier et al., 2015; Talbot & Verrinder, 2014). 'Health for all' continues to be a slogan that reflects the global commitment to social justice. While the WHO recognised that achieving 'health for all people by 2000' was overly ambitious and unrealistic, the commitment to achieving equity of health status has not waned. A target date for achieving this goal was later removed, with member nations agreeing that sustained and concentrated focus would be necessary. The Ottawa Charter affirmed that 'health for all' could be an aspiration, but requires intersectoral approaches that traverse all levels of government and require interagency collaboration to build the capacity of individuals, communities and nations. Five action areas were established to guide nations to refocus and reinforce health-promoting policy and practice.

Ottawa Charter for Health Promotion – an outcome of the first international conference on health promotion. The charter provided a blueprint for achieving 'health for all'.

1. Build healthy public policy.
2. Create supportive environments.

3. Strengthen community action.
4. Develop personal skills.
5. Reorient health services (Francis et al., 2013).

There have been many WHO meetings since the Ottawa meeting that have advanced strategies to achieve health for all.

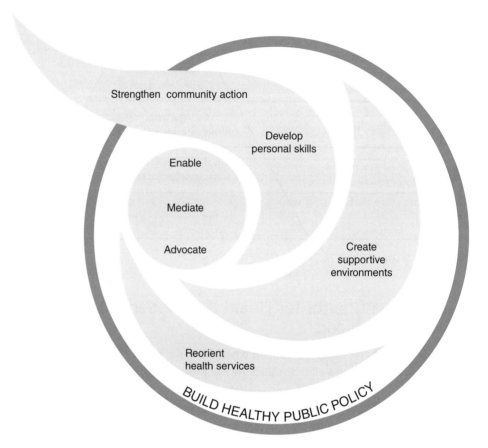

Figure 3.3   The Ottawa Charter for Health Promotion
Source: WHO (1986)

The Australian and New Zealand context

The Australian and New Zealand governments are both signatories to the Alma-Ata agreement, and have continued to embrace policy changes to accommodate primary health care as a model of health care service delivery to reduce inequity and improve the overall health and wellbeing of their populations (Edgecombe & Stephens, 2010). Preventative health care is the most efficient and ethically appropriate method for improving the health status of nations, particularly among vulnerable populations such as Aboriginal and Torres Strait Islander Australians and Māori people of New Zealand. Other vulnerable populations include people who are living with a chronic condition, people living with a disability, mothers/parents and children, young people, people living with a mental illness, and refugees and people from culturally and linguistically diverse backgrounds (Francis et al., 2013; Talbot & Verrinder, 2014). Understanding the factors that impact on health status, the determinants of health (for example, genetics, immunity, lifestyle, education, wealth, ethnicity, environment) and other extrinsic factors, provides focus for preventative interventions to promote optimal health and wellbeing, particularly among the most vulnerable people in society (Australian Institute of Health and Welfare (AIHW), 2018; Standing Council on Health, 2013).

Nurses have a significant role to play in promoting the health and wellbeing of individuals, groups and populations. As direct care providers, nurses have a responsibility to promote safe, healthy environments that support optimal health outcomes. For example, nurses scan the physical environments in which their patients reside to ensure that potential hazards are removed or at least limited. Lowering the height of beds, and removing any fluid spillage on floors and unnecessary clutter from walk areas are strategies that nurses initiate to reduce the falls risk of patients in hospital (Australian Commission on Safety and Quality in Health Care, 2009).

Raising community awareness of environmental concerns and methods that can be adopted to limit risk and improve the health outcomes of individuals and populations is commensurate with nurses' work, particularly those who work in general practice, community health, aged care, occupational health and safety, or with children in educational settings. For example, skin cancer can be avoided if excessive exposure to ultraviolet radiation is limited by wearing sunscreen, protective clothing, hats and sunglasses (Cancer Council Victoria, 2015). Likewise, reminding people who have a respiratory disorder to be aware of and limit exposure to triggers, improves health status and enhances quality of life (National Asthma Council of Australia, 2015).

As frontline health professionals, nurses have a central role in connecting people, families, groups and populations to intersectoral services that can include the health, social, transport, legal, policing and financial services required to ensure positive health and wellbeing outcomes. **Health literacy** is recognised as a central factor influencing an individual's capacity to make informed choices that impact on their health status (Johnson, 2007). Nurses can promote health literacy in their everyday practice. For example, a nurse who is a member of a multidisciplinary health care team working with people who have chronic heart or lung conditions will talk with them about lifestyle modification, medication management, recognising symptoms requiring medical support and developing a plan of action detailing a process to be followed. The nurse may also provide information on activities to improve heart and lung function – such as swimming, walking, yoga or bike riding – and give details of centres and groups that can be contacted for further information (National Heart, Lung and Blood Institute, 2015). Health education and promotion involves building an individual's capacity to make informed choices.

Health literacy – defined as tan individual's capacity to access, understand and process information about their health and available services in order to make informed decisions.

Preventative health care

Preventative health care refers to a broad range of methods that prevent or limit ill health, thus promoting wellbeing (AIHW, 2018; Talbot & Verrinder, 2014). For example, some influenza vaccination programs are offered free to people who are considered at risk, which includes people aged 65 years and over, Indigenous people aged over 15 years, pregnant women, and people aged six months and over with medical conditions that include severe asthma, lung or heart disease, low immunity or diabetes (Standing Council on Health, 2013). Influenza is a contagious disease with varying impacts ranging from mild symptoms – such as fever, tiredness, runny nose, muscle aches and poor appetite – to longer-term problems such as bronchitis, chest and sinus infections, heart, blood system or liver complications and, in some cases, death (Australian Government Department of Health, 2015).

Another example of the impact of preventative health is dealing with obesity. In Australia, two in three people are overweight or obese, with one child in four is overweight or obese (AIHW, 2015). In New Zealand, one in three people over the age of 15 years are obese, and one in ten children are obese (NZMOH, 2015a). Health promotion programs aiming to deal with obesity include the 'Healthy Kids, Eat Well, Get Active' program (NSW Government Healthy Kids, 2015a), which is an initiative of the NSW Ministry of Health, NSW Department of Education, Office of Sport and the Heart Foundation (NSW Division). This program supports teachers, parents, carers, coaches, health professionals, kids and teens to make healthy choices by providing a 'one-stop shop' of current and credible information, resources and support materials about healthy eating and physical activity (AIHW, 2015; Modi, 2015).

Websites such as 'Healthy Kids' are easily accessible and, coupled with localised action-orientated programs such as the 'NSW Premier's Sporting Challenge' (NSW Government Healthy Kids, 2015b) and 'What is Live Well @ School?' (NSW Government Healthy Kids, 2015c), reinforce key messages to promote health and wellbeing of children to proactively address the burden of obesity.

Similarly, in New Zealand, the Health Promoting Schools program is a community-led initiative that targets school-aged children. In this program, a health-promoting school facilitator supports the school community and assists them to develop strategies that address health and wellbeing while developing partnerships that encompass the school, health and social services in that community (NZMOH, 2015b).

SKILLS IN PRACTICE

Childhood obesity

Childhood obesity is a significant chronic condition in Australia and New Zealand. You are a community nurse working with the local public health unit. As part of a joint project between the public health unit and local schools in your area, you have agreed to focus on a health promotion project tackling childhood obesity.

QUESTIONS

1. What information do you think should be included on a fact sheet that could be given to parents?

2. Where could you source this information?

3. Would a fact sheet be different for parents as opposed to one for children? Why?

Community resources

Communities are groups of people united by a commonality such as a shared interest, a culture and language, or through living in a defined geographic area like a street, neighbourhood or township (NSW Government Healthy Kids, 2015a; 2015b; 2015c). Every community has a resource base that can support the quality of life of the community (Community Tool Box, 2015; Francis et al., 2013). Members of the community (human capital), physical structures and infrastructure, services and businesses are resources within communities that support daily life. Not all communities are aware of their resource base, although local governments produce reports that capture information at the community level. Poor or incomplete information, or not knowing where to find information, can limit individuals' or groups' access to available resources. This is particularly so for vulnerable peoples, such as older people who require assistance with activities of daily living, home maintenance or transport.

Community assessment

Understanding the range of resources available in communities is often achieved by undertaking a community assessment. Doing a community assessment involves mapping the resource base, which includes a demographic profile, inventory of assets (schools, health services, aged-care facilities, faith organisations, businesses, welfare services and other amenities), transport links, access to other centres, distances from major capitals, and reviewing available data, such as morbidity and mortality patterns, to generate a community profile. This data can be used by nurses and other health professionals to connect people to the services and resources that they require (Francis et al., 2013).

> **REFLECTION**
>
> The local media in your community continue to report concern about young people using crystal methamphetamines (ice) and the potential impact on them, their families and the community. As a community nurse, you are approached to talk to community groups about this issue. Reflect on the information you would need to ensure that you meet the needs of the community, families and the young people.

Stigmatisation

Stigmatisation refers to the labelling or stereotyping of others as different (Halding, Heggdal & Wahl, 2011). Ethnicity, skin colour, religious affiliation, language, age, sex, physical attributes or disability are common characteristics used as a basis for discrimination and labelling. Studies have found that people who have chronic conditions can be stigmatised. Halding and colleagues (2011) reported that participants in their study who had chronic obstructive pulmonary disease described being stereotyped and discredited because others; including family, community and health care professionals;

accepted prevailing attitudes that the condition was related to tobacco smoking and was, therefore, self-inflicted. Nash (2013) described how physical ill health among people with mental illness can be missed or attributed to their mental health status by health professionals. He claimed that delays in recognising physical ill health among this population increased the possibility of complications occurring. Nash (2013) believed this situation may occur as an outcome of inappropriate attitudes of health professionals and subsequent stigmatisation of people with mental health conditions. A study of women with chronic fatigue syndrome and fibromyalgia reported that the participants felt that some doctors stigmatised them. As a consequence of being labelled, they were 'psychologised' (that is, made to feel that the symptoms they were experiencing were **psychosomatic**), and the physical symptoms they experienced were marginalised (Msibi et al., 2014).

Psychosomatic – a physical ailment or condition that has been caused or aggravated by an underlying psychological issue.

Human rights and anti-discrimination legislation exists to protect the vulnerable and limit the impact of stigma and stigmatisation (Australian Government Department of Health, 2015; Ministry of Business, Innovation & Employment, 2015). Such legislation is incorporated into organisational human resources policies to promote workplaces that are free from discrimination and harassment (Australian Government Department of Health, 2015; Ministry of Business, Innovation & Employment 2015). Employers are required to ensure that all employees are familiar with workplace policies, and that the behaviours of both the individuals and the organisation reflect the principles embedded in the legislation.

Limiting the impact of stigmatisation of others by nurses

Understanding our own values and beliefs is the first step towards recognising the domains for prejudicial thoughts and the bases for behaviours that result in the stigmatisation of others (Halding et al., 2011). It is important to understand and respect others, be aware of one's position as a nurse, and acknowledge that unequal power relationships can exist with other health staff, patients, families and communities. Appreciating how power can be exerted on others is a necessary element of self-insight required by nurses to recognise and curtail prejudice and labelling (Gallagher & Polanin, 2015). Being an advocate for others, irrespective of who they are, is an integral role of all nurses. It is the fundamental right of the people for whom nurses have a responsibility that they are respected and receive quality care which encompasses the physical, spiritual and psychosocial domains of health and wellbeing.

SUMMARY

Learning objective 1: Explain how the meso level of the ICCCF addresses care for the person with a chronic condition.
The meso level of the ICCCF incorporates the health care organisation and the community. Together these combine to provide the health care needs of the individual.

Learning objective 2: Understand how to build a supportive environment with the person with a chronic condition and other health partners.
A health care environment that supports the sharing of information among multiple health providers is essential to the coordination of care. Information systems that provide client follow-ups and recalls are recommended. Health services need to be redesigned so that support for long-term management of care is facilitated, rather than focusing on single episodes of care.

Learning objective 3: Explore aspects of health promotion and education within chronic care nursing.
Health promotion is defined as 'the process of enabling people to increase their control over, and to improve, their health' (Francis et al., 2013). Health is a social and a personal resource that encapsulates social, economic and political determinants (Francis et al., 2013). Enhancing the health literacy of individuals is advocated as an appropriate approach to promote self-efficacy. Health education is an accepted strategy to increase the knowledge that supports individuals to make informed choices about their health.

Learning objective 4: Consider the available resources within the community that support the care of the person with a chronic condition and identify methods to develop future resources within health care organisations.
Every community has a resource base that can support the quality of life of the community. Understanding the range of resources available in communities is often achieved by undertaking a community assessment. This information can be used by nurses and other health professionals to connect people to the services and resources that they require.

Learning objective 5: Describe the impact of stigma in relation to chronic illness.
Reducing stigmatisation, which is based on prejudicial thoughts and beliefs, will support equity and access to health care for marginalised groups such as people with chronic illness or disability. To reduce stigmatisation, health promotion and prevention programs should include raising awareness about chronic illness.

REVIEW QUESTIONS

1. Describe the significance of the Declaration of Alma-Ata and the Ottawa Charter for Health Promotion.
2. Discuss strategies that could be used to generate understanding of community resources.
3. Define health promotion.
4. Describe what constitutes a healthy person.
5. What are some of the factors that influence health and wellbeing?

RESEARCH TOPIC

Select a chronic condition and, on paper, draw a map of the services and health professionals that are available in your local community, and which could be of assistance to someone with that condition.

FURTHER READING

Australian Institute Health and Welfare (AIHW). (2018). *Australia's Health 2018. Australia's Health Series No. 16*. Canberra: AIHW.

Council of Australian Governments. (2011). *National Health Reform Agreement*. Canberra: Council of Australian Governments. Retrieved from www.federalfinancialrelations .gov.au/content/npa/health/_archive/national-agreement.pdf

Francis, K., Chapman, Y., Hoare, K. & Birks, M. (2013). *Australia and New Zealand, Community as Partner: Theory and Practice in Nursing* (2nd edn). Sydney: Lippincott Williams & Wilkins.

New Zealand Ministry of Health (NZMOH). (2016). *New Zealand Health Strategy: Future Direction*. Wellington: Ministry of Health. Retrieved from www.health.govt.nz/ publication/new-zealand-health-strategy-2016

Nuño, R., Coleman, K., Bengoa, R. & Sauto, R. (2012). Integrated care for chronic conditions: The contribution of the ICCC Framework. *Health Policy*, 105(1), 55–64. doi: http://10.1016/j.healthpol.2011.10.006

The World Health Organization (WHO) supports a broad range of initiatives designed to improve the health and wellbeing of all people. Visit the WHO website and read about the work of WHO: www.who.int/en

REFERENCES

Anderson, J. K. & Malone, L. (2015). Chronic care undergraduate nursing education in Australia. *Nurse Education Today*, 35(12), 135–8. doi: http://10.1016/ j.nedt.2015.08.008

Andrews, L., Gajanayake, R. & Sahama, T. (2014). The Australian general public's perceptions of having a personally controlled electronic health record (PCEHR). *International Journal of Medical Informatics*, 83(12), 889–900. doi: http://dx.doi.org/ 10.1016/j.ijmedinf.2014.08.002

Australian Bureau of Statistics. (2015). Coordination of health care. Retrieved from www .abs.gov.au/ausstats/abs@.nsf/Lookup/by Subject/4839.0~2014–15~Main Features~Coordination of health care~6

Australian Commission on Safety and Quality in Health Care. (2009). Preventing falls and harm from falls in older people. *Australian Commission on Safety and Quality in Health Care*. Canberra: Commonwealth of Australia.

Australian Government Department of Health. (2015). Influenza (flu). Retrieved from www .immunise.health.gov.au/internet/immunise/publishing.nsf/Content/immunise-influenza

Australian Institute of Health and Welfare (AIHW). (2015). Overweight and obesity. Retrieved from www.aihw.gov.au/overweight-and-obesity

—— (2018). *Australia's Health 2018. Australia's Health Series No. 16.* Canberra: AIHW.

Cancer Council Victoria. (2015). Be sunsmart. Retrieved from www.cancervic.org.au/preventing-cancer/be-sunsmart

Community Tool Box. (2015). Section 8. Identifying community assets and resources. Retrieved from http://ctb.ku.edu/en/table-of-contents/assessment/assessing-community-needs-and-resources/identify-community-assets/main

Council of Australian Governments. (2011). *National Health Reform Agreement.* Canberra: Council of Australian Governments. Retrieved from www.federalfinancialrelations .gov.au/content/npa/health_reform/national-agreement.pdf

Department of Health and Human Services, Victoria. (2018). Care coordination. Retrieved from www2.health.vic.gov.au/hospitals-and-health-services/patient-care/rehabilitation-complex-care/health-independence-program/care-coordination

Edgecombe, G. & Stephens, R. (2010). Healthy communities: The evolving roles of nursing. In J. Daly, S. Speedy & D. Jackson (eds), *Contexts of Nursing* (3rd edn, pp. 274–86). Sydney: Churchill Livingstone, Elsevier.

Francis, K., Chapman, Y., Hoare, K. & Birks, M. (2013). *Australia and New Zealand, Community as Partner: Theory and Practice in Nursing* (2nd edn). Sydney: Lippincott Williams & Wilkins.

Gallagher, R. W. & Polanin, J. R. (2015). A meta-analysis of educational interventions designed to enhance cultural competence in professional nurses and nursing students. *Nurse Education Today,* 35(2), 333–40. doi: http://10.1016/j.nedt.2014.10 .021

Halding, A.-G., Heggdal, K. & Wahl, A. (2011). Experiences of self-blame and stigmatisation for self-infliction among individuals living with COPD. *Scandinavian Journal of Caring Sciences*, 25(1), 100–7. doi: http://10.1111/j.1471-6712.2010.00796.x

Harris, M. F., Jayasinghe, U. P., Taggart, J. R., Christle, B., Proudfoot, J. G., Crookes, P. A., ... & Powell Davies, G. (2011). Multidisciplinary team care arrangements in the management of patients with chronic diseases in Australian general practice. *Medical Journal of Australia*, 194(5), 236–9.

Johnson, A. (2007). Health literacy, does it make a difference? *Australian Journal of Advanced Nursing*, 31(3), 39–45.

Kim, H. & Xie, B. (2017). Health literacy in the eHealth era: A systematic review of the literature. *Patient Education and Counseling,* 100(6), 1073–82. doi: http://doi.org/10 .1016/j.pec.2017.01.015

Kozier, B., Erb, G. L., Berman, A., Snyder, S., Levett-Jones, T., Dwyer, T., ... & Stanley, D. (2015). *Kozier and Erb's Fundamentals of Nursing, Australian Edition* (vol. 1). Melbourne: Pearson.

Malone, L. M. & Anderson, J. K. (2014). The right staffing mix for inpatient care in rural multi-purpose service health facilities. *Rural Remote Health,* 14(4), 2881.

Ministry of Business, Innovation & Employment. (2015). New Zealand employment legislation. Retrieved from www.business.govt.nz/laws-and-regulations/employment-regulations/new-zealand-employment-legislation

Modi. (2015). Facts & figures, obesity in Australia. Retrieved from www.modi.monash.edu .au/obesity-facts-figures/obesity-in-australia

Moodie, A. R. (2008). *Australia: The healthiest country by 2020. Medical Journal of Australia*, 189(10), 588–90.

Msibi, G. S., Mkhonta, N. R., Nkwanyana, N. R., Mamba, B. & Thembisile, G. (2014). Establishing a national programme for continuing professional development of nurses and midwives in Swaziland. *African Journal of Midwifery & Women's Health*, 14–16.

Nash, M. (2013). Diagnostic overshadowing: A potential barrier to physical health care for mental health service users. *Mental Health Practice*, 17(4), 22–6.

National Asthma Council of Australia. (2015). What is asthma? Retrieved from www.nationalasthma.org.au/understanding-asthma/what-is-asthma-#3

National Heart, Lung and Blood Institute. (2015). What is cardiac rehabilitation? Retrieved from www.nhlbi.nih.gov/health-topics/cardiac-rehabilitation

New Zealand Ministry of Health (NZMOH). (2014). Primary health care. Retrieved from www.health.govt.nz/our-work/primary-health-care

——(2015a). Obesity data and stats. Retrieved from www.health.govt.nz/nz-health-statistics/health-statistics-and-data-sets/obesity-data-and-stats

——(2015b). Welcome to health promoting schools. Retrieved from http://hps.tki.org.nz

——(2016). *New Zealand Health Strategy: Future Direction.* Wellington: Ministry of Health. Retrieved from www.health.govt.nz/publication/new-zealand-health-strategy-2016

NSW Government Healthy Kids. (2015a). Healthy Kids. Retrieved from www.healthykids.nsw.gov.au/home/about-us.aspx

——(2015b). NSW Premier's sporting challenge. Retrieved from www.healthykids.nsw.gov.au/teachers-childcare/healthy-lifestyle-programs-for-primary-schools/nsw-premiers-sporting-challenge.aspx

——(2015c). What is Live Well @ School? Retrieved from www.healthykids.nsw.gov.au/teachers-childcare/live-life-well-@-school.aspx

Nuño, R., Coleman, K., Bengoa, R. & Sauto, R. (2012). Integrated care for chronic conditions: The contribution of the ICCC Framework. *Health Policy*, 105(1), 55–64. doi: http://10.1016/j.healthpol.2011.10.006

Standing Council on Health. (2013). *National Primary Health Care Strategic Framework.* Canberra: Commonwealth of Australia.

Talbot, L. & Verrinder, G. (2014). *Promoting Health: The Primary Health Care Approach* (5th edn). Sydney: Elsevier.

Wagner, E. H., Austin, B. T., Davis, C., Hindmarsh, M., Schaefer, J. & Bonomi, A. (2001). Improving chronic illness care: Translating evidence into action. *Health Affairs*, 20 (6), 64–78. doi: http://10.1377/hlthaff.20.6.64

World Health Organization (WHO). (1986). *The Ottawa Charter for Health Promotion.* Geneva: WHO. Retrieved from http://www.who.int/healthpromotion/conferences/previous/ottawa/en/index.html

——(2002). *Innovative Care for Chronic Conditions: Building Blocks for Action: Global Report.* Geneva: WHO.

——(2015). WHO called to return to the Declaration of Alma-Ata. Retrieved from www.who.int/social_determinants/tools/multimedia/alma_ata/en

Zangerle, C. M. (2017). Engaging clinical nurses in care coordination. *Nursing Management,* 48(3), 10–11.

4

Implementing the micro level of the Innovative Care for Chronic Conditions Framework

Judith Anderson, Linda Deravin
and Kathryn Anderson

LEARNING OBJECTIVES

After studying this chapter, you should be able to:

1. explain how the micro level of the Innovative Care for Chronic Conditions Framework (ICCCF) interacts with other levels to provide care for the person with a chronic condition
2. describe how collaborative client interaction can be fostered between the nurse and the person with a chronic condition
3. understand important aspects of holistic nursing care, including psychosocial aspects, for the person with a chronic condition
4. describe the importance of the nursing role at the micro level of the ICCCF.

Introduction

This chapter introduces the micro level of the ICCCF. This level of the ICCCF focuses on patient interaction and the need to empower patients/clients. The imperative of valuing patient interactions and the role of the nurse in supporting them in self-care strategies is explored. Empowerment as the basis of self-care is described and psychosocial aspects of care are reviewed. Patients/clients and family members are viewed holistically, and their contextual backgrounds (for example, cultural and lifestyle factors) are included in the framework (Epping-Jordan et al., 2004; World Health Organization (WHO), 2002).

Prevention of chronic conditions, early detection, effective management and prevention of complications are all aims of the ICCCF. The micro level focuses on interacting with individuals to meet these aims.

The micro level is at the centre of the ICCCF, with direct contact and interaction between the patient/client, health care team and the community. This level of the ICCCF is also directly supported by the meso level, which includes the wider community and health care services where this interaction takes place (Epping-Jordan et al., 2004).

Describing the micro level

The micro level of the ICCCF attempts to encapsulate the importance of patient behaviour and the value of good-quality interactions with health care workers (see Figure 4.1). The majority of research that has been undertaken in relation to the care of people with chronic conditions has targeted this level and needs to be well incorporated into current practice (WHO, 2002).

At the centre of the ICCCF is the triad of the patient and family, community partners such as advocates and carers, and the health care team. These groups are seen to be most successful when they are all informed, motivated, prepared and working together (Epping-Jordan et al., 2004; WHO, 2002). Although the client is at the centre of the ICCCF, health care professionals also need to communicate and collaborate with each other to provide a seamless approach to chronic care management (Zangerle, 2017).

Nursing care is planned at this level of the ICCCF in consultation with the individual client/groups of clients, their significant others and the interdisciplinary health care team. This planning is undertaken with the client and their family in a holistic and collaborative manner that addresses their psychosocial needs, as well as their physical and spiritual needs. It empowers them to self-care as much as they are able or willing to do at each stage of their condition.

The micro level of the ICCCF is supported by both the meso and macro levels. This is required so that a triad is formed which supports best possible patient outcomes (Epping-Jordan et al., 2004; WHO, 2002).

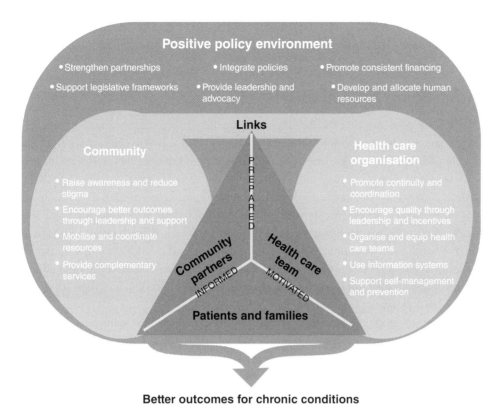

Figure 4.1 Innovative Care for Chronic Conditions Framework: the micro level (coloured section)
Source: WHO (2002)

REFLECTION

What are the key components in the micro level of the ICCCF?

Collaborative client interaction

Clients are highly valued in the ICCCF. As mentioned previously, the interactions with clients and their families are considered to be at the centre of the ICCCF (Epping-Jordan et al., 2004; WHO, 2002). This is consistent with the concept of person- or family-centred care. A **person-centred approach** has been demonstrated to increase client satisfaction, recall of content of health visits, adherence with documented plans, improved health outcomes, health care utilisation and health care provider satisfaction (Wolstenholme et al., 2017). The triad at the centre of the framework represents the collaboration between clients and their families, health care providers and the community. The requirement for each member of this triad to be informed, motivated and prepared with the skills necessary to manage chronic conditions indicates a significant

Person-centred approach – focuses on the client and their family, and their perspectives and wishes.

role for the nurse as a member of the health care team in ensuring that such knowledge and skills are available to the client, their family and community members who may be able to support them (Epping-Jordan et al., 2004; WHO, 2002).

Developing client partnerships

The ICCCF proposes that the development of good-quality relationships with clients, which last over long periods of time, are imperative if health care workers are to make a significant impact on their lives. The ICCCF identifies the need for 'motivated' health care workers, clients, families and community members (Epping-Jordan et al., 2004; WHO, 2002). This requirement for motivation is supported by research that has linked optimism, hope and self-efficacy with better health outcomes for clients with a variety of chronic conditions. However, motivating people can be a difficult task. Motivational interviewing and communication techniques are important skills for the nurse to develop. These skills include open-ended questions, affirming the strengths and efforts of the patient, validating the patient's meaning through reflection, and then summarising what the patient has said (Welch, 2014).

Ensuring that clients have adequate information and skills to manage their conditions is an important aspect to providing an environment where they feel supported in managing their own conditions (Epping-Jordan et al., 2004; WHO, 2002). In order to have an informed client, health care professionals must to be well-informed themselves and have a good understanding of evidence-based practice, as described in Chapter 1. Part of being a well-informed health professional is having an awareness of other health professionals, their roles and methods of communicating.

The discussion on informed clients is often related to health literacy. Health literacy involves being able to obtain, read, understand and act upon health-related information (Kim & Xie, 2017), and has been demonstrated to have a greater impact on a person's health status than age, socioeconomic status, educational level or ethnicity. Health literacy can vary according to a person's cultural and ethnic background, and their ability to understand a second language. Health literacy predicts not only the degree of interaction a client has with their health care provider (the micro level of the ICCCF) but also the health care organisation (the meso level of the ICCCF) (Kim & Xie, 2017). Health literacy within the general population is low, so it is important that nurses, who have provided information to clients, check how well this has been understood by asking clients to explain what has been said to them in their own words, rather than asking them if they have understood. This is sometimes known as a 'teach-back process' and has been demonstrated to be best practice. The teach-back process includes four stages: explaining, assessing, clarifying and understanding (Caplin & Saunders, 2015).

Research demonstrates that clients are frequently not asked about risk factors for chronic conditions during their visits with health care providers. Sensitive topics, such as sexuality, are unlikely to be broached by clients unless the health care provider makes it known that they are interested in discussing them. It is important to discuss risk factors to assist clients to reduce the impact of potential risks and to ensure they are well-informed about their conditions. Using well-known evidence-based tools to assess and monitor clients' progress can facilitate communication across professional boundaries. This presents a united front that clients will find reassuring and less confusing than if each profession uses different terms and makes contradictory suggestions for their care. Key strategies to interacting with people who have chronic conditions include: seeking their perspective, responding to their concerns, informing them, building partnerships with them, engaging them in collaborative decision making, and developing a care plan together (Byron, 2017).

Follow up

There is a significant difference in acute episodic care provision, which is unpredictable and instigated by the client, to the care provision required to effectively manage chronic conditions (Oni et al., 2014). Interactions with clients for health workers who are managing chronic care need to include active follow up. Follow up is essential to further examine or observe a client to monitor the success of an intervention, including any self-care that may have been initiated. This assists in building the relationship and ensuring that clients are not lost to the system, as it is often when clients are least able to seek care that they would benefit from it the most. Active follow up of clients also considers the frequent scenario where people with chronic conditions feel well or, conversely, omit to take preventative actions. An example of this is when a patient ceases to take regular medications. An active follow-up program can assist in maintaining their motivation at these times as they are reminded of the benefits and value of prevention. An active follow-up program can also monitor treatment outcomes and assist with negotiating adjustments that are acceptable to the client, or enable the client to seek further advice and intervention if treatment has not been successful (Davies et al., 2014).

Empowerment

Empowerment is an essential part of the ICCCF. Empowerment is the encouragement of patient/clients by health professionals to become active in exercising control over, and autonomy, in their health care and decision making, rather than being passive recipients of health care (McAllister et al., 2012). While health care professionals should always aspire to empower patients, empowerment is particularly important in the management of people with chronic conditions who need to manage their condition over the long term. Developing independence is essential for clients to maintain quality of life during the progression of the chronic condition and to prevent complications. This is discussed further in Chapter 6.

Empowerment is initiated by involving people with chronic conditions in their treatments – encouraging self-care management, decision making and taking an active role in conversing with the interdisciplinary team. This is assisted through patient education and the development of therapeutic relationships with health professionals (Lawn et al., 2014, pp. 389–90). Empowerment itself is a subjective concept. It is difficult to accurately measure and construct effective mechanisms to ensure that all clients are empowered. For this reason, it is important to check that health care is tailored to empower individuals to manage their conditions. As the health care system moves towards the use of the ICCCF, the emphasis on holistic care, including the empowerment of the person, becomes an integral element (Small et al., 2013). Effective treatment of chronic conditions requires the knowledge and expertise of various members of the interdisciplinary team to devise appropriate treatment and care that is person-centred, and all members need to value empowerment for it to be effective. Disempowerment occurs when health professionals fail to communicate effectively and over-regulate patients, leading to negative health outcomes (Lawn et al., 2014, p. 391).

SKILLS IN PRACTICE

Empowering people with chronic conditions

Joan has type 2 diabetes, which is diet controlled. She has had frequent hospital admissions for poorly controlled blood glucose levels. On her last discharge from an acute care facility, Joan was referred to you, the diabetes clinical nurse consultant at the local community centre, for continued follow up. She has presented for an appointment today after missing three appointments that you made with her. Joan states she could not make the other appointments as she had other health professionals to see. Joan tells you that she is not complying with her diet and forgets to monitor her blood glucose levels. She is going back to see her doctor next week for an ulcer on her foot after seeing the podiatrist to have her toenails cut.

QUESTIONS

Consider the following aspects of Joan's care in relation to the micro level of the ICCCF.

1. What are the issues for this client, regarding both physical and psychosocial concerns?

2. As a nurse, what strategies could you implement to support the care for Joan in the management of her chronic condition?

3. Can you identify some of the barriers that might influence the care of Joan in having to seek a variety of health care services from multiple health providers? Suggest ways to overcome these barriers.

Self-care management

Self-care – an overarching term that includes self-management, and a person taking responsibility for their own health and wellbeing.

Self-management – a person's ability to organise themselves to cope with their difficulties and conditions.

Self-care is an important aspect of the ICCCF. Self-care assists the client and their family to manage their own condition (Block, Tran & McIntosh, 2011). It is based on the belief that people want control over their own lives, including the dignity, respect and independence that this entails. Self-care is an overarching term that includes **self-management** and a person taking responsibility for their own health and wellbeing.

REFLECTION

A person with asthma will need to be educated on developing an asthma management plan. Can you think of other examples where strategies might be needed for nurses to support people with chronic conditions to manage their own care?

Psychosocial aspects of care

Evidence clearly indicates a link between **psychosocial health** and physical health. There are several aspects of this: poor psychosocial health often increases a person's predisposition to chronic conditions, delays detection of chronic conditions, and leads to poor self-management of chronic conditions; chronic conditions themselves often lead to a deterioration of psychosocial health. Psychosocial aspects of care contribute to holistic nursing care, which is seen to address the health issues of the mind, body and spirit of the client. These issues are of equal importance and neglecting one will create issues in others (Selimen & Andsoy, 2011).

Psychosocial aspects of care are strongly linked to a client's family and community, both of which are embedded in the micro level of the ICCCF. The assistance that community organisations and members can and will provide to clients is invaluable. Some services may be more oriented towards physical aspects such as financial support, access to services and equipment; others may be more oriented towards social networking. Together, these services can reduce the sense of isolation, hopelessness and discrimination that many people with chronic conditions feel at some time. To deal effectively with the psychosocial aspects of care, clients may need assistance in stress management, or strategies to develop new habits (Lukewich et al., 2015).

Psychosocial health – considers both psychological and social aspects of health.

Spirituality

Spirituality can be thought of as the aspects of a person's life that give it meaning, purpose and direction. It can be regarded as the very essence of a person's being – how they perceive the world, and their place within the world and how they relate to the world they live in. In the context of the micro level of the ICCCF, nurses need to consider what spirituality means for the person as an individual, and the interrelationships between the person, their family and their community. Spirituality is a complex and multidimensional concept that is also connected with religiosity and personal belief (Lopez et al., 2014). This is not to say that spirituality is solely based on religious beliefs – a person can be spiritual without being religious because religion and the concept of spirituality can be separate; however, the connection between the two is something that needs to be considered.

Barnum (2010) describes religion as being in contrast with spirituality because religion is an organisation that brings together people who share a common purpose, a shared belief and shared rituals. Spirituality is something that is more personal and individualised. Spirituality can also be part of a person's religious beliefs, and nurses will encounter a variety of individual preferences among clients. Nurses need to think, therefore, in terms of being spiritually sensitive and aware that care needs to be delivered in a non-judgemental and non-biased way. People with chronic conditions may experience individual challenges when faced with thoughts about their own mortality, and their journey regarding their own spiritual beliefs is one that nurses should acknowledge and support (Barnum, 2010). Spiritual care should be considered in terms of attitudes and actions within nursing practice. Nursing values, such as the recognition of human dignity, compassion and kindness, are particularly relevant to the care of a person with a chronic condition who is seeking to understand their own health needs while facing an uncertain future (MacLeod et al., 2017).

Suffering

The inner conflict that chronic illness may create commonly results in people finding ways to make meaning out of their circumstances and the consequences for themselves. One of the ways this may be experienced is through suffering.

Suffering is a profound human experience. Cassell defines suffering as 'an anguish that is experienced, not only as a pressure to change, but as a threat to our composure, our integrity and the fulfilment of our intentions' (Ferrell & Del Ferraro, 2012). The internal conflict that someone may face as they go through, not only physical changes, but also self-identity changes, may lead to them experiencing suffering. Chronic illness can undermine an individual's sense of being and identity. Through the progression of their illness, a person's place within relationships, and how they function within their family and community may significantly change (Greenstreet, 2006). Common themes that are often related to suffering include isolation, hopelessness, despair, vulnerability and loss.

Hope

Hope is another concept that is often felt when people face chronic illness and the challenges this brings. Hope is an expectation that good things may happen, and it focuses on an optimistic view of the future. Hope is not the denial of suffering, but rather is incorporated into the experience. The resilience needed to combat suffering also requires hope. To have hope for a cure, for improved health and wellness, and to bring about a change that positively influences the future is often seen as part of the conflict that arises within chronic conditions, and forms part of the coping strategies in dealing with illness (Eliot, 2012).

Sexuality

Sexuality – a person's sexual orientation, their sexual activities and associated feelings, and their ideas and thoughts of a sexual nature. It includes gender role and body image, and the experiences of intimacy and love.

Another important component of psychosocial care is the concept of **sexuality**. Sexuality incorporates a person's self-concept of their own body's needs and wants. The ability of a person with a chronic illness to fulfil this important aspect of their life can be fraught with challenges. Relationships bring meaning to people's lives, and understanding how we connect with fellow human beings is an important aspect of care for the nurse to consider. How a person looks, feels and thinks about themselves affects their relationships. Yet health professionals often find it difficult to talk about sex and the concept of sexuality. Often this stems from preconceived ideas about sex and sexuality that are influenced by such things as cultural beliefs and personal attitudes (Bahouq et al., 2013; Byron, 2017).

Human beings all like to feel accepted and wanted, and perhaps be the object of another person's desire. Chronic illness may change how a person feels about themselves, and it may also affect the person's ability to engage in sexual relations and intimacy. Simultaneously, people who become carers for their partners may experience a change in their desire and energy for sexual activities. Many chronic illnesses have a significant impact on physiological processes and this will impact on a person's ability to engage in sexual activity. As relationships are such an important part of human interaction, the need for intimacy and caring should never be underestimated (Steinke, 2013). It is important for nurses to understand the value of sexual health and sexuality.

Cultural and lifestyle factors

At the micro level, it is important to consider cultural and lifestyle factors in the care of people with chronic conditions. The predisposition for chronic illness can be influenced by lifestyle. Lifestyle factors are modifiable risks in chronic disease and illness and should be taken into consideration when planning care with the client. Cultural factors also play an important role in communication, dietary habits, level of physical activity and, for some, the predisposition to chronic illness. Some ethnic groups are more prone to specific types of chronic illness than others. In some cultures, the more financially rich a person is, the more likely they are to consume foods high in sugar and fat, as consuming these foods is considered to align with social status. In other cultures, however, having more money allows a person to purchase healthier foods. Conversely, people who live in low socioeconomic communities may have poor dietary habits and consume less healthy foods (Bittner & Kulesz, 2015).

Communication styles vary across cultures, so it is essential that nurses apply principles of effective communication that are sensitive to the culture they are presented with. For example, the importance of non-verbal communication and body language can have a different meaning depending on someone's cultural background (Gallagher & Polanin, 2015). Indigenous Australians may consider it rude to make eye contact when speaking to another person. This can be misinterpreted by health professionals as the client not paying attention or disengaging from the conversation. Where language barriers exist, the difficulty in effectively communicating may mean additional time is needed to deliver or communicate patient care needs (Paterson, Nayda & Paterson 2012; Waterworth et al., 2015). Some cultures will express caring, grief and the experience of pain differently to others.

A culturally safe approach to nursing care requires the nurse to be mindful of their own attitudes, values and beliefs regarding gender, race, religion and sexuality. In recent years, the impetus to educate health staff regarding cultural awareness and sensitivity has increased. Cultural awareness is recognising and acknowledging cultural differences. Within health systems, cultural competence embraces cultural diversity, and ensures that policy and services are responsive to the needs of differing cultures. Promoting shared respect for individuals regardless of cultural background; and acknowledging that different cultures can bring to the caring process a wealth of knowledge, meaning and experience; is good practice. Showing cultural respect allows the focus to move towards health equity and improved health outcomes (Gallagher & Polanin, 2015)

SKILLS IN PRACTICE

Cultural safety in practice: Greg

Greg – an Indigenous man – has pancreatic cancer and is at the terminal stage of his condition. He lives with his wife and two children and is considered to be an 'uncle' within his community. He does not want to die in hospital, and would prefer to be surrounded by his extended family and friends.

QUESTIONS

You are the community nurse caring for Greg.

1. What communication considerations do you need to think about in ensuring that Greg receives and understands what care options are available to him?

2. What services or resources are available to help you?

The nurse's role in caring for people with chronic conditions

Nurses working with people who have chronic conditions usually focus on the clinical aspects of their role; that is, monitoring client conditions and treatments, and providing support for them and their families to manage their own care. However, these nurses also need to be able to work collaboratively, not only with other members of the health care team, but also with the clients themselves to assist them in changing their behaviour and managing their own conditions. Each health interaction is an opportunity for any health provider to inform clients about health promotion and disease prevention. Nurses working in the delivery of chronic care need specialised knowledge and expertise to predict the course of chronic conditions (Anderson & Malone, 2015), so that they can provide follow-up care and advice on the prevention of symptoms or complications.

Identification of risk factors is a first step in identifying and informing those who would benefit the most from interactions with health professionals. The WHO (2010) identifies several risk factors as having worldwide implications. These include tobacco use, lack of physical activity, harmful alcohol use and unhealthy diets; and it recommends that these risk factors are targeted to prevent chronic conditions.

Advanced nursing practice

Advanced nursing practice is defined by the International Council of Nursing as 'a registered nurse who has acquired the expert knowledge base, complex decision making skills and clinical competencies for expanded practice, the characteristics of which are shaped by the context and/or country in which s/he is credentialed to practice' (Lowe et al., 2012, p. 680). Six practice domains have been identified as being specific to establish the level of advanced nursing practice. These domains are: direct and comprehensive care, supportive systems, education, research, publication and professional leadership (Chang et al., 2012). The nursing role will be further explored in subsequent chapters and specifically related to individual chronic conditions to provide context.

SUMMARY

Learning objective 1: Explain how the micro level of the ICCCF interacts with other levels to provide care for the person with a chronic condition.

The micro level is at the centre of the ICCCF, with direct contact and interaction between the patient/client, health care team and the community. This level of the framework is directly supported by the meso level, which includes the wider community and the health care services where this interaction takes place. It is mainly through this meso layer that interaction takes place with the macro layer of the external environment, although some influences, such as government benefits and financial support, may have a more direct impact on the patient/client and the interactions that occur at the micro level.

Learning objective 2: Describe how collaborative client interaction can be fostered between the nurse and the person with a chronic condition.

The health care team collaborates with the client to form a partnership and negotiate a care plan that they not only agree to but are also able and willing to implement.

Learning objective 3: Understand important aspects of holistic nursing care, including psychosocial aspects, for the person with a chronic condition.

Holistic nursing care recognises that health issues of the mind, body and spirit are closely linked. Psychosocial aspects of care are just as integral as physical aspects to chronic care for the client.

Learning objective 4: Describe the importance of the nursing role at the micro level of the ICCCF.

The role of nurses working with people who have chronic conditions is usually considered to focus on the clinical aspect; that is, monitoring client conditions and treatments and providing support for them and their families to manage their own care.

REVIEW QUESTIONS

1. Describe how the micro level of the ICCCF relates to the meso level.
2. Describe some strategies that health care providers can use to effectively interact with clients who have chronic conditions.
3. What are some of the key principles that support empowerment for the person with a chronic condition?
4. Explain the difference between spirituality and religion.
5. What cultural barriers might you encounter when engaging with people from other ethnic backgrounds?

RESEARCH TOPIC

The WHO (2010) identifies several risk factors as having worldwide implications. These include tobacco use, lack of physical activity, harmful alcohol use and unhealthy diets. Research and prepare the advice you would give a patient with these risk factors to assist them to prevent chronic conditions or reduce the impact of chronic illness.

FURTHER READING

Epping-Jordan, J. E., Pruitt, S. D., Bengoa, R. & Wagner, E. H. (2004). Improving the quality of health care for chronic conditions. *Quality and Safety in Health Care*, 13(4), 299–305. doi: http://10.1136/qhc.13.4.299

Usher, K., Mills, J., West, R. & Power, T. (2017). Cultural Safety in nursing and midwifery. In J. Daly, S. Speedy & D. Jackson (eds), *Contexts of Nursing: An Introduction* (5th edn, pp. 337–50). Sydney: Elsevier.

Wepa, D. (2015). *Cultural Safety in Aotearoa New Zealand*. Melbourne: Cambridge University Press.

Westera, D. A. (2017). *Spirituality in Nursing Practice: The Basics and Beyond*. New York: Springer Publishing.

REFERENCES

Anderson, J. K. & Malone, L. (2015). Chronic care undergraduate nursing education in Australia. *Nurse Education Today*, 35(12), 135–8. doi: http://10.1016/j.nedt.2015.08.008

Bahouq, H., Allali, F., Rkain, H. & Hajjaj-Hassouni, N. (2013). Discussing sexual concerns with chronic low back pain patients: Barriers and patients' expectations. *Clinical Rheumatology*, 32(10), 1487–92. doi: http://10.1007/s10067-013-2299-y

Barnum, B. S. (2010). *Spirituality in Nursing: The Challenges of Complexity* (3rd edn). New York: Springer Publishing Company.

Bittner, J. V. & Kulesz, M. M. (2015). Health promotion messages: The role of social presence for food choices. *Appetite*, 87, 336–43. doi: https://doi.org/10.1016/j.appet.2015.01.001

Block, R. C., Tran, B. & McIntosh, S. (2011). Integrating the chronic care model into a novel medical student course. *Health Education Journal*, 70(1), 39–47. doi: http://10.1177/0017896910367955

Byron, P. (2017). Friendship, sexual intimacy and young people's negotiations of sexual health. *Culture, Health & Sexuality*, 19(4), 486–500.

Caplin, M. & Saunders, T. (2015). Utilizing teach-back to reinforce patient education: A step-by-step approach. *Orthopaedic Nursing*, 34(6), 365–8.

Chang, A. M., Gardner, G. E., Duffield, C. & Ramis, M. A. (2012). Advanced practice nursing role development: Factor analysis of a modified role delineation tool. *Journal of Advanced Nursing*, 68(6), 1369–79.

Davies, H., McKenzie, N., Williams, T. A., Leslie, G. D., McConigley, R., Dobb, G. J. & Aoun, S. M. (2014). Challenges during long-term follow-up of ICU patients with and without chronic disease. *Australian Critical Care*, 29(1), 27–34.

Eliot, J. (2012). Hope. In M. Cobb, C. M. Puchalski & B. D. Rumbold (eds), *Oxford Textbook of Spirituality in Healthcare* (pp. 119–26). New York: Oxford University Press.

Epping-Jordan, J. E., Pruitt, S. D., Bengoa, R. & Wagner, E. H. (2004). Improving the quality of health care for chronic conditions. *Quality and Safety in Health Care*, 13(4), 299–305. doi: http://10.1136/qhc.13.4.299

Ferrell, B. & Del Ferraro, C. (2012). Suffering. In M. Cobb, C. M. Puchalski & B. D. Rumbold (eds), *Oxford Textbook of Spirituality in Healthcare* (pp. 157–62). New York: Oxford University Press.

Gallagher, R. W. & Polanin, J. R. (2015). A meta-analysis of educational interventions designed to enhance cultural competence in professional nurses and nursing students. *Nurse Education Today*, 35(2), 333–40. doi: http://10.1016/j.nedt.2014.10.021

Greenstreet, W. (2006). Spiritual care. From spirituality to coping strategy: Making sense of chronic illness. *British Journal of Nursing*, 15(17), 938–42.

Kim, H. & Xie, B. (2017). Health literacy in the eHealth era: A systematic review of the literature. *Patient Education and Counseling*, 100(6), 1073–82. doi: https://doi.org/10.1016/j.pec.2017.01.015

Lawn, S., Delany, T., Sweet, L., Battersby, M. & Skinner, T. C. (2014). Control in chronic condition self-care management: How it occurs in the health worker–client relationship and implications for client empowerment. *Journal of Advanced Nursing*, 70(2), 383–94. doi: http://10.1111/jan.12203

Lopez, V., Fischer, I., Leigh, M. C., Larkin, D. & Webster, S. (2014). Spirituality, religiosity, and personal beliefs of Australian undergraduate nursing students. *Journal of Transcultural Nursing*, 25(4), 395–402. doi: http://10.1177/1043659614523469

Lowe, G., Plummer, V., O'Brien, A. P. & Boyd, L. (2012). Time to clarify – the value of advanced practice nursing roles in health care. *Journal of Advanced Nursing*, 68(3), 677–85.

Lukewich, J., Mann, E., VanDenKerkhof, E. & Tranmer, J. (2015). Self-management support for chronic pain in primary care: A cross-sectional study of patient experiences and nursing roles. *Journal of Advanced Nursing*, 71(11), 2551–62. doi: http://10.1111/jan.12717

MacLeod, R., Wilson, D. M., Crandall, J. & Austin, P. (2017). Death anxiety among New Zealanders: The predictive roles of religion, spirituality, and family connection. *OMEGA - Journal of Death and Dying*. doi: http://10.1177/0030222817724307

McAllister, M., Dunn, G., Payne, K., Davies, L. & Todd, C. (2012). Patient empowerment: The need to consider it as a measurable patient-reported outcome for chronic conditions. *BMC Health Services Research*, 12, 157.

Oni, T., McGrath, N., BeLue, R., Roderick, P., Colagiuri, S., May, C. R. & Levitt, N. S. (2014). Chronic diseases and multi-morbidity – a conceptual modification to the WHO ICCC model for countries in health transition. *BMC Public Health*, 14(1), 243–55. doi: http://10.1186/1471–2458-14-575

Paterson, G. A., Nayda, R. J. & Paterson, J. A. (2012). Chronic condition self-management: Working in partnership toward appropriate models for age and culturally diverse clients. *Contemporary Nurse*, 40(2), 169–78. doi: http://10.5172/conu.2012.40.2.169

Selimen, D. & Andsoy, I. I. (2011). The importance of a holistic approach during the perioperative period. *AORN Journal*, 93(4), 482–90. doi: http://10.1016/j.aorn.2010.09.029

Small, N., Bower, P., Chew-Graham, C. A., Whalley, D. & Protheroe, J. (2013). Patient empowerment in long-term conditions: Development and preliminary testing of a new measure. *BMC Health Services Research*, 13(1), 263. doi: http://10.1186/1472-6963-13-263

Steinke, E. E. (2013). Sexuality and chronic illness. *Journal of Gerontological Nursing*, 39(11), 18–27. doi: http://10.3928/00989134-20130916-01

Waterworth, P., Dimmick, J., Pescud, M., Braham, R. & Rosenberg, M. (2015). Factors affecting Indigenous West Australians' health behavior: Indigenous perspectives. *Qualitative Health Research*, 26(1), 55–68. doi: http://10.1177/1049732315580301

Welch, J. (2014). Building a foundation for brief motivational interviewing: Communication to promote health literacy and behavior change. *Journal of Continuing Education in Nursing*, 45(12), 566–72. doi: http://10.3928/00220124-20141120-03

Wolstenholme, D., Ross, H., Cobb, M. & Bowen, S. (2017). Participatory design facilitates person centred nursing in service improvement with older people: A secondary directed content analysis. *Journal of Clinical Nursing*, 26(9–10), 1217–25.

World Health Organization (WHO). (2002). *Innovative Care for Chronic Conditions: Building Blocks for Action: Global Report*. Geneva: WHO.

—— (2010). *Global Status Report on Noncommunicable Diseases 2010*. Geneva: WHO.

Zangerle, C. M. (2017). Engaging clinical nurses in care coordination. *Nursing Management*, 48(3), 10–11.

5

The Australian and New Zealand health care systems

Maureen Miles
and Karen Francis

With acknowledgement to Heather Latham and Jessica Biles

LEARNING OBJECTIVES

After studying this chapter, you should be able to:

1. outline the Australian and New Zealand health care systems
2. identify and describe the health care challenges faced by rural communities in Australia and New Zealand, including Aboriginal and Torres Strait Islander and Māori peoples
3. list the national health priorities and strategies for achieving improved health outcomes in Australia and New Zealand
4. critically analyse health differentials and health inequality, and their interaction on individuals, groups and communities
5. discuss the impact that vulnerability has on individuals and populations, and the importance of resilience.

Introduction

This chapter describes the Australian and New Zealand health care systems, which are both predominantly publicly funded and aim to provide equity in access to health care for all citizens. In Australia, there is also a private market model that provides a significant amount of funding for health care services. In New Zealand, the Treaty of Waitangi underpins all health and social policies, assuring partnership, participation and protection of Māori peoples (New Zealand Ministry of Health (NZMOH), 2014a). As in many countries around the world, the Australian and New Zealand governments and health care systems face the significant challenges of an increasing burden of chronic disease among ageing populations. The Australian *National Strategic Framework for Chronic Conditions* (Australian Health Ministers' Advisory Council, 2017) is a new approach that embraces the prevention and management of chronic conditions, rather than focusing on specific illnesses. This framework utilises a systemic, person-centred approach that considers shared health determinants, risk factors and multi-morbidities (Australian Health Ministers' Advisory Council, 2017, p.2). Partnerships and coordinated approaches to health care underpin the framework (Australian Health Ministers' Advisory Council, 2017). Similarly, in New Zealand, a 'long-term conditions approach' that also comprises a patient-focused, integrated health care partnership program has been implemented (NZMOH, 2016a).

Australia and New Zealand are countries that boast cosmopolitan cities, and vast rural and remote landscapes that are associated with unevenly distributed populations (New Zealand Tourism, 2018; Tourism Australia Corporation, 2018). There is a recognised health differential between the health and wellbeing of Aboriginal and Torres Strait Islander and Māori peoples compared to non-Indigenous peoples of Australia and New Zealand (Australian Institute of Health and Welfare (AIHW), 2016; NZMOH, 2015a). Disparity also exists for both Indigenous and non-Indigenous people who live in rural and remote settings. **Rurality** is classified in Australia according to three systems that determine the level of remoteness and funding available (AIHW, 2004). Whereas in New Zealand the urban/rural profile classification is used (National Health Committee, 2010). Rural and remote populations that include Aboriginal and Torres Strait Islander and Māori peoples experience higher morbidity and mortality compared with people who reside in metropolitan areas (AIHW, 2017a; National Health Committee, 2010). This challenges the governments of both countries to deliver equitable and accessible services reflective of those available in their metropolitan and urban areas.

Rurality – the distance of a community and the associated infrastructure of the community to a major metropolitan centre.

The Integrated Care for Chronic Conditions Framework (ICCCF) provides a model for change to address these challenges. **National health priorities**, developed in response to the World Health Organization's (WHO) 'health for all' global strategy (WHO, 1981), provide guidance for governments in promoting the health of their citizens and addressing the needs of the most vulnerable groups. Health differentials and inequalities are caused by a range of complex factors including: social and economic factors, health behaviours, physical factors, environmental issues, and access to health services and their utilisation. This chapter explores these factors and the role of governments in addressing them, as well as identifying the key role that nurses have in the management of people with chronic conditions.

National health priorities – health goals or targets set by the Australian government in response to the WHO's 'health for all' global strategy (WHO, 1981).

The Australian health care system

Maintaining health care was a part of everyday living for the original custodians of Australia – the Aboriginal and Torres Strait Islander peoples (Australian Indigenous Health*InfoNet*, 2018). Providing food and shelter were primary activities attended to by communities to ensure survival. Learning how to use resources available to treat deterioration in health status were embedded in cultural beliefs and traditions (McKendrick et al., 2014). Due to the effects of colonisation, the universal health care system arose from the traditions of the dominant culture which was based on a biomedical approach (illness focus). Today, a respect for health and wellbeing has largely replaced the illness model with an approach that values promoting health, reducing risk and preventing ill-health (AIHW, 2016). While the Australian health care system is a multifaceted web of public welfare and a private market model that has been in place since 1950 (Willis, Reynolds & Keleher, 2012), there have been successive alterations attempting to address rising health costs and changing demands (Macri, 2016). The increasing burden of chronic disease, together with an ageing population and the associated escalating cost of health care, are among the many challenges that confronts the Australian government. Macri (2016) reports that 21 per cent of the population will be aged 65 years and older by 2053. A reorientation of the health system away from the acute model of care is expected to address these challenges by introducing integrated care strategies and creating health service networks. The guiding principles of the *National Strategic Framework for Chronic Conditions* (Australian Health Ministers' Advisory Council, 2017) foster a universal, person-centred partnership approach to health and the maintenance of wellbeing that is supported by evidence-based decision making, and the promotion of health and reduction of risk; with an emphasis on quality, flexibility, accountability, integration and sustainability (Australian Health Ministers' Advisory Council, 2017). This framework supports the integration and networking of services to enhance accessibility and reduce differentials in health status between socioeconomic groups, particularly Aboriginal and Torres Strait Islander peoples, and those experiencing chronic illness.

The public health care system

Medicare was introduced in 1984 by the Hawke Labor government. Medicare is a compulsory universal health insurance scheme designed to provide equal access to health care for all Australians (AIHW, 2016). The Medicare levy (income tax) provides funding for health care in two ways. First, Medicare provides funding from the Commonwealth to state and territory governments for hospitals. Second, Medicare funds primary care services by direct payments to general practitioners; medical specialists; and some nurses, midwives and allied health professionals (AIHW, 2016) including aged care and disability services (Willis, Reynolds & Keleher, 2012, p. 5). State and territory governments also provide psychiatric/mental health services and community health programs, including home and community care.

The private health care system

While Medicare is the largest component of the Australian health care system, private health insurance provides a significant amount of funding for health care services (AIHW, 2016). The private health care system provides private access to health care by a health professional or doctor in either a public or private hospital, providing the doctor has practising rights at the hospital. Medicare funds 75 per cent of the schedule fee for medical and surgical treatment in private hospitals and some ancillary services (for example, dental and allied health). Private health insurance can cover the remaining gap (Willis et al., 2012, p. 31). Today, a respect for health and wellbeing has largely replaced the illness model with an approach that values promoting health, reducing risk and preventing ill health (AIHW, 2016).

The New Zealand health care system

The New Zealand health care system is predominantly publicly funded, with the Treaty of Waitangi underpinning all health and social policies, and assuring partnership, participation and protection of Māori peoples (NZMOH, 2014a). The New Zealand health care system provides high-quality, accessible and affordable health care through a community-oriented model. New Zealand has a proud history of being an international leader in health, and social policy development and implementation (NZMOH, 2013a). Similar to governments around the world, the New Zealand government now faces significant challenges to sustain and improve the health of the most disadvantaged and vulnerable groups within the community, including Māori and Pacific Islander peoples, who experience poorer education, employment and health outcomes compared with non-Māori and non-Pacific Islander peoples (Marriott & Sim, 2014; NZMOH 2016b). The 'Better, Sooner, More Convenient' primary health care strategy is an initiative to address inequality by providing population-based health services through the alignment, collaboration and participation of teams of multidisciplinary health professionals (Francis et al., 2013, p. 77–8). In 2016, the updated New Zealand Health Strategy was released. The slogan 'all New Zealanders living well, staying well and getting well' reflects the New Zealand government's focus on prevention rather than cure (NZMOH, 2016b).

The health and disability system

The NZMOH has overall responsibility for the management and development of the New Zealand health and disability system. This system is largely funded from general taxation (Vote Health), totalling approximately $14 655 billion in 2013–14. More than three quarters of this funding is allocated to district health boards (DHBs). The allocated funds pay for public hospitals and community services, while the remaining public funds provide national services for disability, targeted screening programs, mental health services, well child and primary maternity services, Māori health services, and postgraduate clinical education and training (NZMOH, 2013b). District health boards are charged with the responsibility of improving, promoting and protecting the health of people and communities. They also promote the integration of primary and secondary health care services to deliver the most effective and efficient health care to the population (NZMOH, 2014b). District health boards fund primary health organisations, which also aim to provide integrated population-based primary health care services to members of the community. A strong feature of the New Zealand health system is direct budget control to contain costs, and achieve efficiency and quality in the delivery of health services (Blank & Burau, 2010, p. 248).

Rurality

People who reside in smaller communities away from metropolitan areas may have limited access to education, support or resources to meet their needs. Rurality has been defined by the AIHW as the distance of a community and the associated infrastructure of the community to a major metropolitan centre (AIHW, 2004). Three classifications systems have been used in Australia to determine resource support: Rural, Remote and Metropolitan Area (RRMA), Accessibility/Remoteness Index of Australia (ARIA) and the Australia Standardised Geographical Classification (ASGC) (AIHW, 2004). Generally, the classification determines the level of remoteness and thus the funding available. While the allocation of funding and resources is imperative to the sustainability of small rural communities, the quality of life that people experience is the overarching interest for health professionals.

Health in rural communities in Australia

There is a link between rurality and poorer health outcomes of populations (AIHW, 2015). The more remotely people live, the higher the mortality and incidence of chronic disease. The major contributors to death in rural areas include coronary heart disease, motor vehicle accidents and chronic obstructive pulmonary disease. The cycle of reduced access to health services, hazardous environmental exposure (for example, driving long distances) and health risk factors (such as alcohol consumption and smoking) is higher in rural areas, and leads to an alarming suite of risks for rural communities (AIHW, 2017a).

Health in rural communities of New Zealand

Although only 25 per cent of New Zealanders live in rural areas, a high percentage of these are children, older people and Māori families. It is a priority of the NZMOH to ensure that rural communities have access to publicly funded services, and so infrastructure has been created through mobile and telehealth services (O'Connor, 2013). New Zealand has seen success in empowering local rural communities as a means to ensuring that socioeconomic disadvantage, rurality and access to health care are not always contributors to poorer health. The allocation of funding to DHBs supports unique community goals that are addressed through funded primary health care services (McMurray & Clendon, 2015).

Aboriginal and Torres Strait Islander communities

An estimated 25 per cent of Aboriginal and Torres Strait Islander peoples live in rural areas. The impact of rurality is even greater in Aboriginal and Torres Strait Islander communities given the huge disparity in overall health status compared to non-Indigenous Australians. Several schools of thought link the overall health disparity to learned socioeconomic disadvantage, a lack of culturally responsive health resources, Western models of health care dominating health environments, and the non-willingness of Aboriginal and Torres Strait Islander clients to access mainstream health settings due to direct and indirect racism by health care providers (Durey et al., 2016). It is also reported that Aboriginal and Torres Strait Islander peoples experience high costs related to transport and travel, which are also factors impacting access to health services (Daly, Speedy & Jackson, 2014).

In 2008, the Australian government launched the 'Closing the Gap' initiative to reduce disadvantage among Aboriginal and Torres Strait islander peoples. The areas of disadvantage targeted in this strategy included life expectancy, child mortality, access to early childhood education, educational achievement and employment options, and included time frames for achieving stated changes. A report released by the Australian government in 2018 stated that only three of the target areas were on track. This report acknowledged that renewed commitment was necessary and must involve a 'refreshed agenda', supported by stronger collaboration between Indigenous Australians, the state and federal governments and the non-government and private sectors, if the reform agenda was to be achieved (Commonwealth of Australia, Department of the Prime Minister and Cabinet, 2018; Deravin, Francis & Anderson, 2018).

Māori communities

He Korowai Oranga is the overarching framework that guides the government of New Zealand to achieve the best health outcomes for Māori communities. It encompasses three major elements; Māori ora (healthy individuals), Whanau ora (healthy families) and Te Puni Kokiri Wai ora (healthy environments) and is the responsibility of all peoples. This initiative has been developed to combat overall higher mortality and morbidity rates in Māori communities. Significant gains have been made over the past 10 years in preventative health. Currently, in Māori communities, immunisation figures are at a much higher standard than their non-Māori counterparts. This is seen as an outcome of individuals empowering themselves through the He Korowai Oranga. Significant work is still under way in rural New Zealand communities as community groups and health professionals enact the He Korowai Oranga (NZMOH, 2014c).

REFLECTION

By understanding and reflecting on how our views have been influenced and shaped, we can gain insight into other's perceptions around rurality. How do you define rurality and what is its impact on rural nursing?

National health priorities

The promotion of the health and wellbeing of the Australian and New Zealand populations is vital for ongoing sustainable health outcomes based on prevention. The national social **determinants of health**, equity principles and health priorities form the basis for identifying populations at risk, and the targets for governments, communities and local populations to achieve.

Determinants of health – a range of complex factors including biological, genetic, behavioural, social and economic that interact on individuals, groups and communities.

The national health priorities are health goals set by governments and are intended to be realised by collaborative action within countries. Governments across the world were prompted to respond to the WHO's global strategy 'Health for All by the Year 2000' (WHO, 1981) and to set ongoing health initiatives into the future. The motivation to work towards achieving these priorities is to reduce the social and financial cost burdens of chronic conditions on society.

Australia

In 1995, the Australian government, through bipartisan agreement, responded to the WHO's global strategy and developed the National Health Priority Areas initiative based on collaborative action between the state, territory and Commonwealth governments, non-government agencies, health experts, organisations, clinicians and consumers. The initiative identified specific diseases and conditions that were seen as being high prevalence and costly. It was also believed that if priorities were set, there would be improved financial savings and health outcomes for individuals. Cardiovascular health was one of the first priorities, and was added to the initiative in 1996, along with cancer control, injury prevention and control, and asthma in 1999. In 2002, arthritis and musculoskeletal conditions were added to the list, while mental health, diabetes mellitus and obesity were added in 2008 and in 2012, respectively. The dementia crisis declared in Australia (Hunter & Doyle, 2014) has seen dementia included as a significant health burden and it was added to the national health priority list in 2013.

The Australian national health priorities are:

- arthritis and musculoskeletal conditions
- asthma
- cancer control
- cardiovascular health
- dementia
- diabetes mellitus
- injury prevention and control
- mental health
- obesity (AIHW, 2017b).

It is believed that, through the modification of behaviours, the prevalence of disease and conditions can be lowered and, thereby, the health status of Australians can be improved and health inequities reduced.

The National Health Priority Areas initiative aims to improve health outcomes in each of the health priority areas and seeks to do the following.

- Monitor health outcomes and progress towards set targets.
- Identify the most appropriate and cost-effective points of intervention.

- Identify the most appropriate roles for government and non-government organisations in fostering the adoption of best practice.
- Investigate some basic determinants of health, such as education, employment and socioeconomic status (AIHW, 2017b).

The *National Strategic Framework for Chronic Conditions* (Australian Health Ministers' Advisory Council, 2017) provides direction for a multi-sectoral response to the prevention and management of chronic conditions that continue to impact adversely on the health of the nation, particularly Aboriginal and Torres Strait Islander peoples (Australian Health Ministers' Advisory Council, 2017).

New Zealand

New Zealand has had a similar journey to Australia, in that its health care system is complex, but at the heart of its national health priorities is a strong commitment to the improvement of people's health beginning with its response to the WHO call for 'Health for All by the Year 2000' (NZMOH, 2001). However, as in Australia, New Zealand has suffered fiscal problems and has needed to develop priorities that could be demonstrated in quantifiable outcomes and cost-effectiveness. To this end, the New Zealand government has focused on the development of a primary health care system, with the prime objective being to improve the health of New Zealanders and, in particular, tackle inequalities in health (NZMOH, 2001).

The NZMOH (2001, p. vii) has discussed the specific contribution primary health care can make to improved health outcomes and this has informed the new direction. New Zealand supports health targets that lead to improvement and outcomes at local and national levels. Accountability to achieve these targets is aimed at community and hospital settings, with a strong focus on prevention and patient access to services to address health and the social determinants of health. New Zealanders review their health targets annually to ensure they align with the nation's health priorities. New Zealand government health targets are:

- better help for smokers to quit
- faster cancer treatment
- improved access to elective surgery
- increased immunisation
- more heart and diabetes checks
- shorter stays in emergency departments (NZMOH, 2015b).

The paper implementing the New Zealand health strategy and intent (NZMOH, 2015b) called on doctors, nurses, community health workers and others in primary health care to work together with communities to reduce health inequalities and to address the causes of poor health status.

Health determinants

Health differentials and health inequalities are caused by a range of complex factors. These factors then impact on the choice, power and control of individuals, groups and communities. Determinants of health can be described as biological, genetic, behavioural, social and economic (DeLaune et al., 2016). It is known that often there is more than one determinant that impacts on people's lives. For example, many individuals who have a mental health illness will also have a physical illness, social illness or other comorbidity. The focus on social determinants highlights social and economic factors, health behaviours, physical conditions (including chronic illness and impairment), environmental factors, and access to health services and their utilisation.

For Australians and New Zealanders, socioeconomic status, race and ethnicity, and gender are significant to their social fabric. Less is known about the importance of 'place' and belonging to 'country' to health and wellbeing. In terms of health equality, health services and accessibility, the importance of place will depend on whether a person lives in a rural, remote or urban environment (Francis, Chapman & Davies, 2014). For the Indigenous populations of New Zealand and Australia, there are complex and multiple factors relating to culture and history that have substantially impacted on health outcomes. There have been significant changes in terms of access to services, recognition and acknowledgement of traditional culture requirements over the past two decades, but there remains a gap in the health between the Indigenous and non-Indigenous populations (King, Smith & Gracey, 2009).

The social measures for good health are reliant on:

- socioeconomic status
- health behaviours and lifestyle risks
- physical/environmental factors
- access to services and services fit for their purpose
- social capital and social support
- health professionals, including nurses, whose roles are in improving inequality.

Social determinants can be understood as the conditions into which people are born, grow, live, work and age (WHO, 2015). The Robert Wood Johnson Foundation (2010) states that '[t]his concept can be turned around to provide a platform for improved health. That is, health starts where we live, learn, work and play.'

REFLECTION

Identify a marginalised community and the social determinants of health that impact on the wellbeing of community members. In your role as a nurse, consider how you might collaborate with others to initiate preventative and interventionalist strategies to limit the impact of these social determinants.

Vulnerable populations

As social determinants impact on populations, the groups become vulnerable and are often described as more likely to: be susceptible to the development of poor health, have limited access to health care services or depend on others for care. Social determinants, therefore, can explain some of the factors that make groups vulnerable to being at risk. Examples of vulnerable population groups include the homeless, older people, individuals living in poverty, those in abusive relationships, people with mental health issues, substance abusers and new immigrants (Crisp & Potter, 2013).

Vulnerable populations are, however, more than groups. The WHO (2002) defined vulnerability as individuals, organisations or populations 'who are unable to anticipate, cope with, resist and recover from the impacts of disasters'. The WHO was referring specifically to national emergencies and environment disasters, but this definition can, as McMurray and Clendon (2015) assert, incorporate individuals and populations at relative and potential risk. Vulnerable populations are those that are identified as being at greater risk of developing health problems. Sociocultural status, limited access to resources, or characteristics such as age and gender suggest a level of vulnerability and therefore a potential risk. Using the concept of risk also suggests that anyone can potentially be at risk of ill health and therefore vulnerability (Francis et al., 2014).

Understanding vulnerability is much more challenging than just identifying groups and individuals. De Chesnay and Anderson (2012) assert that nurses need to work to understand vulnerability, and develop skills to assist those who are different. There is also a danger that if nurses understand vulnerability as being fragile, insecure, in danger and unable to manage, their practice could result in doing 'for' the person or doing 'to' the person. However, if instead the concepts of vulnerability, resilience, information sharing and partnerships in practice are understood, nurses can address vulnerabilities on various levels. These may include activating awareness campaigns, identifying policies that need to be adapted to meet individual and group needs, and modifying health care settings to address inequalities. If health professionals, including nurses, choose not to develop an awareness or understanding of these issues, they risk ignoring the strength and resilience of the individual (Hegney et al., 2007).

SKILLS IN PRACTICE

Gender and vulnerability

Plunket nurse – a registered nurse in New Zealand with specialist postgraduate qualifications in child health.

Sally, 27 years old, lives in Ohura, an isolated town in New Zealand. When she was 22, she was diagnosed with multiple sclerosis. Recently she gave birth to a baby boy who is now eight weeks old. While Sally is visiting her **Plunket nurse**, Rebecca; who travels to Sally's community once per month; Sally discloses feeling very lonely at home with her baby boy and often finds herself crying. Sally tells Rebecca that she has a very small community of friends in her home town and her husband travels frequently for work, leaving her and their baby for long periods of time each month.

QUESTIONS

If you were Sally's nurse, consider the following.

1. What data do you deem to be a high priority?

2. What support options does Sally have in a rural town? What other resources could you consider sharing with Sally?

3. What are the challenges faced by women living with a chronic illness in regional, rural and remote communities?

Resilience

Norman Garmezy, in the 1970s, brought the concept of **resilience** to psychology (Rolf, 1999). He defined 'resilience' as a condition that presents as personal growth and adaptation in spite of significant catastrophes. Rutter (1987), in the 1990s, added to the concept by suggesting that resilience came from the wish 'to inject some hope and optimism into the dispiriting story of stress and adversity'.

One of the key components that enables individuals to adapt in positive ways to adverse circumstances is the development of resilience. Resilience is described as a protective factor that can provide a positive impact on health outcomes (Hegney et al., 2007). These protective factors include the individual's spiritual, behavioural, cognitive, emotional and physical states. Hegney and colleagues (2007) have suggested that valuing close friendships and a broader social network are characteristics of resilient people. For Aboriginal and Torres Strait Islanders, and Māori peoples, connection to the land is important and has a positive influence on how these populations deal with adversity. Nurses play an important role in providing care that enables resilience to flourish through information sharing; joint decision making and health promotion; and encouraging creativity, humour and self-belief (Hegney et al., 2007).

> **Resilience** – a process of adaptation and growth despite experiences of significant trauma or suffering.

SKILLS IN PRACTICE

Resilience

Shane lives in Brunswick, Melbourne. He is 63 years old and has been married to Jill for 40 years; they have three teenage children. Prior to his recent stroke, Shane had been running a very successful graphic design company. The haemorrhagic stroke he experienced left him with some weakness on the right side of his body, making caring for himself and walking challenging. His speech is slurred and he has difficulties in selecting the right words. He is often tired, confused and frustrated.

QUESTIONS
As Shane's nurse consider the following.

1. What are the long-term challenges that Shane and his family will encounter?

2. What assistance might Shane and his family require to maintain optimal health and wellbeing?

3. The *Australian National Strategic Framework for Chronic Conditions* 2017 talks about prevention and management. What assistance and support could be available through this initiative?

4. How can you help Shane and Jill navigate the health system to successfully access services to meet their immediate and ongoing needs?

SUMMARY

Learning objective 1: Outline the Australian and New Zealand health care systems.
An overview of the Australian and New Zealand health care systems has highlighted the benefits of the public welfare system in providing equal access to health care for all citizens. The need for new directions in health policy has been identified to meet future challenges and sustain accessibility to health care services on an equitable basis.

Learning objective 2: Identify and describe the health care challenges faced by rural communities in Australia and New Zealand, including Aboriginal and Torres Strait Islander and Māori peoples.
Challenges faced by rural communities in Australia and New Zealand include limited access to education, support and resources, which contribute to poorer health outcomes.

Learning objective 3: List the national health priorities and strategies for achieving improved health outcomes in Australia and New Zealand.
The national health priorities are health goals or targets set by the governments of Australia and New Zealand. The social determinants of health and equity, and health priorities have been examined as the basis for identifying populations at risk and strategies to achieve improved health outcomes.

Learning objective 4: Critically analyse health differentials and health inequality, and their interaction on individuals, groups and communities.
A range of complex factors contribute to health differentials, health determinants and health inequality for Australians and New Zealanders, including socioeconomic status, race, ethnicity and gender. Access to culturally appropriate health services is a key factor in addressing equity in health care.

Learning objective 5: Discuss the impact that vulnerability has on individuals and populations, and the important of resilience.
A brief introduction to issues of vulnerability and resilience has been presented as vulnerability is often dependent on health determinants, along with potential and relative risks for poor health. All individuals are at risk of being in a vulnerable state of health. Resilience has been described as a concept that needs to be fostered as a means to deal with adversity and disadvantage.

REVIEW QUESTIONS

1. Discuss the challenges facing governments in Australia and New Zealand in the provision of health care to vulnerable populations with complex chronic conditions.
2. Compare and contrast rural communities in Australia and New Zealand. In your response consider the following factors: morbidity and mortality, major diseases, application of a primary health care model, and current infrastructure to ensure access to health for all.
3. Analyse how governments will address their national health priorities.
4. Describe how social and economic factors, health behaviours, physical and environmental factors, access to health services and their utilisation impacts on the health of individuals and populations.
5. Identify the various factors that might render a person or population vulnerable.

RESEARCH TOPIC

Investigate the health needs of a specific rural community in Australia or New Zealand. Discuss the role of the nurse in conjunction with the associated competencies that are required when working with this community, and the strategies the nurse could employ to address poor health outcomes.

FURTHER READING

Australian Health Ministers' Advisory Council. (2017). *National Strategic Framework for Chronic Conditions*. Canberra: Australian Government.

Deravin, L., Francis, K. & Anderson, J. (2018). Closing the gap in Indigenous health inequity – Is it making a difference. *International Nursing Review*. doi: http://10.1111/inr.12436

Mills, J. & Francis, K. (2012). Rural and remote communities. In W. St John & H. Keleher, *Community Nursing Practice: Theory, Skills and Issues*. Sydney: Allen & Unwin.

National Aboriginal Community Controlled Health Organisation. (2015). *NACCHO – Aboriginal Health in Aboriginal Hands*. Retrieved from www.naccho.org.au

New Zealand Ministry of Health (NZMOH). (2016). *New Zealand Health Strategy: Future Directions*. Wellington: Ministry of Health.

REFERENCES

Australian Health Ministers' Advisory Council. (2017). *National Strategic Framework for Chronic Conditions*. Canberra: Australian Government.

Australian Indigenous Health*InfoNet*. (2018). Aboriginal and Torres Strait Islander concept of health. Retrieved from https://healthinfonet.ecu.edu.au/learn/cultural-ways/aboriginal-and-torres-strait-islander-concept-of-health/

Australian Institute of Health and Welfare (AIHW). (2004). *Rural, Regional and Remote Health: A Guide to Remoteness Classifications. Rural Health Series No. 4*. Cat. no. PHE 53. Canberra: AIHW. Retrieved from www.aihw.gov.au/publication-detail/?id=6442467589

—— (2015). *National Health Priority Areas*. Retrieved from www.iahw.gov.au/national-health-priority-areas/

—— (2016). *Australia's Health 2016. Australia's Health Series No.15*. Cat. no. AUS 199. Canberra: AIHW.

—— (2017a). Rural and remote health. Canberra: AIHW. Retrieved from www.aihw.gov.au/reports/rural-health/rural-remote-health/contents/rural-health

—— (2017b). National Health Priority Areas. Retrieved from www.aihw.gov.au/getmedia/336ed4ed-1ead-404f-96d5-3f8f31a480e1/Health-priority-areas-Sept-2017.pdf.aspx

Blank, R. & Burau, V. (2010). *Comparative Health Policy* (3rd edn). New York: Palgrave MacMillan.

Commonwealth of Australia, Department of the Prime Minister and Cabinet. (2018). *Closing the Gap: Prime Minister's Report 2018*. Canberra: Commonwealth of Australia.

Crisp, J. & Potter, P. (2013). *Potter and Perry's Fundamentals of Nursing* (4th ANZ edn). Sydney: Mosby.

Daly, J., Speedy, S. & Jackson, D. (2014). *Contexts of Nursing* (4th edn). Melbourne: Oxford University Press.

De Chesnay, M. & Anderson, B. A. (2012). *Caring for the Vulnerable: Perspectives in Nursing Theory, Practice, and Research* (3rd edn). Burlington, MA: Jones & Bartlett Learning.

DeLaune, S., Ladner, P., McTier, L., Tollefson, J. & Lawrence, J. (2016). *Australian and New Zealand Fundamentals of Nursing* (1st edn). Melbourne: Cengage Learning Australia.

Deravin, L., Francis, K. & Anderson, J. (2018). Closing the gap in Indigenous health inequity – Is it making a difference. *International Nursing Review.* doi: http://10.1111/inr.12436

Durey, A., McEnvoy, S., Swift-Otero, V., Taylor, K., Katzenellenbogen, J. & Bessarab, D. (2016). Improving healthcare for Aboriginal Australians through effective engagement between community and health services. *BMC Health Services Research*, 16(1), 1. doi: http://org/10.1186/s12913-016-1497-0

Francis, K., Chapman, Y. & Davies, C. (2014). *Rural Nursing: The Australian Context.* Melbourne: Cambridge University Press.

Francis, K., Chapman, Y., Hoare, K. & Birks, M. (2013). *Australia and New Zealand Community as Partner: Theory and Practice in Nursing* (2nd edn). Sydney: Wolters Kluwer.

Hegney, D., Buikstra, E., Baker, P., Rogers-Clark, C., Pearce, S. & Ross, H. (2007). Individual resilience in rural people: A Queensland study. *Australia. Rural and Remote Health*, 7, 620.

Hunter, C. & Doyle, C. (2014). Dementia policy in Australia and the 'social construction' of infirm old age. *Health and History*, 16(2), 44–62. doi: http://10.5401/healthhist.16.2.0044

King, M., Smith, A. & Gracey, M. (2009). Indigenous health part 2: The underlying causes of the health gap. *Lancet*, 374, 76–85.

Macri, J. (2016). Australia's health sytem: Some issues and challenges. *Journal of Health and Medical Economics*, 2(2), 1–3.

Marriott, L. & Sim, D. (2014). *Indicators of inequity for Maori and Pacific people: Working papers in public finance.* Wellington: Victoria University of Wellington.

McKendrick, J., Brooks, R., Hudson, J, Thorpe, M. & Bennet, P. (2014). *Aboriginal and Torres Strait Islander Health Programs: A Literature Review.* Canberra: Healing Foundation. Retrieved from http://healingfoundation.org.au//app/uploads/2017/02/Aboriginal-and-Torres-Strait-Islander-Healing-Programs-A-Literature-Review.pdf

McMurray, A. & Clendon, J. (2015). *Community Health and Wellness: Primary Health Care in Practice.* Sydney: Elsevier Health Sciences.

National Health Committee. (2010). *Rural Health: Challenges of Distance, Opportunities for Innovation.* Wellington: National Health Committee.

New Zealand Ministry of Health (NZMOH). (2001). *The Primary Health Care Strategy.* Wellington: Ministry of Health. Retrieved from www.moh.govt.nz

—— (2013a). *Implementing the New Zealand Health Strategy 2013.* Wellington: Ministry of Health.

——(2013b). New Zealand Health Strategy: Future direction. Retrieved from www.health.govt.nz/new-zealand-health-system

——(2014a). Treaty of Waitangi principles. Retrieved from www.health.govt.nz/our-work/populations/maori-health/he-korowai-oranga/strengthening-he-korowai-oranga/treaty-waitangi-principles

——(2014b). District health boards. Retrieved from www.health.govt.nz/new-zealand-health-system/key-health-sector-organisations-and-people/district-health-boards

——(2014c). *The Guide to He Korowai Oranga: Māori Health Strategy 2014.* Wellington: Ministry of Health.

——(2015a). Tatau Kahukura: Māori Health Statistics. Retrieved from www.health.govt.nz/our-work/populations/maori-health/tatau-kahukura-maori-health-statistics

——(2015b). *Statement of Intent 2015 to 2019: Ministry of Health.* Wellington: Ministry of Health. Retrieved from www.health.govt.nz/publications/health

——(2016a). Long-term conditions. Retrieved from www.health.govt.nz/our-work/diseases-and-conditions/long-term-conditions

——(2016b). *New Zealand Health Strategy: Future Directions.* Wellington: Ministry of Health.

New Zealand Tourism. (2018). Welcome to New Zealand. Retrieved from www.newzealand.com

O'Connor, T. (2013). Telehealth bridges the great divide. *Kai Tiaki Nursing New Zealand,* 19(6), 14–15.

Robert Wood Johnson Foundation. (2010). A new way to talk about the social determinants of health. Retrieved from www.rwjf.org/content/dam/farm/reports/reports/2010/rwjf63023

Rolf, J. E. (1990). Resilience. An interview with Norman Garmezy. In M. D. Glantz & J. L. Johnson (eds), *Resilience and Development. Positive Life Adaptations* (pp. 5–14). New York: Kluwer Academic/Plenum.

Rutter, M. (1987). Psychosocial resilience and protective mechanisms. *American Journal of Orthopsychiatry,* 57, 316–31.

Tourism Australia Corporation. (2018). *Welcome to Australia.* Retrieved from www.australia.com/en

Willis, E., Reynolds, L. & Keleher, H. (2012). *Understanding the Australian Health Care System* (2nd edn). Sydney: Churchill Livingstone.

World Health Organization (WHO). (1981). *Global Strategy for Health for All by the Year 2000.* Geneva: WHO.

——(2002). *Environmental Health in Emergencies and Disasters: A Practical Guide.* Geneva: WHO.

——(2015). Social determinants of health. Retrieved from www.who.int/social_determinants/en

6

Self-management and empowerment

Michelle Baird, Sally Bristow
and Amanda Moses

LEARNING OBJECTIVES

After reading this chapter, you should be able to:

1. describe self-management and its underlying principles
2. explain the term 'empowerment' in the context of nurses and the person self-managing
3. describe the models of self-management by comparing their similarities, differences and underlying principles
4. explore self-management interventions, enablers and barriers
5. describe the nurse's role in self-management across a variety of settings.

Introduction

Chronic disease management requires coordination, engagement, education and evaluation by the individual and health care professional to create a relationship that encourages person-centered goals that foster self-management (Holman & Lorig, 2000; Lenzen et al., 2017).

This chapter explores the concept of self-management of chronic conditions. The concept of self-management has evolved worldwide, with research supporting its efficacy (Reed et al., 2018). The origin of self-management is embedded in Albert Bandura's social learning theory, which explores **self-efficacy** and its impact on self-management. The concept of self-management was further explored by Wagner and Lorig, who defined the principles of self-management from which current models are derived (Holman & Lorig, 2000). As the concept of self-management has evolved, it has developed into a treatment modality, complementary to biomedical models (Bodenheimer et al., 2002), influencing the person's ability to self-manage and thus shaping their quality of life.

Self-efficacy – an individual's belief in their capacity to implement behaviour necessary to achieve a specific outcome.

The Innovative Care of Chronic Conditions Framework (ICCCF) was developed by the World Health Organization (WHO, 2002) in response to the increasing prevalence and impact of chronic disease. This framework integrates three levels of management – micro, meso and macro — in the management and prevention of chronic disease.

In Australia, as the prevalence and burden of chronic disease impacts significantly on the health care system, the *National Strategic Framework for Chronic Conditions* has identified the need for change in managing chronic disease, to ensure a sustainable health system that is equipped to manage the everchanging impact of chronic disease (Australian Health Ministers' Advisory Council, 2017).

As chronic conditions become more widespread and complex in nature, coordination between health care professionals, people with chronic conditions, their families and carers are essential (Novak et al., 2013). Multiple chronic health conditions contribute to a person's frailty and disability, causing functional limitations with activities of daily living, and challenging an individual's engagement in self-management interventions (Grey et al., 2015; Ko, Bratzke & Roberts, 2018; New Zealand Ministry of Health (NZMOH), 2016). For these individuals, access to health care, the ability to self-manage, and the reliance on caregivers is greater and more complex (Parekh et al., 2011). Self-management should be tailored to the individual's needs to optimise their quality of life. However, it should be acknowledged that there are varying levels of self-management and that not all individuals have the ability to self-manage.

Self-management and empowerment

Thomas Creer first used the term self-management in 1976, based on his studies of children with chronic disease and their rehabilitation. These studies were founded on Bandura's self-efficacy theory (Novak, et al., 2013). Self-efficacy theory is an individual's belief in their own ability to achieve goals. Albert Bandura defines it as a personal judgement of 'how well one can execute courses of action required to deal with prospective situations' (Bandura 1982, p. 122). Individuals with a high self-efficacy will apply the necessary determination to succeed, while those with a low self-efficacy usually cease to make an effort early and fail to achieve their goals (Lenzen et al., 2017).

Other theories that underpin the concept of self-management include:

- social learning theory – concerned with learning and social behaviour suggesting that new behaviors are developed through observation, direct instruction and copying others (Rosenstock, Strecher & Becker, 1988)
- behavioural theory – a theory of learning based on the theory that all behaviours are attained through conditioning (Hupp, Reitman & Jewell, 2008).

Forty years on, chronic disease self-management strategies and interventions are essential to our health care systems, and have become routine clinical practice in the management of people with chronic conditions. This has been demonstrated to improve outcomes for the person who is at the centre of care (Newham et al., 2017; NZMOH, 2016).

Self-management, from the health professional's perspective, refers to a person's engagement in activities that promote, prevent, interact, monitor, implement and manage health, and emotional and physical symptoms. It encompasses relationships that support the person with chronic disease to maintain functional capacity through a collaborative process of person-centered goal-setting (Holman & Lorig, 2000; Lenzen et al., 2017; Reed et al., 2018). Baird and Gullick (2018) explored the meaning of self-management through the eyes of people with chronic obstructive pulmonary disease (COPD). They defined self-management as 'the person's ability to manage day-to-day activities with the sole intention of being self-reliant, not interfering with others' lives, and creating purpose and a sense of worth' (p.10).

A number of chronic disease self-management programs have been developed and implemented globally to meet the needs of a rapidly growing number of people with chronic conditions. These programs, based on social learning theory, self-efficacy and behavioural theories, support individuals and their families/carers to develop self-management skills to manage their chronic conditions. According to the *Australian Primary Health Care Research Institute Annual Report 2008* (Australian National University, 2008), effective strategies for self-management include group-based programs delivered in community settings. The location of the program delivery allows for cultural safety and supports culturally specific delivery of content by incorporating interventions that target lifestyle and motivational changes, and addressing cultural barriers to care (Zwar et al., 2006). Similarly, self-management can be provided on an individual basis, tailoring the education and focusing on person-centred goals (Reed et al., 2018).

Empowerment is a key component of effective self-management because it increases the self-efficacy of a person with chronic disease. Empowerment of individuals requires the health care practitioner to be cognisant of that individual's values and beliefs, which may impact on their willingness to engage in interventions that promote optimum health outcomes (Lenzen et al., 2017).

Self-management is a collaborative, respectful approach, incorporating two essential core elements – individualised appropriate interventions and person-centered care – which have been demonstrated to support a reduction in hospitalisations and an improved quality of life (Lenzen et al., 2017; NZMOH, 2016).

Principles of self-management

To support individuals, families and carers to self-manage chronic conditions, Lorig and Holman (2003) identified six principles of self-management behaviours that a person must develop:

1. problem solving
2. decision making
3. resource utilisation
4. forming a relationship with a provider
5. taking action
6. self-tailoring.

Problem solving

People with chronic conditions must be able to develop problem-solving skills. Problem solving involves nurses supporting the individual, their family and carer in managing the condition through self-management education, and developing problem-solving skills that focus on early symptom recognition and treatment management. When individuals can solve and identify problems, they can modify their behaviour accordingly, allowing them to be able to self-manage their chronic condition. By accepting responsibility for their chronic condition, individuals are empowered to become intrinsically motivated to self-manage, rather than be extrinsically motivated in pleasing others, particularly health care professionals (Bodenheimer et al., 2002).

Decision making

Self-care decision making in chronic conditions is person-centred, revolving around symptom management, risk factor modification and generalised health management decisions. **Empowerment** of individuals with chronic conditions is essential to make short-term and long-term decisions in relation to managing their condition. People make decisions about their care dependent on their understanding of the disease (information and knowledge), confidence and experience of managing symptoms, their readiness to change their own lifestyle choices, and the social context in which they live (Flinders University, Flinders Human Behaviour & Health Research Unit, 2007; Paterson, Thorne & Russell, 2016). For many patients, the challenge of managing their chronic condition requires planning, negotiating competing demands and goal setting, enabling the individuals and their families/carers to prioritise their own health care needs.

Empowerment – measures taken to increase a person's autonomy, so they are fully informed on their condition, treatment options and cantake the appropriate course of action.

Resource utilisation

For effective self-management to occur, a person must have the ability to access the services they require and/or information to support them in managing their chronic condition (Miller et al., 2015). This necessitates a person-centric focus that recognises the individual's context in which they live, including: their social situation (family, community, location, culture and ethnicity) and financial resources. Interventions that are provided to individuals must be adaptable to the person's environment.

Forming a relationship with a provider

It is important for individuals with chronic conditions, their families and carers to be able to collaborate with health care professionals and build rapport to foster a relationship around self-management activities. Placing individuals/their families/carers and the health care professional in partnership, creates a positive relationship that provides support and encouragement, enabling the process of decision making and problem solving to occur. A strong relationship between the health care team and individual facilitates trust, respect and communication. The approach is person-focused and allows choice, ultimately resulting in an optimal outcome for the individual (Novak et al., 2013).

Taking action

Individuals must take action to be able to self-manage their condition. This includes making behaviour and lifestyle modifications. For behaviour change to occur, a person must be inspired to make change and be ready for change. Health care practitioners must be able to assess the individual's 'readiness to change', which is often referred to within the stages of the transtheoretical model of health behaviour change (see Figure 6.1) (Prochaska & DiClemente, 1986; Prochaska, DiClemente & Norcross, 1992). This model integrates numerous psychotherapy models and provides the framework for behaviour change.

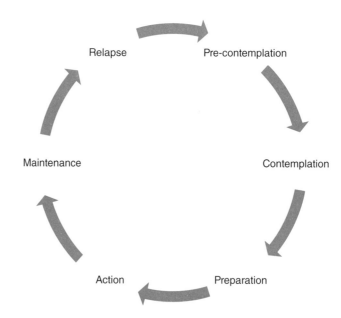

Figure 6.1   Transtheoretical model of health behaviour change
Source: Adapted from Prochaska & Velicer (1997)

Person-centred care – an approach to providing health care that considers a person's preferences, respects their situation and includes their decision making and treatment choices.

Self-tailoring

To be successful in self-management, individuals must have the confidence in their abilities to engage in self-management behaviours. Emotional support is essential for individuals and their families/carers, to ensure **person-centred care** is provided. This approach to care acknowledges the individual's differences in lifestyle choices, psycho-social status, culture and spirituality. Individuals all have different goals, courses of disease and life circumstances so tailoring and allowing for self-management programs to be individually tailored is important (Novak et al., 2013).

Models of self-management

Supporting individuals in self-management is the key component of many models of care for chronic conditions and results in optimising a person's quality of life (Parekh et al., 2011).

Chronic disease self-management programs are tailored to the individual and their goals. It is important to recognise that not all people with chronic conditions are able to self-manage and that various models of self-management may be used to enable goals to be met. Goals are a collaborative, person-directed process that may be short or long term. Goals are expressed in the form of SMART goals: Specific, Measurable, Achievable, Realistic and Timely (MacLeod, 2012).

For example, a SMART goal for a person with osteoporosis may be stated as: 'I will exercise daily for 30 minutes (Specific, Measurable, Achievable, Realistic), monitor and record my times and activities, and review it in a fortnight (Timely) with my chronic care nurse.'

Programs are delivered individually, such as the Flinders Program and Health-Change Australia, or are group-based such as the Stanford Chronic Disease Self-Management Program. Programs can be generic in nature or disease-specific. For example, registered nurses ensure that type 2 diabetes patients have a specific understanding of their disease and are able to monitor its progress, including being aware of any complications and symptoms, and sick-day management. Patients are also educated to make healthy lifestyle changes to their diet and take regular exercise (Vita et al., 2016). Programs like this bring about lifestyle changes through using motivational techniques to improve confidence (self-efficacy) and providing education to guide behaviour change (Markle-Reid et al., 2018).

The Chronic Care Model

The Chronic Care Model (CCM) (described in more detail in Chapter 1) places emphasis on enhancing health professionals' skills in self-management support by promoting processes in which people with chronic conditions are informed, engaged and activated within their encounters with health care professionals. This model identifies six essential elements required by the health care system to deliver high-quality chronic health care. These elements are:

1. community resources and policies
2. health system
3. self-management support
4. delivery system design
5. decision support
6. clinical information systems.

These elements assist in forming partnerships between the health care professional and individuals, and their families and carers, to ensure that people with chronic conditions are informed and can participate actively in their care. The CCM can be adapted and applied to numerous chronic conditions, health care settings and target populations (Wagner et al., 2001).

Stanford Chronic Disease Self-Management Program

The Stanford Chronic Disease Self-Management Program aims to support individuals' self-efficacy in managing their chronic conditions. It is a peer-led community-based course, run on a weekly basis for six weeks, involving people with different chronic conditions. The sessions are interactive and focus on encouraging the person's self-confidence in managing their health problems, including early symptom recognition and management, regardless of their condition. People are provided with support in developing skills and coping strategies such as:

- problem solving
- decision making
- techniques
- behaviour changes (e.g. diet and exercise)
- medication use
- evaluation of new treatments.

The program focuses on general skills and health behaviours (Lawn & Schoo, 2010; Lorig et al., 2001).

The Flinders Program

The Flinders Program is a generic model of chronic disease self-management based on cognitive behavioural therapy. Individuals are invited to complete the Partners in Health Scale, which provides the health care professional with the person's self-assessment of their understanding and current management of their chronic condition. A Cue and Response Interview is then conducted by the health care professional, assessing a person's self-management behaviour and problem identification. In a collaborative approach of goal setting, an individualised written care plan is developed and reviewed as needed (Lawn et al., 2018). The Flinders Program can be adapted to numerous chronic health conditions, settings and populations. It is informed by the CCM, which places an emphasis on enhancing health professionals' skills in self-management support (Lawn & Schoo, 2010).

The Patient-Centred Medical Home (PCMH) model of care

The Patient-Centred Medical Home (PCMH) model of care is used in primary health care, and ensures that care is coordinated and integrated. It is underpinned by the integration of health care professional services – such as the individual's local doctor, practice nurse and health care team – in consultation with the individual and their family/carers, to coordinate care for individuals with multiple chronic conditions (Baird et al., 2014). The PCMH model relies on the individual, their families and carers implementing the recommended treatment plans provided by their health care practitioners. These treatment plans enable the individual to acquire specific skills, which vary in complexity, so that they can manage their condition independently. Some examples of this include: home dialysis, home oxygen therapy, medication administration, or applying a manual and mechanical chest percussion vest to loosen and thin mucus in the lungs. Some of the more complex treatment regimens require disease-specific self-management programs to assist individuals and their families in adapting to their chronic health condition, and adjusting to lifestyle changes that affect their finances, time, resources, family, work and friends (Grey, et al., 2015; NZMOH, 2016).

HealthChange Australia

HealthChange Australia (HCA) is committed to supporting health professionals in working with the individual to promote behaviour change and improve adherence to treatment regimes. Through the support in lifestyle change and disease management, this approach can improve the individual's symptom management and quality of life, with less health care service utilisation. The methodology utilised by HCA is based on a person-centred approach; it ensures that health literacy is addressed, and that the individual is involved in all decision making and is fully informed. The basis of the approach is goal setting and self-management, which is derived from evidence-based practice. The methodology uses a seven-step process that begins with evidence-based practice and person-centred care, through to behaviour change and on to developing a documented, personalised self-management plan. The acronym RICk measures the individual's ability to attain their goals (Gale, 2012; HealthChange Australia, 2018):

- R – readiness to change
- I – information
- C – confidence
- k – knowledge.

SKILLS IN PRACTICE

Creaky bones: osteoporosis

Eleanor is a 68-year-old Indigenous woman who lives with her daughter and three grandsons in a remote town in northern Australia. Eleanor has a BMI of 32 and generalised osteoarthritis that limits her ability to exercise. Due to her daughter working long hours and the encouragement of the boys, she admits that they consume a diet high in fast food and soft drinks. Eleanor has a long-standing history of asthma that has been managed with inhaled medications, including corticosteroids, but she has experienced many exacerbations that have resulted in admissions to hospital with intravenous corticosteroid use. Recently Eleanor presented to the local hospital after slipping on the kitchen floor, which resulted in a fractured wrist. Eleanor is upset by the injury as she is leaving to go back to country in the next month and is looking forward to visiting her mob. She fears she may not be able to travel or will be an inconvenience for her daughter. She was referred for a bone mineral density test, the results of which indicate osteoporosis.

QUESTIONS

1. What aspects, which are individual to Eleanor, would you need to take into consideration when assisting her to develop self-management skills to reduce her risk of injury and promote healthy bones? This could include the social determinants of health that you can identify from her story (refer to Chapter 3).

2. What strategies could you consider in support of Eleanor self-managing her condition?

3. Which model of self-management would be the most appropriate. Why would you choose it?

Interventions used in self-management

Self-management for people with multiple chronic health conditions requires health care practitioners to consider new approaches that need collaborative interactions between the individual and health care providers. Nurses should be equipped with and have knowledge of approaches that support chronic disease self-management programs.

Motivational interviewing (MI) is a collaborative intervention between the health care practitioner (nurse) and the individual/family/carer (who is living with or self-managing chronic conditions), which promotes and supports a person's self-management. Droppa and Lee (2014, p. 40) state that 'MI is a vehicle for mapping out a personal plan for behavior change based on patient preferences and priorities'. Motivational interviewing is grounded in five principles:

1. express empathy
2. determine discrepancy
3. avoid argumentation
4. roll with resistance
5. support self-efficacy (Droppa & Lee, 2014).

Empathy is expressed through a non-judgemental approach and the use of reflective listening, to ensure the person's concerns are accurately heard. It is often noted that there is a discrepancy between the person's current behaviour and the goal they wish to achieve. By assisting them to determine this, success in goal achievement may be improved. Remembering that the purpose is to identify the person's priorities, which may well differ to that of the health professional's, will help to avoid arguments (Huffman, 2010). Resistance to change may also be identified; it is more successful to work with this resistance, than to argue for change. Self-efficacy is supported through encouragement, and continually confirming belief in the person's ability to change (Droppa & Lee, 2014).

Nurses are in the unique position, as frontline health care practitioners, to identify, guide and review the outcomes of self-management interventions. Nurses are privileged in their position as the individual's advocate, enabling smooth transition in an individual's behaviour change and adaption of self-management interventions.

The 5As

One intervention to support an individual in goal setting and increased self-management is known as the '5As' (Agency for Healthcare Research and Quality, 2014), which is a brief intervention tool. It is easy to remember – Ask, Assess, Advise, Assist, and Arrange – and guides health professionals through a quick process of identifying individual concerns, goals and needs for changing health behaviours (Lawn & Schoo, 2010). Utilising the techniques of MI, the person is asked about their understanding of their health and an assessment of their goals is undertaken. The health care practitioner can then provide some advice on ways to achieve these and assist in setting SMART goals. The final step is to arrange for referrals and follow up to optimise the person's ability to achieve the goals identified (Anderson, 2017).

The 5As tool was originally developed for smoking cessation but has been found useful in supporting individuals in making lifestyle changes for numerous conditions, including chronic disease. This intervention technique has been found to be easily implemented by members of different health care professions, is easily understood by the individual and, when utilised appropriately, places the individual at the centre of care by acknowledging their expertise in their own health and behaviours (Lawn & Schoo, 2010). The 5As approach has been shown to align with identifying a person's readiness for change, along with ensuring adequate support is implemented ('Arrange') and the individual's autonomy is promoted (Pollack et al., 2016). It is necessary to understand the utilisation of the acronym; evidence shows that it is important to ensure that all the areas are addressed, as frequent exclusion of the areas 'Assist' and 'Arrange' has been noted to occur, which reduces the efficacy of the intervention (Dosh et al., 2005).

REFLECTION

Consider a person you know with a condition that requires better management such as obesity, smoking or poor fitness. How could you use the 5As approach to assist this person in setting a SMART goal that would improve their wellbeing?

Self-management enablers and barriers

The process of learning to self-manage has been described as protracted (Russell et al., 2018). Optimising individuals' outcomes requires nurses to be skilful in identifying enablers and barriers in supporting people to self-manage (see Table 6.1).

People with chronic disease, who are faced with managing their long-term condition, are often overwhelmed. Managing chronic disease requires a holistic approach to overcome barriers and promote enablers in supporting an individual to self-manage. The empowerment of an individual harnesses self-efficacy, which fosters the attainment of SMART goals.

Table 6.1   Enablers and barriers to self-management

Enablers	Barriers
Person with chronic disease (micro level): • readiness for change • engagement • knowledge and understanding of chronic disease • self-efficacy	Person with chronic disease (micro level): • readiness for change • engagement • comorbidities • acceptance of disease • health literacy
Health care professional (meso level): • self-management models • reflective practice • skills and knowledge • cultural awareness • communication	Health care professional (meso level): • rigid models of care • resources • cultural awareness • communication • understanding of role in supporting self-management • traditional versus holistic (patients' personal beliefs versus health care professional beliefs)
Health system (macro level): • self-management models of care • funding/resource allocation evidence-based practice • appropriate health care professional training	Health system (macro level): • rigid models of care funding/resource allocation • implementation of evidence-based practice

Sources: Australian Health Ministers' Advisory Council; 2017; Carr et al., 2014; Russell et al., 2018

REFLECTION

Living with a chronic condition is challenging when navigating the health care system. Consider the enablers and barriers in managing a chronic condition such as chronic kidney disease and what your role as a nurse would encompass.

Innovation in self-management

Telemonitoring – the use of technology and equipment (set up in the person's home), which allows for monitoring and evaluation of the individual's health status.

A relatively recent innovation that is proving valuable in assisting individuals in self-management is the use of **telemonitoring**. Telemonitoring involves the provision of easy-to-use equipment that allows the individual to take vital signs such as pulse, blood pressure, blood glucose and heart activity (through an ECG); it also involves the answering of a simple, specific questionnaire. This information is then sent to a central point and monitored by an appropriately qualified nurse. Any deviations from acceptable parameters can be promptly followed up and suitable intervention initiated. This not only ensures early intervention of any change in symptoms, but also provides the person with reassurance that they are being monitored and supported (Celler et al.,

2016). For people who are geographically isolated, or experience mobility issues, this approach can increase contact with health care professionals and reduce the need for travel (Lorentz, 2008). While studies are lacking due to limited utilisation, evidence is showing a reduction in hospitalisation (along with a reduction in the length of stay for those who do need admission), an increase in health care utilisation and an increase in the patient's satisfaction (Celler et al., 2016; Shany et al., 2017).

If telemonitoring is to progress, be a suitably educated nursing workforce needs to be trained so that they can support the technology and clients appropriately (Van Houwelingen et al., 2016). Wade and colleagues (2011) identify a need for more general practitioners to consider using telemonitoring, as well as participate in tele-monitoring projects, which they are currently reluctant to do. To support a person to use telemonitoring, it is necessary to ensure that the equipment provided is easy for them to use. Evidence suggests that more work needs to be done in this area (Middlemass, Vos & Siriwardena, 2017).

According to Devitt (2017), and Celler and colleagues (2016), there is excellent potential for the use of telemonitoring to improve an individual's outcomes and experience of living with a chronic illness, and to reduce the financial burden of chronic disease management on the health budget. This results from the increased ability of the individual to self-manage and the early intervention of any deterioration.

Measures of self-management

Health care services recently changed from volume measures (that is, length of stay) to new measures – such as Patient Reported Outcome Measures (PROMS) and Patient Reported Experience Measures (PREMS) – that provide health care practitioners with a more holistic individual assessment and outcome (Agency for Clinical Innovation, 2017).

The ICCCF describes three core levels in the management of chronic disease. Self-management measures at the micro level are tailored towards the individual and their engagement in risk factor modification or reduction of behaviours through goal-setting. These goals may be as simple as getting dressed daily and can be measured by the person. Baird and Gullick (2018) concluded that measures of success for people with COPD were tangible (able to walk 1000 steps) and intangible (self-reported self-reliance).

At the meso level, measuring successful self-management may be related to a decrease in the use of health care provision – such as hospital admission, length of stay or appropriately trained staff – and, in general practice, measuring successful self-management may be related to an increase in the use of chronic disease management planning, thereby empowering the person to self-manage.

Policies and guidelines contribute to self-management at the macro level. While these are indirectly measured, they provide guidance and support to clinicians to enable individuals to self-manage (see Figure 6.2).

Cultural considerations in self-management

There are many factors that need to be considered when supporting individuals in managing a chronic condition. Not least of these is their cultural background. While we commonly think of culture as the ethnic diversity of our society, we need to keep in

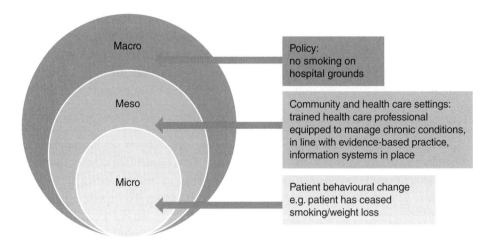

Figure 6.2   Innovative Care for Chronic Conditions Framework model of chronic disease management: integration of self-management measures
Sources: Adapted from Nuno et al. (2012); WHO (2002)

mind that individual experiences of life create understandings that affect how people perceive, engage with and embrace health care approaches (Griswold, Lesko & West-fall, 2013).

To improve effective outcomes of self-management, it is necessary for nurses to approach implementation in a culturally appropriate manner, which incorporates several aspects. First, understanding one's own beliefs and values, and how these might influence interactions, will allow for the development of an ability to accept and acknowledge cultural differences that are encountered. Second, it is necessary to understand that there is no one formula that will work for every individual requiring care and, by acknowledging these differences, diversity in care provision is made possible. Finally, maintaining person-centered care and working in collaboration with the individual ensures that their specific beliefs, values and situation are considered (Laresen & Rice, 2019).

Self-management focuses on improving symptom management and quality of life. It must be recognised, therefore, that the capacity of the person to engage in this approach, and their perception of quality of life, is very individual (Funnell, 2010). The social situation of the individual must also be considered and how it may influence their ability to engage in self-management (Browne et al., 2017). In addition, it is necessary to consider the ethnic diversity of the clients to whom care is provided, and how this may influence the acceptance of the Westernised medicine approach to self-management (Laresen & Rice, 2019). Self-management programs need to be delivered appropriately to provide cultural safety for all participants, and their family and carers (Battersby et al., 2018). Resources used in the programs must reflect the local community, culture or ethnic group, and may include images, voice recording, language and videos. The NZMOH (2016) provides a brief summary of a program that is specific to the Indigenous Māori population of New Zealand.

For Māori, a programme underpinned by kaupapa Māori approaches enriches the environment for effective learning. It focuses on:

- tinorangatiratanga – self determination
- taonga tuku iho – cultural aspirations
- ako Māori – culturally preferred ways of learning
- whānau – the extended family members and their influence and support
- kaupapa – the collective philosophy of the members of the group (Smith & Reid, 2000, pp 9–11).

The nurse's role in self-management

Nursing plays a key role in assisting and empowering individuals and their families to self-manage. Individuals and their families who engage in chronic disease self-management strategies and work in collaboration with health care professionals are known to have improved health outcomes (Ryan & Sawin, 2009; Zimmermann et al., 2016). Self-management for people with chronic conditions is crucial because it enables them to be active participants in their own care. Individuals with chronic conditions, and their families, must acquire self-efficacy skills and confidence to make specific changes to their behaviours, thus encouraging them to take responsibility for their care (Grey et al., 2015; Miller et al., 2015).

Nurses acknowledge that each disease has unique attributes. This may influence chronic disease self-management programs as there are disease-specific medical regimens that a person must learn to control their condition (Zwerink et al., 2014). Disease-specific programs require individuals to develop and learn new skills, and may include medical management and performing medicalised procedures within their own home, such as renal dialysis (Novak et al., 2013).

Partnerships between individuals and nurses are essential to foster support for individuals in their ability to engage in the management of their condition. The role of nurses in self-management is not to do, but to encourage people to be active participants in their own care, because those that need care need to learn how to manage a condition that they may have a limited understanding about. This requires people with chronic conditions to develop the knowledge, skills and behaviours necessary to manage their disease and treatments. Nurses are empowered and equipped to support individuals to self-manage through the nurses' acquisition of knowledge and skills such as MI (Droppa & Lee, 2014).

Nurses work with individuals and their families in a variety of roles and settings to promote health behaviour change. For example, nurses working within community health settings and primary health care are ideally positioned to introduce and run lifestyle intervention programs encouraging lifestyle changes. Nurses can deliver one-to-one or group chronic disease self-management programs, as well as deliver interventions to individuals, their families or carers.

Successful self-management involves patients/families/carers actively participating in their own everyday care; including symptom recognition, management and monitoring, and medical treatments; to prevent progression of their chronic health condition (Novak et al., 2013). Self-management strategies for patients with multiple chronic conditions require a person-centred and integrated approach to ensure all conditions are managed (NZMOH, 2016). Nurses are at the forefront of patient engagement and management. They require the skills and knowledge to provide opportunistic intervention and support in the planning, implementation and evaluation of self-management interventions.

SKILLS IN PRACTICE

Complex chronic health conditions and self-management

Julie is a 45-year-old mother and lives on a cropping farm, run as a family business, with her husband and his brother. Julie has three children: Sam, aged 14; Katie, aged 12; and James, aged 8. The two older children attend boarding school and return home for the holidays. James is at home and attends the local primary school 50 km away. Both Julie's boys have type 1 diabetes that she manages.

Julie has lived with her diabetes for 37 years and has many comorbidities due to both her diabetes and celiac disease, which she developed as a teenager. Julie has stage 3 chronic kidney disease, poor eyesight and osteoporosis. She is currently trying to give up smoking after having smoked since the age of 16.

Julie currently sees her endocrinologist in a large metropolitan hospital every three months at the outpatient clinic. It takes her five hours to drive by car to the appointment in the city – a journey that she takes with her husband. Her nephrologist is based at a regional hospital about two hours' drive from home. Julie engages with a diabetes educator via phone and face-to-face monthly. The local hospital is 50 km away, and is a small, rural hospital, with a locum doctor and regular nursing staff, who cover the acute in-patient ward, and a community registered nurse. She attends a community chronic disease self-management program at the local church hall run by the community registered nurse once a week in town and does her weekly groceries.

Julie has expressed to the diabetes educator that she needs more assistance with managing her own condition. She is concerned that her sons, who have type 1 diabetes, may end up with the same comorbidities as her because she has an autoimmune chronic condition.

QUESTION

Julie has multiple chronic health conditions. Consider the health care teams and services involved in Julie's care. How would you, as a nurse caring for Julie, engage the health care team to provide collaborative support to Julie in self-managing her multiple chronic conditions? Identify the enablers and barriers that may be relevant for this case study.

SUMMARY

Learning objective 1: Describe self-management and its underlying principles.

Self-management is an individual's ability to promote, prevent, monitor and manage their chronic health conditions. Effective self-management is supported by six underlying principles: problem solving, decision making, appropriate resource utilisation, the individual–health care practitioner relationship, taking action and tailored plans for the individual.

Learning objective 2: Explain the term 'empowerment' in the context of nurses and the person self-managing.

Empowerment is the process of strengthening and increasing an individual's belief and ability to make changes. Empowerment includes the nurses' acquisition of skills and knowledge in relation to chronic disease management to increase their self-confidence in supporting a person to self-manage. The empowerment of the person to self-manage is supported by education and skills acquisition, as well as a positive person–nurse relationship.

Learning objective 3: Describe the models of self-management by comparing their similarities, differences and underlying principles.

Self-management models can be delivered individually (e.g. the Flinders Program, HCA and the PCMH model of care), with an orientation to disease-specific interventions such as diabetes; the models can also be group-based (Stanford Chronic Disease Self-Management Program), which provides generic interventions to manage chronic conditions. The Stanford model is a peer-led, community-based program, whereas models such as the Flinders Program, HCA and PCHM model of care are delivered by the health care practitioner. When choosing a model of self-management, nurses should consider the individual, their readiness for change, and their cultural and social background. All programs are based on the premise of empowering individuals and increasing their self-efficacy to attain their goals.

Learning objective 4: Explore self-management interventions, enablers and barriers.

Some of the interventions which have been found to be effective in promoting self-management are MI, telemonitoring and the 5As.

Motivational interviewing is a skill that nurses engage in to support a person to self-manage by:

1. expressing empathy
2. determining discrepancy
3. avoiding argumentation
4. rolling with resistance
5. supporting self-efficacy.

Telemonitoring, a recent innovation in health care delivery, allows individuals real-time interaction and monitoring with a health care practitioner. It encompasses the use of easy-to-use equipment and the knowledge that data is reviewed by a trained health professional, thus increasing access to services and early detection of changes in vital signs, such as blood pressure and pulse.

The 5As approach is used widely in smoking cessation and has been found to be useful in supporting other lifestyle changes. The 5As stand for: Ask, Assess, Advise, Assist and Arrange. The technique enables the nurse to identify a person's concerns, goals and behaviours that may need to be modified to facilitate change. Measures of self-management can be assessed at the micro, meso and macro level to provide an evaluation of individualised health outcomes.

Learning objective 5: Describe the nurse's role in self-management across a variety of settings.

Nurses work across a variety of settings: acute, community and primary health care.

Within the acute setting, nurses are able to promote a person's self-management through the reflective process of what led the person to present to hospital; nurses can identify if the person implemented an action plan or if the person was able to identify new symptoms and their management.

The community health setting is an integral part of supporting self-management. Post-discharge follow up and the explanation of changes to management and new regimes encourage behaviour change. Nurses are able to identify and assess if an individual is able to implement change and address their concerns.

A primary health care nurse is integral to a person's ability to self-manage their chronic condition. The nurse develops chronic disease management plans in consultation with the individual and general practitioner, and provides linkages and referrals to the appropriate health care professional.

REVIEW QUESTIONS

1. Outline the benefits of supporting individuals to engage in self-management interventions for themselves and the health care system.
2. Why is it necessary to understand the principles of self-management and how can you apply them to the models of self-management?
3. Explain the difference between person-centred care and a medical model of care? Are these models interchangeable and if so how?
4. Nurses work in a variety of settings. Are skills learned in different settings transferrable when supporting a person to self-manage? Give an example.
5. Can enablers be barriers, or barriers be enablers, when self-managing? Give an example.

RESEARCH TOPIC

As chronic conditions increase in prevalence and complexity, explain how the ICCCF can be implemented in chronic disease self-management for an individual with more than one chronic condition.

FURTHER READING

Feyer, A. M., McDonald, A., Billot, L., Cass, A., Turnbull, F., Corcoran, K., . . . & Zwar, N. (2014). *State-Wide Evaluation. NSW Health Chronic Disease Management Program. Final Report. October 2014.* Sydney: NSW Health. Retrieved from www.health.nsw.gov.au/cdm/Documents/CDMP-evaluation-report-2014.pdf

HealthChange Australia. (2018). Health Change® methodology. Retrieved from www.healthchange.com/About_HealthChange_Methodology

Lawn, S. & Schoo, A. (2010). Supporting self-management of chronic health conditions: Common approaches. *Patient Education and Counseling*, 80(2), 205–11. doi http://10.1016/j.pec.2009.10.006

New Zealand Ministry of Health (NZMOH). (2016). *Self-Management Support for People with Long-Term Conditions* (2nd edn). Wellington: Ministry of Health.

Willams, R. & Curtis, S. (2004). Aunty Jean's Good Health Team: Celebrating a successful model of an intervention for Indigenous peoples with chronic diseases. *The Chronicle*, 8(3), 1, 3–5.

Young, J., Eley, D., Patterson, E. & Turner, C. (2016). A nurse-led model of chronic disease management in general practice: Patients' perspectives. *Australian Family Physician*, 45(12), 912.

REFERENCES

Agency for Clinical Innovation. (2017). Leading Better Value Care Program. Retrieved from http://eih.health.nsw.gov.au/bvh/about/leading-better-value-care-program

Agency for Healthcare Research and Quality. (2014). Chapter 3: Getting patients excited about crossing the bridge. In *Integrating Primary Care Practices and Community-Based Resources to Manage Obesity*. Rockville, MD: US Department of Health and Human Services. Retrieved from www.ahrq.gov/professionals/prevention-chronic- care/improve/community/obesity-pcpresources/obpcp3.html

Anderson, G. (2017). Tobacco cessations: A quality improvement project using the 5 A's models. University of Kansas. Retrieved from https://kuscholarworks.ku.edu/handle/1808/26920

Australian Health Ministers' Advisory Council. (2017). *National Strategic Framework for Chronic Conditions*. Canberra: Australian Government.

Australian National University. (2008). *Australian Primary Health Care Research Institute Annual Report 2008*. Canberra: Australian National University. Retrieved from http://files.aphcri.anu.edu.au/publications/annual-reports/2008.pdf

Baird, M., Blount, A., Brungardt, S., Dickinson, P., Dietrich, A., Epperly, T., ... & McDaniel, S. (2014). Joint principles: Integrating behavioral health care into the patient-centered medical home. *The Annals of Family Medicine*, 12(2), 183–5.

Baird, M. & Gullick, J. (2018). *Harnessing hope, instilling belief: COPD self-management*. *Respirology*, 23(S1), 21–103. Retrieved from https://onlinelibrary.wiley.com/doi/full/10.1111/resp.13267

Bandura, A. (1982). Self-efficacy mechanism in human agency. *American Psychologist*, 37(2), 122.

Battersby, M., Lawn, S., Kowanko, I., Bertossa, S., Trowbridge, C. & Liddicoat, R. (2018). Chronic condition self-management support for Aboriginal people: Adapting tools and training. *Australian Journal of Rural Health* 26(4), 232.

Bodenheimer, T., Lorig, K., Holman, H. & Grumbach, K. (2002). Patient self-management of chronic disease in primary care. *Journal of the American Medical Association*, 288 (19), 2469–75.

Browne, C. V., Ka'opua, L. S., Jervis, L. L., Alboroto, R. & Trockman, M. L. (2017). United States indigenous populations and dementia: Is there a case for culture-based psychosocial interventions? *Gerontologist*, 57(6), 1011–19. doi: http://10.1093/geront/gnw059

Carr, S. M., Paliadelis, P., Lhussier, M., Forster, N., Eaton, S., Parmenter, G. & Death, C. (2014). *Looking after yourself: Clinical understandings of chronic-care self-management strategies in rural and urban contexts of the United Kingdom and Australia*. SAGE Open Medicine, 2: 2050312114532636. doi: http://10.1177/2050312114532636

Celler, B., Varnfield, M., Sparks, R., Li, J., Nepal, S., Jang-Jaccard, J., . . . & Jayasena, R. (2016). *Monitoring of Chronic Disease for Aged Care: Final Report.* Australia. CSIRO.

Devitt, A. (2017). Nursing reflections on a pilot project: Improving outcomes in chronic disease management using nurse-led home telemonitoring. *The Hive*, 19, 28–9.

Dosh, S. A., Summers Holtrop, J., Torres, T., Arnold, A. K., Baumann, J. & White, L. L. (2005). Changing organizational constructs into functional tools: An assessment of the 5 A's in primary care practices. *Annuls of Family Medicine*, 3(2), S50–2. doi: http://10.1370/afm.357

Droppa, M. & Lee, H. (2014). Motivational interviewing: A journey to improve health. *Nursing*, 44(3), 40–5. doi: http://10.1097/01.NURSE.0000443312.58360.82

Flinders University, Flinders Human Behaviour & Health Research Unit. (2007). *Flinders Model, Chronic Condition Self-Management Education and Training Manual.* Adelaide: Flinders University. Retrieved from www.flindersprogram.com.au

Funnell, M. (2010). Peer-based behavioural strategies to improve chronic disease self-management and clinical outcomes: Evidence, logistics, evaluation considerations, and needs for future research. *Family Practice – An International Journal*, 27, i17–22.

Gale, J. (2012). *A Practical Guide to Health Behaviour Change Using the HCA Approach.* Bomaderry, NSW: HealthChange Australia.

Grey, M., Schulman-Green, D., Knafl, K. & Reynolds, N. R. (2015). A revised self-and family management framework. *Nursing Outlook*, 63(2), 162–70.

Griswold, K. S., Lesko, S. E. & Westfall, J. M. (2013). Communities of solution: Partnerships for population health. *The Journal of the American Board of Family Medicine*, 26(3), 232–8.

Health Change Australia. (2018). HealthChange® methodology. Retrieved from www.healthchange.com

Holman, H. & Lorig, K. (2000). Patients as partners in managing chronic disease: Partnership is a prerequisite for effective and efficient health care. *The British Medical Journal*, 320(7234), 526.

Huffman, M. H. (2010). Health coaching: A fresh approach to improving health outcomes and reducing costs. *American Association of Occupational Health Nurses Journal*, 58(6), 245–52.

Hupp, S. D., Reitman, D. A. & Jewell, J. D. (2008). Cognitive behavioral theory. In M. Hersen & A. M. Gross (eds), *Handbook of Clinical Psychology* (vol. 2, 2nd edn, Chapter 9). New York: John Wiley & Sons.

Ko, D., Bratzke, L. C. & Roberts, T. (2018). Self-management assessment in multiple chronic conditions: A narrative review of literature. *International Journal of Nursing Studies*, 83, 83–90.

Laresen, P. D. & Rice, S. K. (2019). Culture and Diversity. In P. Larsen (ed.) *Lubkins Chronic Illness: Impact and Intervention* (10th edn). Burlington, VT: Jones and Bartlett Learning.

Lawn, S. & Schoo, A. (2010). Supporting self-management of chronic health conditions: Common approaches. *Patient Education and Counseling*, 80(2), 205–11. doi: http://10.1016/j.pec.2009.10.006

Lawn, S., Zabeen, S., Smith, D., Wilson, E. Miller, C., Battersby, M. & Masman, K. (2018). Managing chronic conditions care across primary care and hospital systems: Lessons from an Australian Hospital Avoidance Risk Program using the Flinders Chronic Condition Management Program. *Australian Health Review*, 42(5), 542–9. doi: https://doi.org/10.1071/AH17099

Lenzen, S. A., Daniëls, R., van Bokhoven, M. A., van der Weijden, T. & Beurskens, A. (2017). Disentangling self-management goal setting and action planning: A scoping review. *PLOS ONE*, 12(11), e0188822. doi: http://10.1371/journal.pone.0188822

Lorentz, M. (2008). Telenursing and home healthcare. *Home Healthcare Nurse*, 26(4), 237–43. doi: http://10.1097/01.NHH.0000316702.22633.30

Lorig, K. R. & Holman, H. R. (2003). Self-management education: History, definition, outcomes, and mechanisms. *Annals of Behavioral Medicine*, 26(1), 1–7.

Lorig, K. R., Ritter, P., Stewart, A. L., Sobel, D. S., Brown Jr, B. W., Bandura, A., . . . & Holman, H. R. (2001). Chronic disease self-management program: 2-year health status and health care utilization outcomes. *Medical Care*, 39(11), 1217–23.

MacLeod, L. (2012). Making SMART goals smarter. *Physician Executive*, 38(2), 68–70, 72.

Markle-Reid, M., Ploeg, J., Fraser, K. D., Fisher, K. A., Bartholomew, A., Griffith, L. E., . . . & Upshur, R. (2018). Community program improves quality of life and self-management in older adults with diabetes mellitus and comorbidity. *Journal of the American Geriatrics Society*, 66(2), 263–73.

Middlemass, J., Vos, J. & Siriwardena, A. N. (2017). Perceptions on use of home telemonitoring in patients with long term conditions – concordance with the Health Information Technology Acceptance Model: A qualitative collective case study. *BioMed Central*, 17(89). doi: http://10.1186/s12911-017-0486-5

Miller, W. R., Lasiter, S., Ellis, R. B. & Buelow, J. M. (2015). Chronic disease self-management: A hybrid concept analysis. *Nursing Outlook*, 63(2), 154–61.

New Zealand Ministry of Health (NZMOH). (2016). *Self-Management Support for People with Long-Term Conditions* (2nd edn). Wellington: Ministry of Health.

Newham, J. J., Presseau, J., Heslop-Marshall, K., Russell, S., Ogunbayo, O. J., Netts, P., . . . & Kaner, K. (2017). Features of self-management interventions for people with chronic obstructive pulmonary disease associated with improved health-related quality of life and reduced emergency department visits: A systematic review of reviews with meta-analysis. *International Journal of Chronic Obstructive Pulmonary Disease*, 12, 1705–20.

Novak, M., Costantini, L., Schneider, S. & Beanlands, H. (2013). Approaches to self-management in chronic illness. *Seminars in Dialysis*, 26, 188–94. doi: http://10.1111/sdi.12080

Nuno, R., Coleman, K., Bengoa, R. & Sauto, R., (2012). Integrated care for chronic conditions: The contribution of the ICCC framework. *Health Policy*, 105, 55–64.

Parekh, A. K., Goodman, R. A., Gordon, C., Koh, H. K. & HHS Interagency Workgroup on Multiple Chronic Conditions. (2011). Managing multiple chronic conditions: A strategic framework for improving health outcomes and quality of life. *Public Health Reports*, 126(4), 460–71.

Paterson, B., Thorne, S. & Russell, C. (2016). Disease-specific influences on meaning and significance in self-care decision-making in chronic illness. *Canadian Journal of Nursing Research Archive*, 34(3).

Pollack, K. I., Tulsky, J. A., Brvender, T., Ostbye, T., Lyna, P., Dolor, R. J., . . . & Alexander, S. C. (2016). Teaching primary care physicians the 5A's for discussing weight with overweight and obese adolescents. *Patient Education and Counselling*, 99(10), 1620–5. doi: http://10.1016/j.pec.2016.05.007

Prochaska, J. O. & DiClemente, C. C. (1986). Toward a comprehensive model of change. In W. R. Miller & N. Heather (eds), *Treating Addictive Behaviors* (pp. 3–27). Boston, MA: Springer.

Prochaska, J. O., DiClemente, C. C. & Norcross, J. C. (1992). In search of the how people change: Applications to addictive behaviors. *American Psychologist*, 47(9), 1102–14.

Prochaska, J. O. & Velicer, W. F. (1997). The transtheoretical model of health behavior change. *American Journal of Health Promotion*, 12(1), 38–48.

Reed, R. L., Roeger, L., Howard, S., Oliver-Baxter, J. M., Battersby, M. W., Bond M. & Osborne, R. H. (2018). A self-management support program for older Australians with multiple chronic conditions: A randomised controlled trial. *Medical Journal of Australia*, 208(2), 69–74.

Rosenstock, I. M., Strecher, V. J., & Becker, M. H. (1988). Social learning theory and the health belief model. *Health Education Quarterly*, 15(2), 175–83.

Russell, S., Ogunbayo, O. J., Newham, J. J., Heslop-Marshall, K., Netts, P. Hanratty, B., . . . & Kaner, E. (2018). Qualitative systematic review of barriers and facilitators to self-management of chronic obstructive pulmonary disease: Views of patients and healthcare professionals. *NPJ Primary Care Respiratory Medicine*, 28(1), 2.

Ryan, P. & Sawin, K. J. (2009). The individual and family self-management theory: Background and perspectives on context, process, and outcomes. *Nursing Outlook*, 57(4), 217–25.

Shany, T., Hession, M., Pruce, D., Roberts, M., Basilakis, J., Redmond, S., . . . & Schreier, G. (2017) A small-scale randomised controlled trial of home telemonitoring in patients with severe chronic obstructive pulmonary disease. *Journal of Telemedicine and Telecare*, 23(7), 650–56. doi: http://10.1177/1357633X16659410

Smith, L. T. & Reid P. (2000). *Kaupapa Maori principles and practices: A literature review*. Auckland: International Research Institute for Maori and Indigenous Education.

Van Houwelingen, C. T. M., Barakat, A., Best, R., Boot, W. R., Charness, N. & Kort, H. S. M. (2016). Dutch nurse's willingness to use home telehealth: Implications for practice and education. *Journal of Gerontological Nursing*, 41(4),47–56.

Vita, P., Cardona-Morrell, M., Bauman, A., Singh, M. F., Moore, M., Pennock, R., . . . & Colagiuri, S. (2016). Type 2 diabetes prevention in the community: 12-month outcomes from the Sydney Diabetes Prevention Program. *Diabetes Research and Clinical Practice*, 112, 13–19.

Wade, M. J., Desai, A. S., Spettell, C. M., McGowan-Stackewicz, V., Kummer, P. J., Maccoy, M. C. & Krakauer, R. S. (2011). Telemonitoring with case management for seniors with heart failure. *American Journal of Managing Care*, 17(3), 71–9.

Wagner, E. H., Austin, B. T., Davis, C., Hindmarsh, M., Schaefer, J., & Bonomi, A. (2001). Improving chronic illness care: Translating evidence into action. *Health Affairs*, 20(6), 64–78.

World Health Organization (WHO). (2002). *Innovative Care for Chronic Conditions: Building Blocks for Action: Global Report.* Geneva, WHO.

Zimmermann, T., Puschmann, E., van den Bussche, H., Wiese, B., Ernst, A., Porzelt, S., . . . & Scherer, M. (2016). Collaborative nurse-led self-management support for primary care patients with anxiety, depressive or somatic symptoms: Cluster-randomised controlled trial (findings of the SMADS study). *International Journal of Nursing Studies*, 63, 101–11.

Zwar, N., Harris, M., Griffiths, R., Roland, M., Dennis, S., Powell Davies, G. & Hasan I. (2006). *A Systematic Review of Chronic Disease Management.* Canberra: Australian Primary Health Care Research Institute, The Australian National University.

Zwerink, M., Brusse-Keizer, M., van der Valk, P. D., Zielhuis, G. A., Monninkhof, E. M., van der Palen, J., . . . & Effing, T. (2014). *Self-management for patients with chronic obstructive pulmonary disease. Cochrane Database of Systematic Reviews*, 3, CD002990.

PART 2

Nursing care of clients with chronic conditions

7

Cancer control

Kylie Ash, Kate Cameron,
Tracey Doherty and Marion Eckert

*With acknowledgement to Amy Vaccaro
and Lee Hunt (personal cancer journey)*

LEARNING OBJECTIVES

After studying this chapter, you should be able to:

1. describe the impact of cancer as a chronic condition
2. describe the targeted responses required to prevent and mitigate the impact of chronic cancer at a population level
3. discuss how nurses can promote supportive care pathways
4. discuss the potential contribution of all nurses in meeting chronic care needs for the person affected by cancer
5. describe advanced practice roles in cancer within the chronic condition framework.

Introduction

Cancer – describes a range of diseases in which abnormal cells divide without control and can invade nearby tissues. Cancer cells can also spread to other parts of the body through the blood and lymph systems.

Cancer is a disease in which the usual controls of cell division are lost following a series of mutations, and uncontrolled cell growth occurs. Cancer can be experienced as an acute illness but is recognised from a health system policy perspective as a chronic condition (Australian Health Ministers' Advisory Council, 2017; Department of Health, 2015a). Cancer is the leading causes of morbidity and mortality in Australia, accounting for 19 per cent of the total disease burden (Australian Institute of Health and Welfare (AIHW), 2017).

Prevalence and survival

Despite significant improvements in prevention and screening, the overall incidence of cancer is increasing, largely due to improved screening participation and the ageing population. Modifiable lifestyle factors are also contributing to cancer incidence. Collectively, overweight and obesity, physical inactivity and unhealthy eating are second only to tobacco as preventable risk factors for cancer (Cancer Council Australia, 2015). In Australia, there were approximately 134 174 new cases of cancer in 2017 (excluding basal and squamous cell carcinoma of the skin) (AIHW, 2017). It is estimated that there will be 16 948 new cases of cancer nationally by 2024, based on an average annual increase of 3.3 per cent per year from 2010 (AIHW, 2014a). Current trends predict that one in two Australians will be diagnosed with cancer by the age of 85. Similarly, in New Zealand cancer is the biggest cause of illness, disability and premature mortality (17.5 per cent) within the context of an ageing population (New Zealand Ministry of Health (NZMOH), 2014a). The incidence of cancer is expected to increase with age; AIHW has identified that 71 per cent of new cases in males and 54 per cent of females over the age of 60 are diagnosed (AIHW, 2017).

Cancer is estimated to be a leading cause of the burden of disease in Australia, contributing 19 per cent of the total disease burden (AIHW, 2014a). In 2015, cancer was the most common cause of death in Australia, accounting for 28.9 per cent of all deaths, and the most common in New Zealand, accounting for 30.2 per cent of all deaths (New Zealand Government, 2018).

In 2017, the leading cause of cancer death in Australia was lung cancer (9021 deaths), followed by bowel cancer (4114), prostate cancer (3452), breast cancer (3087) and pancreatic cancer (2976) (AIHW, 2017). In New Zealand, in 2013 the most common causes of cancer deaths were lung cancer (2037), colorectal cancer (3075), breast cancer (3046), prostate cancer (3129) and melanoma (2366) (NZMOH, 2016).

Survival prospects from cancer are increasing in response to effective population-based screening programs, earlier detection rates, better diagnostic methods, lifestyle modifications and advances in treatments. More people are surviving cancer today than ever before. In Australia, five-year relative survival rates for people diagnosed with cancer increased from 48 per cent in 1984–8 to 68 per cent in 2009–13 (AIHW, 2017). In New Zealand, the five-year survival rate is 63 per cent (NZMOH, 2015a).

Cancer survivors often face emotional, physical and financial challenges as a result of the detection, diagnosis and treatment of cancer. The increase in the number of people diagnosed with and surviving cancer creates greater demand and pressures across the specialist and primary care systems. In 2013, the World Economic Forum identified that 'growing demand for healthcare is driven primarily by four factors: an ageing population, an explosion of so-called lifestyle disease, a rise in public expect-ations, and a lack of value-consciousness among consumers and as a result, healthcare systems across the world are adapting to meet the challenges' (World Economic Forum, 2013). The burden of chronic disease management scales across all of these factors and reflects the degree of complexity that health care providers must consider when caring for people with cancer.

With the significantly high number of people diagnosed with cancer, there will be an increased demand on the health system due to the disease burden. This will impact primary health care systems to support the needs of individuals living with cancer or in the shadow of cancer. It is important to understand that many other people are also affected indirectly when a family member or someone else close to them has cancer. This can take a substantial toll on social and economic impacts for individuals, families and community.

The impact of cancer: one disease, many types

While the focus in this text is on chronic aspects of disease, it is useful to develop an understanding of how cancer develops at a cellular level. You may find it useful to review what you have previously learned about cancer, including cell biology, the cell cycle and the processes involved in the development of cancer. For the purpose of this text, the key concepts to be aware of are outlined below.

- There are as many different cancer types as there are cell types in the body, and the predicted course and outcomes of the disease depend on many factors including personal characteristics (for example, comorbidities, age), the organ/s involved, and the stage and grade of the cancer.
- The treatments used vary widely depending on the factors above, with variation consequently in administration, side effects and outcomes.

Whether a cancer is predicted to follow an acute or a chronic course is determined through **staging** and **grading**. Staging provides information about where the cancer is located, its size and extent of spread (AIHW, 2017), and is identified usually through a series of tests or procedures — such as biopsy or excision of the suspected cancer and any lymph nodes or surrounding tissue that may be involved — along with scopes, scans and X-rays. As well as determining cancer stage, it is important to identify cancer grade, meaning how the cells are behaving or how quickly the cancer is likely to grow (AIHW, 2012; Cancer Australia, n.d.). Histopathological testing is used to determine this.

A diagnosis of cancer can affect a person's physical, psychological, spiritual and social wellbeing. Some of these effects will be resolved over time due to individual personal coping resources, and social and professional support. Some needs emerge later or increase over time, but it is important to be aware that at least 50 per cent of survivors suffer from some late effects of cancer treatment (Valdivieso et al., 2012).

Staging – reveals the size and extent of the cancer, including where the cancer is within the person's body.

Grading – refers to the histopathological identification of the cancer cells' degree of malignancy, or how little the cells resemble the normal tissue from which they arose.

Potential health needs for individuals after a diagnosis of cancer include:

• psychosocial issues — such as anxiety, depression, isolation and negative impacts on self-identity or self-image (Davies, Thomas & Batehup, 2010)

• physical effects — such as pain, musculoskeletal issues, fatigue, breathlessness, urinary/bowel problems, lymphoedema, premature menopause, cognitive deficits, infertility and sexual dysfunction (Davies et al., 2010)

• second cancers that are more common in cancer survivors due to genetic susceptibilities, shared etiologic exposures and mutagenic effects of cancer treatments (National Comprehensive Cancer Network (NCCN), 2015)

• fear of recurrence or second cancers. These fears are normal and very common among cancer survivors due to the multiple stressors, vulnerabilities and challenges they face. Fear of recurrence can lead to anxiety related to ongoing surveillance and physical symptoms that may or may not be related to the diagnosis (NCCN, 2015).

Some of the potential cancer pathways can be seen in Figure 7.1.

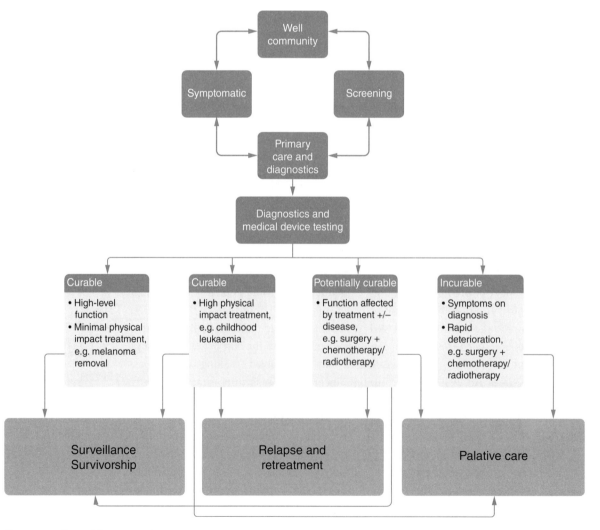

Figure 7.1   Potential cancer pathways
Source: Adapted from WA Cancer and Palliative Care Network (2008), p. 15

Indigenous peoples

In both Australia and New Zealand, significant disparities exist between Indigenous and non-Indigenous populations in relation to cancer outcomes despite the younger age profile in Indigenous populations.

Indigenous Australians were diagnosed with cancer an average of 1279 times in each year between 2009 and 2013. Between 1998 and 2013, the age-standardised incidence rate for all cancers combined increased for Indigenous Australians from 398 to 500 per 100 000, compared with an increase for non-Indigenous Australians of 387 to 423 per 100 000 (AIHW & Australasian Association of Cancer Registries (ACCR), 2015). Diagnosis at an earlier age, geographical isolation and cultural language diversity reflects the potential for more complex pathways for Indigenous peoples. Comorbidities at diagnosis increased the risk of cancer death in addition to risks associated with remoteness and disease stage at diagnosis (Banham, Roder & Brown, 2017; Reilly et al., 2018). The gap between survival rate is still significant. Targeted population health campaigns and further investment into barriers and enablers to screening participation across Australia and New Zealand are constantly being reviewed by community, public health policy and health service providers to improve diagnosis and survival rates (Banham et al., 2017).

Mortality rates are 1.5 times higher in Indigenous than non-Indigenous Australians (AIHW, 2013). Between 1998 and 2015, the age-standardised mortality rate for all cancers combined increased from 195 to 246 per 100 000 for Indigenous Australians, compared to a decrease in the rate for non-Indigenous Australians from 194 to 164 per 100 000 (AIHW & ACCR, 2015). Between 2010 and 2014, the most common cause of death for Indigenous peoples was lung cancer followed by liver cancer, cancer of unknown primary site and breast cancer in females (AIHW, 2017).

Cancer is underreported in Indigenous peoples and, as a consequence, survival after a cancer diagnosis is significantly lower for Indigenous peoples than non-Indigenous Australians (Cancer Australia, 2014). Geography can also play a role; for example, approximately a quarter of Aboriginal and Torres Strait Islander peoples live in remote or very remote areas of Australia (AIHW, 2013), and overall cancer mortality rates are significantly higher for those living in remote and very remote areas when compared with people living in major cities (Cancer Australia, 2014). Significantly, higher rates of liver, lung and cervical cancer in Indigenous Australians may be related to high prevalence of cancer-related modifiable risk factors such as smoking, alcohol consumption, lower participation in cancer screening and hepatitis B infection (AIHW, 2017). The challenges associated with providing health care in rural and remote areas are well known, and present a significant barrier in meeting health needs and reducing cancer morbidity and mortality in these populations (Standing Council on Health, 2012).

For Māori peoples, the registration rate of cancer is 26 per cent higher and the cancer death rate 1.7 times higher than in the non-Māori population (NZMOH, 2015b). Socioeconomic indicators reported higher rates of smoking and lower cancer screening coverage (NZMOH, 2015c).

Targeted programs that are intended to support a reduction in disparities of cancer outcomes in Aboriginal and Torres Strait Islander peoples and Māori include smoking cessation support services and targeted screening programs.

Cancer detection and management

Cancers may be detected through screening when the individual is asymptomatic, through routine health checks (skin) or through investigation of symptoms. Australia currently has three population screening programs targeting breast, cervical and bowel cancers. The bowel cancer screening program is expanding with full implementation of biennial screening due by 2020. Evidence does not support population screening for prostate cancer and melanoma (Department of Health, 2015b). New Zealand similarly offers screening for cervical cancer and breast cancer (NZMOH, 2014b), and a bowel cancer screening program is currently being piloted (Coleman, 2015).

The rise in cancer incidence rates in the Australian Indigenous population can be partly attributed to improved access to and participation in screening services, particularly mammography and cervical cancer screening in rural and remote communities. While participation rates are still significantly less than in non-Indigenous Australians, the implementation of culturally sensitive cancer awareness and screening programs, which include involvement of Indigenous health workers, may have increased Indigenous peoples' awareness and participation in early detection programs (Australian Health Ministers' Advisory Council, 2017).

At diagnosis, the cancer may be determined to be confined to the local area of origin, to have spread to adjoining tissue or nodes or to have spread to another site (metastasised). Cancers that can be completely surgically excised or definitively treated with radiotherapy generally have a greater chance of cure.

When cancer has metastasised, the likelihood of cure decreases significantly. The focus and goal of treatment may need to change to one of disease and symptom control through use of systemic therapies such as chemotherapy, hormone therapy or targeted biologic therapies. Radiotherapy is also used to target specific areas of disease burden or to alleviate localised cancer symptoms such as pain, bleeding or nerve compression. Such therapies can potentially achieve control for prolonged periods of time and may be administered either intermittently, as needed, or continuously. The duration of initial response to treatment is usually a good indicator of the likelihood of a more prolonged response to treatment. Some cancers, including testicular cancer and lymphoma, may be successfully managed with curative intent even with a diffuse spread of the disease beyond the local area of origin at diagnosis, thus signifying the differences in natural history of disease dependent on the type of cancer (Krege et al., 2008). Even when cancer is treated effectively and there is no clinical, pathological or radiological evidence of residual disease, there can be significant long-term adverse effects from the treatments used or from the irreparable damage caused by the cancer itself (Numico et al., 2015).

Predictable needs

The impact of cancer as a chronic disease varies, but some psychosocial aspects are common and predictable. Two areas identified by patients where there are unmet needs are fear of the cancer recurring and fear of it spreading (White et al., 2012). Financial cost 'toxicity' is also an issue commonly identified, as many cancer treatments are expensive due to direct costs or their impact on the person's ability to work. Distress levels due to the impact of cancer as a chronic disease can be screened for by using a tool such as the Distress Screening Tool, as recommended by the NCCN (2013a). This supports nurses in both specialist and community settings to facilitate referrals to the appropriate service provider, ensuring symptoms and side effects are managed (VanHoose et al., 2015).

Some impact may also be related to specific cancers, particularly those that are associated with lifestyle risk factors such as lung cancer and its association with smoking. The person with cancer may feel guilty or at fault for having contracted the disease, exacerbating the distress already resulting from the diagnosis. For smokers, as well as non-smokers, the frequent assumptions people make about them having been a smoker may be felt as a sense of stigma and shame around the diagnosis (Chambers et al., 2012). These perceptions have been associated with delays in seeking treatment and a sense of nihilism or fatalism about whether treatment will help. There may also be a perception that it is not worth trying to stop smoking when cancer has been diagnosed, despite recommendations from health care providers to reduce smoking. Cutting back or quitting smoking is likely to help the person cope better with the impact of cancer treatment and also reduces the risk of cancer recurrence or a second primary diagnosis in the future (Cancer Australia, 2015).

SKILLS IN PRACTICE

Psychosocial needs assessment

Emilio is a 57-year-old husband, father of two and grandfather of two. His primary occupation was farming, but 10 years ago he sold his farm and moved into town and currently works as a salesman. Emilio is an aviation enthusiast; he has his pilot's licence and his own plane.

Five years ago, Emilio's wife Rita decided it would be a good idea 'at their age' to go to the local skin cancer clinic for a check-up. A melanoma was discovered on Emilio's left lateral chest region. It was removed and classed as stage 1. Emilio continued with regular monitoring with the dermatologist and his general practitioner.

After three years, Emilio found a lump in his left axilla. It was thought to be a cancerous lymph node, so four days prior to Christmas he had an axillary clearance and the pathology performed on the removed lymph nodes revealed melanoma cells — a progression to stage 4.

Emilio was commenced on a clinical trial two months after the surgery. This meant that on exactly the same scheduled days each month he needed to attend clinic appointments with the oncology team, a three-and-a-half-hour drive from home. He was required to keep a journal to document any significant side effects of the medications being used for treatment and was advised to abstain from sexual inter-course over the 12-month duration of the trial.

Emilio left his job as a state and territory sales manager to work for a small, local company, which meant a significant reduction in salary. He also had to cut short a planned overseas holiday. Emilio had never had significant exposure to the health care system, had never been in hospital and only saw the doctor periodically for his high blood pressure. Emilio regularly attended his appointments on his own due to Rita's work commitments.

At the final appointment, a CT scan revealed two spots on Emilio's lungs. Despite this, and throughout the experience of the disease process, Emilio had remained physically fit and well.

After such a prolonged and challenging cancer journey, with so much hope and expectation placed on treatment in the form of a clinical trial, a result such as this can lead the person and their family to experience feelings of futility and disappointment. The importance resetting goals, setting of realistic expectations and maintaining a sense of hope throughout the stages of care are important roles of the cancer nurse.

It is also important to recognise the feelings of grief that are likely at this and other times in the cancer journey. Grief and loss can fluctuate over time and have the potential to become destructive or overwhelming. Recognition and assessment of these signs by a skilled nurse can ensure that appropriate access to counselling or to a clinical psychologist can occur, and strategies put in place to better manage unwanted feelings and responses.

Collaborating with the cancer patient in setting self-management strategies to maintain physical and mental fitness and independence can empower a person to regain or maintain some sense of control. This is particularly useful for those who are fit, well, motivated and able to actively participate in such strategies.

QUESTIONS

1. How could you, as the nurse looking after Emilio, assess how he and his family are coping with the metastatic cancer diagnosis, and which nursing supports might be suitable?

2. What advice would you give to Rita about dealing with the emotional stress of her husband being diagnosed with stage 4 melanoma?

3. What are the implications of Emilio and his family having to travel a long way to access treatment for his melanoma?

Population health and cancer prevention

The health of individuals and the broader population are influenced by many factors. These determinants of health can be social, economic, environmental, behavioural (for example, tobacco use or diet), biomedical (for example, blood pressure or obesity) or genetic factors (AIHW, 2014b). They are predictors for rates of cancer and many other chronic diseases, such as heart disease and diabetes. Any actions to prevent cancer are likely to help reduce the risk for other chronic diseases and improve general health outcomes.

Reducing the risk of chronic disease can be achieved via primary prevention through reducing exposure to risk factors for cancer such as: smoking, poor nutrition, excessive alcohol intake, insufficient physical activity, too much exposure to sun and environmental toxins (Cancer Council Australia, 2015). Secondary prevention involves early detection of cancer and interventions to stop or slow an existing disease. Improving diet, increasing exercise, quitting smoking, participating in screening programs and reducing alcohol intake also assist with secondary prevention (Cancer Council Australia, 2015). Health promotion strategies recommended for the well population to prevent cancer are equally important after a diagnosis of cancer (Davies et al., 2010). Prevention also requires targeted additional effort where specific populations and communities have increased chronic disease and cancer risk. Further, nurses and all health care professionals are important health role models in their communities. The general community looks to health care professionals as sources of information about cancer risk and cancer prevention.

Promoting behaviour change

Evidence is building to support the use of self-care management programs in people with chronic conditions, such as cancer survivors (McCorkle et al., 2011). An example of a self-care management program for cancer in Australia is the Living with Cancer Education Program.

Supporting self-care management skills encourages an awareness and active participation by the person in their cancer experience to minimise the consequences of treatment, and to promote survival, health and wellbeing (National Cancer Survivorship Initiative, 2010). A collaborative partnership between the person and the health professional helps to empower individuals to take on responsibility for their health and wellbeing. The national roll-out of My Health Record in Australia in July 2018, provides an opportunity to centralise health correspondence and management, and support individuals who are managed between health care facilities, community and self. New Zealand has adopted a national computerised health care reporting system in the effort to improve the health of all communities.

Nurses have a role in promoting self-care management behaviours in all people affected by cancer. Central to self-care management are strategies to promote 'wellness'. A wellness approach acknowledges the following points.

- A large proportion of people affected by cancer have significant comorbidities and engage in lifestyle behaviours that have adverse consequences for health; for example, smoking, poor diet and limited physical activity (NCCN, 2013b).
- A healthy lifestyle during and after cancer is associated with improved physical and psychological wellbeing, reduced risks of side effects or late effects of treatment, enhanced self-esteem, reduced risk of recurrence and improved survival (Davies et al., 2010).
- The post-treatment phase is a significant period of opportunity for health professionals to support and motivate survivors to take action to reduce their modifiable cancer risk factors (Lotfi-Jam, Schofield & Jefford, 2009).

Returning to work may fulfil a range of needs for the survivor; it is often regarded as an important psychological step to recovery and may enhance wellness through provision of:

- a regular source of income
- meaning and self-worth
- a social-support network
- an indication to the survivor, their family and work colleagues that recovery from cancer is possible, and life is returning to normal (Eva et al., 2012).

Survivorship

Survivorship refers to a cancer survivor from the time of diagnosis, through to the balance of his or her life (National Cancer Institute, 2014). Survivorship is a dynamic process as there is no clear 'end' to the cancer illness and it is artificial to consider survivorship as a sequential stage in a cancer journey. Instead, survivorship issues need to be addressed throughout the illness experience (Olver, 2011).

The nurse's role in caring for people with cancer

People affected by cancer are supported by a range of health and support services across all levels of care. Registered nurses play an essential role across the cancer continuum of care and across settings. Core capabilities for nurses caring for individuals affected by cancer have been developed (Aranda & Yates, 2009). The Australian *National Professional Development Framework for Cancer Nursing* (EdCaN Framework) establishes expectations of all nurses working in cancer control and is consistent with the Innovative Care for Chronic Conditions Framework (ICCCF). For example, the EdCaN Framework:

Cancer control – all actions that aim to reduce the burden of cancer on individuals and the community. Cancer control encompasses the impact of diagnosis, active treatment, follow up, survivorship, and supportive and palliative care.

- promotes a person-centred approach
- recognises that people affected by cancer have many, and often complex, needs requiring a multidisciplinary approach to which nurses can make important contributions.

The model presented in Figure 7.2 describes the contributions that nurses provide in all phases of the cancer continuum and highlights that all nurses, regardless of practice setting, can support people affected by cancer. This model has been endorsed for application in the *New Zealand Knowledge and Skills Framework for Cancer Nursing* (NZMOH, 2014c). The model of care aligns to the Whanau ora approach and the Māori value of 'Mana Tupuna'; that is, the role of the whanau (extended family) in decision making as determined by the person.

Nursing roles in cancer control vary widely; however, key cancer care concepts have been identified as relevant for all nurses entering practice, including: beginning-level communication; psychological, social and emotional support; conceptualisation of the meaning of cancer; and a basic understanding of carcinogenesis (Aranda & Yates, 2009).

Carcinogenesis – describes the formation of cancers, including how normal cells transform into cancer cells.

Supportive care is an approach used in cancer care to prevent or minimise the effects of cancer and its treatment across all phases of a person's cancer experience. Supportive care refers to the provision of the relevant services for those living with or affected by cancer to meet their physical, emotional, social, psychological, informational, spiritual and practical needs during the diagnostic, treatment and follow-up phases; it encompasses issues of survivorship, palliative care and loss (Fitch, 1994).

The principles of supportive care are aligned with the ICCCF. Nurses contribute to effective supportive care by:

- reducing the risk of developing unmet supportive care needs
- detecting unmet supportive care needs early
- implementing interventions to address supportive care needs, during and following treatment, and at end of life
- timely referral to other professionals, individuals and services if required (Fitch, 2008; Victorian Government Department of Human Services, 2009).

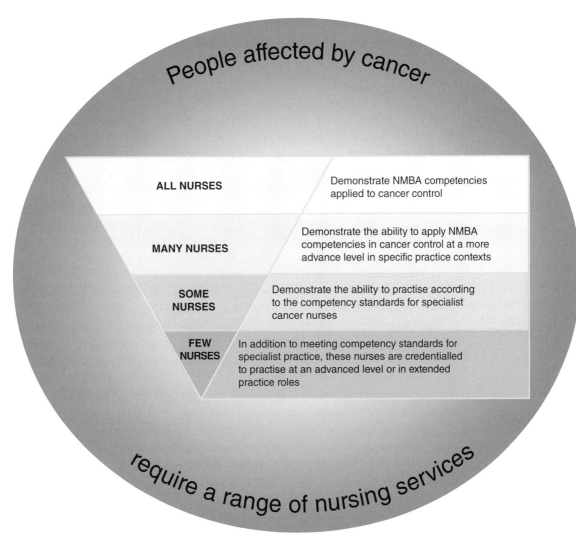

Figure 7.2   Professional development model for nursing in cancer control
Note: NMBA = Nursing and Midwifery Board of Australia
Source: Aranda & Yates (2009), p. 13.

Interventions may include self-management support, information, psychological support, symptom control, social support, rehabilitation, spiritual support, palliative care and bereavement care (Victorian Government Department of Human Services, 2009). Tools such as the Distress Screening Tool can be valuable aids in identifying unmet needs across the psychosocial spectrum (VanHoose et al., 2015).

REFLECTION

How would skills and attributes differ for nurses caring for people with cancer across different settings?

SKILLS IN PRACTICE

A personal cancer journey

At age 53, Lee discovered the lump that was to turn her world upside down. It was a shock as four months earlier her mammogram showed no evidence of cancer. Lee's general practitioner (GP) referred her for a fine needle biopsy and an appointment with a leading breast surgeon. Lee had always been grateful for the care she received from her GP and for giving her the best possible chance of surviving cancer.

The surgeon confidently told Lee that he felt it hadn't spread. He would be able to operate the next day, but he would need to have nuclear medicine tests to identify the sentinel lymph nodes. Pathology from the site of the tumour revealed the cancer was contained and only needed a lumpectomy and sentinel node removal.

The clinical team of surgeon, oncologist and radiation oncologist worked out Lee's care plan. She had utmost faith in their expertise, knowledge and experience. Lee was diagnosed with HER2+ breast cancer, a grade 3 tumour; she noted that HER2+ cancers tend to be more aggressive and harder to treat.

Lee's treatment consisted of chemotherapy – Adriamycin and Cyclophosphamide (AC) – a course of radiation therapy, and if she chose, a new drug at the time, Herceptin. She was warned her lung would be burnt by the radiation, her hair would fall out and she would need a cocktail of drugs to combat the nausea of chemotherapy. Unfortunately, she was not in a strong emotional state to comprehend how the therapy would impact on her life.

Lee's family were devastated and together they struggled through 18 months of therapy. She suffered badly during chemotherapy. Lee's hair started to fall out in the second week. Her husband shaved her hair off. At first Lee cried, as no hair was a visual sign that she had cancer. She then picked herself up, put on a scarf in the morning and never again looked at her bald head in the mirror.

Lee's weight dropped to 42 kgs. She knew she had to eat, but it was difficult to push herself. She lived on vegemite toast and Coca-Cola. They were the only smells she could bare. A massive ulcer developed on the side of her tongue preventing Lee from swallowing. An alternative therapy, oil of cloves, anaesthetised the site of the ulcer allowing her to swallow and eat a meal.

She vividly remembers switching channels on the TV to watch every news broadcast available to help get through the day. She was too ill to read or undertake simple activities. Her head was so sensitive she couldn't touch it. She was very lonely as her daughter was at university, and her husband and friends at work. She became chronically constipated from the anti-nausea drugs. Just after the fourth cycle, she collapsed and woke to her daughter cradling her between her legs on the floor.

Having survived chemotherapy, Lee felt the following treatments would be a breeze in comparison. How wrong was she in making this assumption. Following six weeks of radiation therapy, Lee commenced 17 cycles of Herceptin. At this time, it had not been approved for funding under the Pharmaceutical Benefits Scheme in Australia. Lee would have to fund the treatment at $3000 per cycle. It was financially crippling.

One side effect of Herceptin is a reduction in the heart's ability to pump blood efficiently. This only happens to a small percentage of patients. Unfortunately, Lee was part of this small percentage. She proceeded well on the drug for six cycles. Testing revealed that her heart was affected.

Physical exhausted raised adrenalin levels, which was trying to keep her heart pumping, preventing Lee from sleeping. One morning, after another night of no sleep, she collapsed with exhaustion. It was at this point that she mentally hit rock bottom. The inability to sleep, even though she was so tired she could hardly walk, temporarily destroyed her will to live. It was really hard to push through the feeling that she couldn't take any more treatment or go on the way she was feeling.

Four years later, Lee experienced late onset symptoms. An excruciating pain would travel from the base of her oesophagus upwards to the throat. An endoscope examination revealed that Lee's oesophagus was rigid in sections. The gastroenterologist believed this was caused by radiation burns.

Another symptom emerged where she would suddenly faint. Ongoing heart problems had been linked to Herceptin. Testing revealed that Lee's left ventricle wasn't affected, however her heart muscle was damaged by the AC chemotherapy. The drugs were critical to Lee's survival, but they were very toxic to the body. As further side effects developed, such as loss of strength in the hands, she learned to modify her life.

Lee is presently undergoing treatment for a reoccurrence of cancer. Her experiences have given her the confidence to ask for specific details from clinicians to help her cope with the ongoing cancer journey.

Every step and stage of the cancer journey challenges the mind, body and soul. Recognition and assessment of these signs by a skilled nurse can ensure that appropriate access to counselling or to a clinical psychologist can occur and strategies put in place to better manage unwanted feelings and responses.

Working in partnership with the person with cancer in setting self-management strategies to maintain physical and mental fitness and independence can empower a person to regain or maintain some sense of control. This is particularly useful in those who are fit, well, motivated and able to actively participate in such strategies.

QUESTIONS

1. How could you, as the nurse looking after Lee, assess how she and her family are coping with the cancer diagnosis and which nursing supports might be suitable?

2. What advice would you give to Lee's family about dealing with the emotional stress of being diagnosed with cancer?

3. What are the implications for Lee and her family having to deal and manage with the financial impact of the cancer?

Advanced nursing practice

Nurses working in advanced practice roles provide a high level of skill to a variety of complex and chronic clients, including the person with cancer. The nature of the position that the nurse holds, and the setting within which they practice, is likely to result in variability in the advanced practice role, its focus and its levels of activity within advanced practice domains such as direct comprehensive care, support of systems, education, research, publication and professional leadership (Chang, et al., 2012; Gardner et al., 2016a; 2016b).

Within the cancer nursing context, advanced practice roles in nursing continue to develop to meet the needs of people at risk of and affected by cancer, and can reduce the impact of cancer as a chronic disease. Nurses in these roles may work independently or collaboratively with other members of the health care team. The EdCaN Framework includes competency standards to support practice at the specialist cancer nurse level (Aranda & Yates, 2009). The *New Zealand Knowledge and Skills Framework for Cancer Nursing* also identifies key capabilities required at specialist and advanced levels of practice (NZMOH, 2014c). These frameworks provide a guide to assist nurses to deliver consistent and safe care in cancer control at an advanced level (Aranda & Yates, 2009; NZMOH, 2014c).

Table 7.1 outlines some examples of advanced nursing roles in a range of contexts and at different stages of the disease trajectory.

Table 7.1 Advanced nursing roles to meet the chronic care needs for specific groups of people affected by cancer

Supporting public health initiatives for screening	
Job title	**Roles**
Nurse endoscopists	Advanced practice nurses are trained to deliver safe and efficient screening for colorectal cancer (Duffield et al., 2017; Joseph, Vaughn & Strand, 2015; Limoges-Gonzalez et al., 2011). Reported benefits include: increased screening rates, lower cost and improved access (Brotherstone et al., 2007). Care provided by nurse endoscopists is associated with high levels of patient satisfaction and positive patient experiences of care (Duffield et al., 2017).
Advanced practice nurse in genetics	Within hereditary cancer programs, these nurses work with individuals and families. They undertake risk assessments, counselling sessions and education, and make recommendations for prevention and screening. They may also evaluate the suitability for families to participate in clinical trials to identify a hereditary susceptibility gene (Mahon, 2013).
Nurse practitioner (NP)	Community-based NPs focus on the psychosocial implications of cancer care, manage comorbid conditions and long-term sequelae of cancer treatments, and provide referral of cancer patients to specialty care providers including oncology NPs. Primary care NPs can expand to provide support across various models of cancer care with an emphasis on collaboration during and throughout the transition period from specialist back to primary care (a potentially uncoordinated period of health care) (Cooper, Loeb & Smith, 2010).

Supporting public health initiatives for screening	
Job title	Roles
	NPs in acute care settings, such as in-patient, outpatient and same day services, have been shown to increase access to timely and appropriate cancer care (Bishop, 2009; Cox, et al., 2013). They are recognised as experts in the management of side effects and symptoms related to cancer and cancer treatments, including chemotherapy and targeted therapies (Bishop, 2009).
	The NP role in oncology and haematology continues to expand globally with positive outcomes emerging in geriatric oncology (Morgan & Tarbi, 2016; Puts et al., 2018) and cancer survivorship (Bishop, 2009; Faithfull et al., 2016)

Meeting the chronic care needs for specific groups of people affected by cancer	
Job title	Roles
Cancer-specific nurse specialists and coordinators	Specialist cancer nurse roles have been implemented to coordinate patient care, address unmet needs and provide continuity of care (Yates, 2004).
	Breast care nurses have well-established roles and have become core members of the multidisciplinary team. Their role includes provision of physical and psychological support, coordination of care from diagnosis to therapy, and strengthening communication between the person with cancer and the treatment team (National Breast Cancer Centre, 2005).
	Prostate cancer is another prevalent cancer in Western countries and specialist prostate cancer nurse coordinator roles have been implemented in some settings. The role is still developing, but nurses in these roles directly support men with cancer and contribute positively to the multidisciplinary treatment team (Morgan et al., 2015).
	Some cancers are less common but have more complex and intense treatments, and leave the person affected with lifelong effects; for example, head and neck cancer, which is often treated with surgery, radiotherapy and chemotherapy. It is recommended that these patients have access to specialist nurses and psychosocial support throughout treatment, and attention is increasingly turning towards nursing management of survivorship care (Wells, Semple & Lane, 2015).
	Other groups for which there may be specialist nurse coordinator roles are according to age group; for example, adolescent and young adult, paediatric or geriatric.

Table 7.1 (cont.)

Meeting the chronic care needs for specific groups of people affected by cancer	
Job title	**Roles**
Treatment-specific nursing roles	Highly complex forms of treatment such as haematopoietic cell transplantation (used in haematological malignancies such as leukaemias) are often provided with the support of a specialist nurse coordinator. This type of support is even more important for those coming from rural and regional areas (Bray et al., 2011).
Late effects advanced practice nurse (APN)	A range of roles have been described in the literature, such as: • Telephone counselling by an APN, in addition to printed survivorship care plans, has been shown to increase cardiomyopathy screening in at-risk paediatric cancer survivors (Hudson et al., 2012). • In late effects APN for Hodgkin lymphoma, the APN role, situated within a multidisciplinary late effects haematology team, offers a new model of cancer survivorship care that may prove to be applicable to other patient groups with chronic illness in the future (Gates, Seymour & Krishnasamy, 2012).

SUMMARY

Learning objective 1: Describe the impact of cancer as a chronic condition.
Cancer is a leading cause of mortality in Australia and New Zealand and, despite improvements in screening, treatments and care, is increasing in significance largely due to the ageing populations in both countries. A diagnosis of cancer can affect a person's physical, psychological, spiritual and social wellbeing, and at least 50 per cent of those diagnosed with cancer will be affected by late and/or continuing effects.

Learning objective 2: Describe the targeted responses required to prevent and mitigate the impact of chronic cancer at a population level.
Interventions to reduce the risk of cancer are similar to those for other chronic diseases such as diabetes and cardiac conditions. Promoting a healthy lifestyle will both reduce the risk of cancer and mitigate its effects as a chronic condition. Nurses are important role models in the community.

Learning objective 3: Discuss how nurses can promote supportive care pathways.
Nurses have the knowledge and expertise to support the person with cancer, offering suitable support and health care services. Empowering people with cancer to self-manage their care supports their ability to make healthy lifestyle changes and choices that can have a significant impact on their wellbeing regardless of the status of their cancer.

Learning objective 4: Discuss the potential contribution of all nurses in meeting chronic care needs for the person affected by cancer.
All nurses are expected to have an understanding of cancer as a condition and the supportive care needs of those with cancer and their families. The nurse's ability to assess levels of distress, refer to support services and to support a self-management approach are key in all settings.

Learning objective 5: Describe advanced practice roles in cancer within the chronic condition framework.
Advanced practice roles have been developed for some cancer types such as breast care nurses, and settings such as primary care nurse practitioners.

REVIEW QUESTIONS

1. What are the characteristics of cancer that lead it to be identified as a chronic condition?
2. How would you identify if a person affected by cancer was distressed?
3. How would the nursing care you provide for a 20-year-old person diagnosed with cancer differ from that for an 80-year-old?
4. In what settings would you see people with cancer being cared for?
5. How does your role as a nurse impact on the person with cancer and their family?

RESEARCH TOPIC

Select a commonly occurring cancer in Australia or New Zealand. Take the time to learn more about the chosen cancer in detail, such as the main risk factors, any prevention measures, what treatments may be used, the expected survival rates and a possible trajectory of care, as well as considered late effects, including the role of the registered nurse.

FURTHER READING

Australian Institute of Health and Welfare (AIHW). (2012). *Cancer Survival and Prevalence in Australia: Period Estimates from 1982 to 2010. Cancer Series No. 69*. Cat. no. CAN 65. Canberra: AIHW. Retrieved from https://www.aihw.gov.au/getmedia/ da7bff73-5b78-4cf8-a719-5903a75fcc9a/13953.pdf.aspx?inline=true

—— (2014). *Cancer in Australia: An Overview 2014. Cancer Series No. 90*. Cat. no. CAN 88. Canberra: AIHW. Retrieved from www.aihw.gov.au/publication-detail/?id= 60129550047

Breast Cancer Network Australia. Retrieved from www.bcna.org.au

Cancer Council. Optimal cancer care pathways. Retrieved from www.cancer.org.au/health-professionals/optimal-cancer-care-pathways.html

Mukherjee, S. (2010). *The Emperor of All Maladies: A Biography of Cancer*. New York: Simon & Schuster.

New Zealand Ministry of Health (NZMOH). (2015). *Cancer: New Registrations and Deaths 2012*. Wellington: Ministry of Health.

Skloot, R. (2010). *The Immortal Life of Henrietta Lacks*. New York: Random House Inc.

REFERENCES

Aranda, S. & Yates, P. (2009). *A National Professional Development Framework for Cancer Nursing* (2nd edn). Canberra: The National Cancer Nursing Education Project (EdCaN), Cancer Australia. Retrieved from http://edcan.org.au/professional-development/edcan-framework

Australian Health Ministers' Advisory Council. (2017). *National Strategic Framework for Chronic Conditions*. Canberra: Australian Government.

Australian Institute of Health and Welfare (AIHW). (2012). *Cancer Survival and Prevalence in Australia: Period Estimates from 1982 to 2010. Cancer Series No. 69*. Cat. no. CAN 65. Canberra: AIHW. Retrieved from www.aihw.gov.au/WorkArea/Download Asset.aspx?id=10737422721

—— (2013). *Cancer in Aboriginal and Torres Strait Islander Peoples of Australia: An Overview. Cancer Series No. 78*. Cat. no. CAN 75. Canberra: AIHW. Retrieved from: www.aihw.gov.au/WorkArea/DownloadAsset.aspx?id=60129544698

—— (2014a). *Cancer in Australia: An Overview 2014. Cancer Series No. 90*. Cat. no. CAN 88. Canberra: AIHW. Retrieved from www.aihw.gov.au/WorkArea/DownloadAsset .aspx?id=60129550202

—— (2014b). *Australia's Health 2014. Australia's Health Series No. 14*. Cat. no. AUS 178. Canberra: AIHW. Retrieved from www.aihw.gov.au/WorkArea/DownloadAsset .aspx?id=60129548150

—— (2017). *Cancer in Australia 2017. Cancer Series No.101*. Cat. no. CAN 100. Canberra: AIHW.

Australian Institute of Health and Welfare & Australasian Association of Cancer Registries (AIHW & AACR). (2015). *Australian Cancer Incidence and Mortality (ACIM) Books: All Cancers Combined*. Retrieved from www.aihw.gov.au/acim-books

Banham, D., Roder, D. & Brown, B, (2017). Comorbidities contribute to the risk of cancer death among Aboriginal and non-Aboriginal South Australians: Analysis of a matched cohort study. *Cancer Epidemiology*, 52, 75–82.

Bishop, C. S. (2009). The critical role of oncology nurse practitioners in cancer care: Future implications. *Oncology Nursing Forum*, 36(3), 267–9. doi: http://10.1188/09.ONF.267-269

Bray, L., Jordens, C. F. C., Rowlings, P., Bradstock, K. & Kerridge, I. (2011). The long haul: Caring for bone marrow transplant patients in regional Australia. *Australian Journal of Advanced Nursing*, 29(1), 5–13.

Brotherstone, H., Vance, M., Edwards, R., Miles, A., Robb, K. A., Evans, R. E. C., . . . & Atkin, W. (2007). Uptake of population-based flexible sigmoidoscopy screening for colorectal cancer: A nurse-led feasibility study. *Journal of Medical Screening*, 14(2), 76–80.

Cancer Australia. (n.d.). *Cancer Australia Glossary*. Retrieved from https://canceraustralia.gov.au/publications-and-resources/glossary#G

—— (2014). *Cancer Australia Strategic Plan 2014–2019*. Retrieved from http://canceraustralia.gov.au/sites/default/files/publications/cancer-australias-strategic-plan-2014-2019/pdf/2014_strategic_plan.pdf

—— (2015). Supportive care needs during treatment. Retrieved from http://edcan.org.au/edcan-learning-resources/case-based-learning-resources/lung-cancer/active-treatment/supportive-care-needs

Cancer Council Australia. (2015). National Cancer Control Policy. Retrieved from http://wiki.cancer.org.au/policy/National_Cancer_Prevention_Policy

Chambers, S. K., Dunn, J., Occhipinti S., Hughes, S., Baade, P., Sinclair, S., . . . & O'Connell, D. L. (2012). A systematic review of the impact of stigma and nihilism on lung cancer outcomes. *BMC Cancer*, 12(184).

Chang, A. M., Gardner, G. E., Duffield, C. & Ramis, M. A. (2012). Advanced practice nursing role development: Factor analysis of a modified role delineation tool. *Journal of Advanced Nursing*, 68(6), 1369–79. doi: http://10.1111/j.1365-2648.2011.05850.x

Coleman, J. (2015). Consultation on next steps for bowel screening programme. Wellington: New Zealand Government. Retrieved from www.beehive.govt.nz/release/consultation-next-steps-bowel-screening-programme

Cooper, J. M., Loeb, S. J. & Smith, C. A. (2010). The primary care nurse practitioner and cancer survivorship care. *Journal of the American Academy of Nurse Practitioners*, 22, 394–402.

Cox, K., Karikios, D., Roydhouse, J. K. & White, K. (2013). Nurse-led supportive care management: A 6-month review of the role of a nurse practitioner in a chemotherapy unit. *Australian Health Review*, 37, 632–5.

Davies, N. J., Thomas, R. & Batehup, L. (2010). Advising cancer survivors about lifestyle. A selective review of the evidence. London: Macmillan Cancer Support.

Department of Health. (2015a). Chronic disease. Retrieved from www.health.gov.au/internet/main/publishing.nsf/content/chronic-disease

—— (2015b). Cancer screening. Retrieved from www.cancerscreening.gov.au

Duffield, C., Chapman, S., Rowbotham, S. & Blay, N. (2017). Nurse-performed Endoscopy: Implications for the nursing profession in Australia. *Policy Politics & Nursing Practice*, 18(1), 36–43. doi: http://10.1177/1527154417700740

Eva, G., Playford, D., Sach, T., Barton, G., Risebro, H., Radford, K. & Burton, B. (2012). Thinking positively about work. Delivering work support and vocational rehabilitation for people with cancer. London: Macmillan Cancer Support, Department of Health and University College London.

Faithfull, S., Samuel, C., Lemanska, A., Warnock, C. & Greenfield, D. (2016). Self-reported competence in long term care provision for adult cancer survivors: A cross sectional survey of nursing and allied health care professionals. *International Journal of Nursing Studies*, 53, 85–94. doi: https://doi.org/10.1016/j.ijnurstu.2015.09.001

Fitch, M. I. (1994). *Providing Supportive Care for Individuals Living with Cancer (Task Force Report)*. Toronto: Ontario Cancer Treatment and Research Foundation.

—— (2008). Supportive care framework. *Canadian Oncology Nursing Journal*, 18(1), 6–24.

Gardner, G., Duffield, C., Doubrovsky, A. & Adams, M. (2016a). Identifying advanced practice: A national survey of a nursing workforce. *International Journal of Nursing Studies*, 55, 60–70. doi: http://10.1016/j.ijnurstu.2015.12.001

—— (2016b). Identifying advanced practice: A national survey of a nursing workforce. *International Journal of Nursing Studies*, 55, 60–70. doi: https://doi.org/10.1016/j.ijnurstu.2015.12.001

Gates, P., Seymour, J. F. & Krishnasamy, M. (2012). Insights into the development of a nurse-led survivorship care intervention for long-term survivors of Hodgkin lymphoma. *Australian Journal of Cancer Nursing*, 13(1), 4–10.

Hudson, S., Miller, S., Hemler, J., Ferrante, J., Lyle, J., Oeffinger, K. & DiPaola, R. (2012). Adult cancer survivors discuss follow-up in primary care: 'Not what I want, but maybe what I need'. *Annals of Family Medicine*, 10(15), 418–27.

Joseph, J., Vaughn, R. & Strand. H. (2015). Effectiveness of nurse-performed endoscopy in colorectal cancer screening: A systematic review. *Gastrointestinal Nursing*, 13(4), 26–33.

Krege, S., Beyer J., Souchon, R., Albers, P., Albrecht, W., Algaba, F., . . . & von der Maase, H. (2008). European Consensus Conference on diagnosis and treatment of germ cell cancer: A report of the Second Meeting of the European Germ Cell Cancer Consensus Group (EGCCCG): Part II. *European Urology*, 53, 497–513.

Limoges-Gonzalez, M., Mann, N. S., Al-Juburi, A., Tseng, D., Inadomi, J. & Rossaro, L. (2011). Comparisons of screening colonoscopy performed by a nurse practitioner and gastroenterologists: A single-center randomized controlled trial. *Gastroenterology Nursing*, 34(3), 210–16.

Lotfi-Jam, K., Schofield, P. & Jefford, M. (2009). What constitutes ideal survivorship care? *Cancer Forum*, 33(3), 171–4.

Mahon, S. M. (2013). Allocation of work activities in a comprehensive cancer genetics program. *Clinical Journal of Oncology Nursing*, 17(4), 397–404.

McCorkle, R., Ercolano, E., Lazenby, M., Schulman-Green, D., Schilling, L. S., Lorig, K. & Wagner, E. H. (2011). Self-management: Enabling and empowering patients living with cancer as a chronic illness. *CA: A Cancer Journal for Clinicians*, 61(1), 50–62.

Morgan, B. & Tarbi, E. (2016). The role of the advanced practice nurse in geriatric oncology care. *Seminars in Oncology Nursing*, 32(1), 33–43. doi: http://10.1016/j.soncn.2015.11.005

Morgan, M., Butow, P., Maddern, R. & Shaw, J. (2015). The role of the prostate cancer nurse coordinator: Nurses' perspectives of barriers and challenges. *International Journal of Urology Nurses*, 9(1), 22–8.

National Breast Cancer Centre. (2005). *Specialist Breast Nurse Competency Standards and Associated Educational Requirements*. Sydney: National Breast Cancer Centre.

National Cancer Institute – Division of Cancer Control and Population Sciences. (2014). Retrieved from https://cancercontrol.cancer.gov/ocs/statistics/definitions.html

National Cancer Survivorship Initiative. (2010). Priorities for research on cancer survivorship. Retrieved from www.ncsi.org.uk/wp-content/uploads/NCSI-Research-Priorities-Report.pdf

National Comprehensive Cancer Network (NCCN). (2013a). NCCN distress thermometer for patients. Retrieved from www.nccn.org/patients/resources/life_with_cancer/pdf/nccn_distress_thermometer.pdf

—— (2013b). *NCCN Clinical Practice Guidelines in Oncology (NCCN Guidelines) Survivorship Version 1*. Fort Washington, PA: NCCN.

—— (2015). *NCCN Clinical Practice Guidelines in Oncology (NCCN Guidelines) Survivorship Version 2*. Fort Washington, PA: NCCN.

New Zealand Government. (2018). Mortality 2015 data tables. Retrieved from www.health.govt.nz/publication/mortality-2015-data-tables

New Zealand Ministry of Health (NZMOH). (2014a). *Briefing to the Incoming Minister of Health 2014*. Wellington: Ministry of Health.

—— (2014b). *Screening*. Retrieved from www.health.govt.nz/our-work/preventative-health-wellness/screening

—— (2014c). *New Zealand Knowledge and Skills Framework for Cancer Nursing*. Retrieved from http://file://sagrahf20/canusers/kcamer05/Downloads/KSFCN_2014_FINAL%20formatted.pdf

—— (2015a). *Cancer Patient Survival: 1994 to 2011*. Wellington: Ministry of Health.

—— (2015b). *Cancer: New Registrations and Deaths 2012*. Wellington: Ministry of Health.

—— (2015c). *Tatau Kahukura: Maori Health Chart Book 2015* (3rd edn). Wellington: Ministry of Health.

—— (2016). *Cancer: New Registrations and Deaths 2013*. Wellington: Ministry of Health. Retrieved from www.health.govt.nz/publication/cancer-new-registrations-and-deaths-2013

Numico, G., Longo, V., Courthod, G. & Silvestris, N. (2015). Cancer survivorship: Long-term side-effects of anticancer treatments of gastrointestinal cancer. *Current Opinion in Oncology*, 27, 351–7.

Olver, I. (2011). *The MASCC Textbook of Cancer Supportive Care and Survivorship*. New York: Springer, pp. 3–7.

Puts, M. T. E., Strohschein, F. J., Del Giudice, M. E., Jin, R., Loucks, A., Ayala, A. P. & Alibhai, S. H. M. (2018). Role of the geriatrician, primary care practitioner, nurses, and collaboration with oncologists during cancer treatment delivery for older adults: A narrative review of the literature. *Journal of Geriatric Oncology*, 9(4), 398–404. doi: http://10.1016/j.jgo.2018.04.008

Reilly, R., Micklem, J., Yerrell, P., Banham, D., Morey, K., Stajic, J., . . . & Brown, A. (2018). Aboriginal experiences of cancer and care coordination: Lessons from the Cancer Data and Aboriginal Disparities (CanDAD) narratives. *Health Expectations*, 2–10.

Standing Council on Health. (2012). *National Strategic Framework for Rural and Remote Health*. Canberra: Commonwealth of Australia. Retrieved from www.ruralhealthaustralia.gov.au/internet/rha/publishing.nsf/Content/EBD8D28B517296A3CA2579FF000350C6/$File/NationalStrategicFramework.pdf.

Valdivieso, M., Kujawa, A. M., Jones, T. & Baker, L. H. (2012). Cancer survivors in the United States: A review of the literature and a call to action. *International Journal of Medical Science*, 9, 163–73.

VanHoose, L., Black, L., Doty, K., Sabata, D., Twumasi-Ankrah, P., Taylor, S. & Johnson, R. (2015). An analysis of the Distress Thermometer problem list and distress in patients with cancer. *Support Care Cancer*, 23, 1225–32.

Victorian Government Department of Human Services. (2009). *Providing Optimal Cancer Care: Supportive Care Policy for Victoria*. Melbourne: Metropolitan Health and Aged Care Services Division. Retrieved from www.supportivecancercarevictoria.org/PDF/supportive_care_policy.pdf

WA Cancer & Palliative Care Network. (2008). *Model of Care for Cancer*. Perth: Department of Health.

Wells, M., Semple, C. J. & Lane, C. (2015). A national survey of healthcare professionals' views on models of follow-up, holistic needs assessment and survivorship care for patients with head and neck cancer. *European Journal of Cancer Care*, 24, 873–83.

White, K., D'Abrew, N., Katris, P., O'Connor, M. & Emery, L. (2012). Mapping the psychosocial and practical support needs of cancer patients in Western Australia. *European Journal of Cancer Care*, 21, 107–16.

World Economic Forum. (2013). Sustainable health systems: Visions, strategies, critical uncertainties and scenarios. Retrieved from www3.weforum.org/docs/WEF_SustainableHealthSystems_Report_2013.pdf

Yates, P. (2004). Cancer care coordinators: Realising the potential for improving the patient journey. *Cancer Forum*, 28(3), 128.

8

Chronic cardiovascular conditions

Amali Hohol, Michelle Baird
and Melissa Johnston

LEARNING OBJECTIVES

After studying this chapter, you should be able to:

1. demonstrate knowledge of the underlying pathogenesis of cardiovascular conditions and their associated risk factors
2. discuss the importance of prompting health and reducing risk in the management of chronic cardiovascular conditions
3. understand the concepts of person-centred care and care coordination in relation to chronic cardiovascular conditions
4. identify the nurse's role in the care of chronic cardiovascular conditions
5. identify the characteristics of the role of a nurse who practises at an advanced level in cardiovascular health.

Introduction

Cardiovascular disease (CVD) is considered one of the main contributors of death and disease burden in Australia and New Zealand. In 2012, CVD accounted for approximately 30 per cent of all deaths recorded within both nations (Department of Health, 2015; National Heart Foundation of New Zealand, 2015). Patients suffering from CVD are found across a variety of care environments. Nurses who provide care to these individuals are required to possess skills and knowledge that will enable optimal health outcomes. The successful management of CVD requires the implementation of a number of key strategies including behavioural change, prevention, risk factor identification and reduction, and ongoing monitoring and support (Loades, 2017).

The term 'cardiovascular disease' is used in reference to health conditions that affect the heart and blood vessels. This includes coronary heart disease (also known as ischaemic heart disease), acute myocardial infarction, heart failure and cardiomyopathy, hypertension, peripheral vascular disease and stroke (Department of Health, 2015). It is important to realise that CVDs are largely preventable. Increasing and improving health care access, in conjunction with early identification and reduction of CVD risk factors, may lead to a decrease in the health burden to which this collection of chronic conditions contributes (Loades, 2017).

This chapter focuses on several key issues relating to chronic CVD. The pathophysiology of the differing disease processes associated with CVD is outlined, as well as the importance of promoting health, and primary and secondary disease prevention in relation to CVD. The concepts of person-centred care and care coordination in relation to the CVD patient, and the nurse's role across a variety of health care settings is explored, with an emphasis on establishing a therapeutic nurse–client relationship and advocating self-care management. Advanced nursing practice is also highlighted, focusing on how nurses with advanced cardiovascular nursing skills are involved in the care of the individual with chronic CVD.

Differentiating the pathophysiology of cardiovascular conditions

Atherosclerosis is the main factor in the development of several CVDs, including coronary heart disease. Atherosclerosis is a process that occurs over time and involves the abnormal build-up of lipids and other fatty materials in the internal lumen of arteries (see Figure 8.1). As these atherosclerotic **plaque** increase in size, the internal vessel diameter narrows and reduces blood flow. Plaque rupture may occur, initiating a cascade of events which results in **thrombus** formation and subsequent tissue ischaemia, injury or acute myocardial infarction (Farrell, 2017).

Plaque – a build-up of fatty substances, cholesterol, calcium, cellular waste products and fibrin within the arterial wall.

Thrombus – a blood clot that is created in a vessel and remains there, creating a partial or total blockage.

Stroke

Strokes (also termed cerebral vascular accident, or CVA) are classified as either ischaemic or haemorrhagic. Ischaemic stroke can be further categorised into being thrombotic or embolic in nature. A thrombotic stroke occurs when the cranial arteries become narrowed as a result of atherosclerosis. As atherosclerotic changes progress, thrombus formation may occur and result in partial to full occlusion of the artery

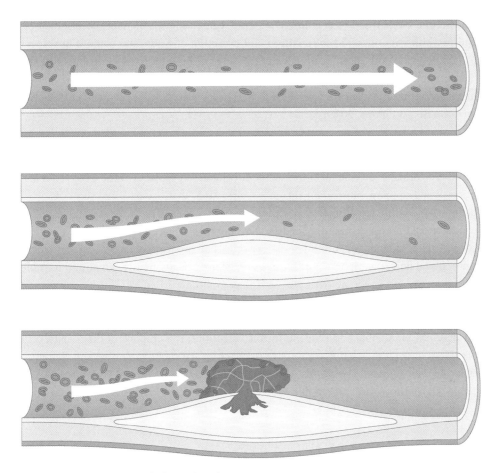

Figure 8.1   Development of atherosclerosis

(Massaro, 2013). An embolic stroke is most often the result of a cardiogenic event, whereby the emboli is formed within the heart and is circulated to the cerebral vasculature and interrupts cerebral blood flow (Farrell, 2017). Haemorrhagic stroke is characterised by bleeding into either the subarachnoid space, or in the brain, secondary to the rupturing of an aneurysm or small artery (Stroke Foundation, 2018).

Cardiomyopathy and heart failure

Cardiomyopathies are CVDs that affect the heart muscle or myocardium. The myocardium becomes progressively dilated, thickened or stiffened and this decreases the pumping ability of the heart, leading to heart failure as the heart becomes unable to meet metabolic demand. Chronic heart failure is the subsequent inability of the heart to maintain adequate systemic tissue perfusion (McCartan et al., 2012). This is the result of structural changes or myocardial dysfunction, whereby the ability of the ventricles to fill with, or eject blood, is diminished (Davidson & Ferguson, 2014).

Hypertension

Hypertension is diagnosed when either the systolic or diastolic blood pressure (BP) is elevated. There are several mechanisms that are involved with BP regulation, including arterial baroreceptors, atrial naturetic peptide, endothelins, and the renin-angiotensin-aldosterone system. This collection of systems regulates levels of systemic vasodilation and vasoconstriction, and the retention and excretion of water and sodium in respect to circulating blood volume. Impairment of any of these systems contributes to the development of hypertension. Alterations in the vasculature of blood vessels, such as increased arterial stiffness, can increase systemic vascular resistance and further increase BP (Williams, 2015).

Peripheral vascular disease

Peripheral vascular disease (also termed peripheral artery disease) is the atherosclerotic plaque build-up, and subsequent thrombus formation, that occurs to vessels outside of the heart and brain, resulting in end organ ischaemia. Involved in the development of this condition is a complex interplay of vascular endothelial cells, vascular smooth muscle cells, platelets, fibroblasts and inflammatory cells. The progressive narrowing and block-age of blood flow to peripheral limbs causes tissue hypoxia, tissue ischaemia, and possible limb necrosis and gangrene (Krishna, Moxon & Golledge, 2015).

While there is no singular cause for CVD, it is important to recognise the associated risks factors so that prevention strategies can be implemented. Risk factors are divided into modifiable and non-modifiable categories. It is important that health care providers understand that several CVD risk factors are silent in nature and therefore lack obvious clinical symptoms (National Heart Foundation of Australia, 2015). Table 8.1 outlines the modifiable and non-modifiable risk factors associated with CVD as stated by the World Heart Federation (2015).

Table 8.1   Risk factors associated with cardiovascular disease

Non-modifiable	Modifiable
Age	Tobacco smoking
Ethnicity	Alcohol
Family history	High-fat diet
Gender	Hyperlipidaemia
	Hypertension
	Diabetes mellitus
	Physical inactivity
	Obesity
	Depression
	Social isolation

SKILLS IN PRACTICE

Living with a chronic cardiovascular condition

Edward, a 64-year-old male, has a complex and chronic comorbid health history that includes diabetes, peripheral vascular disease, alcoholic cardiomyopathy, hypertension, depression and biventricular heart failure. Edward's father died at 56 of a heart attack.

Edward and his wife divorced several years ago. He has two adult children – a son and a daughter – who live nearby. His daughter, Alison, is actively involved in her father's care and commonly accompanies him to his medical appointments. However, Edward would prefer to self-manage his chronic conditions as he does not like doctors much. Edwards feels that doctors are too bossy and are always telling him what he can and cannot do.

Edward has recently been discharged from an acute care facility following an admission for acute pulmonary oedema and uncontrolled blood glucose levels secondary to excessive alcohol consumption. This was Edward's third admission in the past 12 months for the same health issue. Upon discharge the heart failure nurse practitioner, Kate, met with Edward to coordinate his outpatient management plan.

Secondary prevention strategies were put in place, in conjunction with cardiovascular rehabilitation services, to assist Edward in his day-to-day activities. The education and support provided by the cardiac rehabilitation service has empowered Edward to engage in self-care activities, and enabled him to recognise and better manage his cardiac symptoms when they worsen. Kate meets with Edward on a regular basis and, as a result of her higher-level nursing skills, Edward does not need to see the doctor as frequently. Through the implementation of person-centred care, facilitated by advanced nursing practice, Edward has been able to reduce his incidence of hospitalisation and improve his quality of life.

QUESTION

Given the complexity of Edward's health history, how will his cardiovascular conditions, and their associated risk factors, impact on his self-care management plan?

Promoting cardiovascular health and reducing risk: an international concern

Cardiovascular disease contributes to death and disability worldwide. The World Health Organization (WHO, 2013) recognises that CVD health promotion and disease prevention should not be limited to preventing reoccurrence of a CVD event (secondary prevention), but also should be opportunistic in predicting and preventing the first occurrence of a CVD event (primary prevention). Health promotion and prevention in CVD is synonymous with optimum patient outcomes through prevention, early detection, and modification of lifestyle and risk factors, thus reducing hospitalisations and cost both to the health care system and the patient. Nurses; be they acute or community-based, public or privately employed; are in an excellent position to provide opportunistic education and intervention.

The three-tiered approach of the Innovative Care of Chronic Conditions Framework (ICCCF) in managing and preventing chronic disease – micro (patient level), meso (community and health care organisation) and macro (policy) (Nuño et al., 2012) – incorporates horizontal and vertical integration of an interdisciplinary service delivery. Cardiovascular disease prevention at the micro level primarily involves assisting the patient to set goals to modify risk factors through healthy food choices,

Secondary prevention – is concerned with reducing the impact of a disease or illness after it has occurred.

Primary prevention – is concerned with preventing disease or illness prior to it occurring.

regular physical activity, awareness of risk factors and strategies to reduce the impact of modifiable risk factors (National Heart Foundation of Australia and Cardiac Society of Australia and New Zealand, 2012). Core organisations, such as the Australian and New Zealand National Heart Foundations, and the Australian National Stroke Foundation are instrumental at the meso level of CVD reduction through awareness campaigns. Policies developed by the Australian Department of Health and the New Zealand Ministry of Health (macro level) guide clinicians in their management of CVD, as well as promote prevention of risk factors such as smoking, with the enforcement of no-smoking policies in public places.

Primary prevention

The Absolute Cardiovascular Disease Risk (Australia) and the publication *Cardiovascular Disease Risk Assessment and Management for Primary Care* (New Zealand) are tools used in general practice to predict a person's risk of a CVD event occurring within five years (National Vascular Disease Prevention Alliance, 2012; New Zealand Ministry of Health (NZMOH), 2018). The *Cardiovascular Disease Risk Assessment and Management for Primary Care* is a measurement tool for people aged 30–74 years of age without pre-existing CVD (NZMOH, 2018). Identifying people who are at greater risk of CVD either through modifiable lifestyle choices (diet, inactivity, poor medication use) or non-modifiable factors (gender, genetic predisposition) can encourage the prevention and management of risk factors to reduce the likelihood of a CVD event. Regular check-ups with general practitioners can identify a person's early risk factors. It is recommended that New Zealanders who identify as Indigenous (Māori) or have CVD risk factors be assessed using the CVD risk assessment tools from age 30 for men, and 40 for women. Non-Indigenous individuals should be assessed from age 45 for men and from age 55 for women (NZMOH, 2018). Similarly, in Australia, Indigenous peoples are assessed from age 35 and the general population, regardless of gender, from age 45 (National Vascular Disease Prevention Alliance, 2012).

Secondary prevention

Once a CVD event has occurred, it is even more important to modify risk factors to reduce the occurrence of subsequent events. Strategies utilised in managing secondary prevention encompass all primary prevention strategies as well as cardiac rehabilitation, or in the case of stroke, rehabilitation. Medications such as antiplatelet, beta-blockers and angiotensin-converting enzyme (ACE) inhibitors are an integral part of secondary prevention of CVD (National Vascular Disease Prevention Alliance, 2012).

Cardiac rehabilitation

Cardiac rehabilitation has been shown to improve patients' quality of life and psychological wellbeing, reduce hospital admissions and, most importantly, reduce CVD risk factors to slow down disease progression (Dalal, Doherty & Taylor, 2015; Price et al., 2016). Cardiac rehabilitation is a program designed to promote return to an active and complete lifestyle for individuals who have suffered a CVD event such as a heart attack or post-revascularisation. It can be hospital-, community- or home-based and is run over a 4–12-week period, incorporating six core components:

1. assessment
2. risk-factor modification
3. individualised exercise programs
4. education and counselling
5. behaviour-modification strategies
6. self-care management (National Heart Foundation of Australia, 2010).

After completing a CR program, individuals are encouraged to exercise and adopt a healthy lifestyle (Price et al., 2016).

Stroke rehabilitation

Stroke rehabilitation commences in the acute setting and continues upon discharge in the community or a stroke rehabilitation service. It is a multidisciplinary service with the patient and family/carer at the centre. The aim of this service is to obtain maximum functional and cognitive capacity for the client. Members of the rehabilitation team include doctors, dieticians, nurses, occupational therapists, pharmacists, physiotherapists, psychologists, social workers and speech pathologists (Stroke Foundation, 2017).

Rehabilitation, with its focus on maximising function after a chronic condition has been diagnosed, is also described as tertiary prevention. It aims to prevent further deterioration and complications from the chronic condition, and to assist people in adjusting to their new situation in the most effective manner possible. Table 8.2 outlines the management of the main risk factors.

Table 8.2   Cardiovascular disease management of risk factors

Risk factor	Management
Smoking	• Cessation: Australia – 5As (Ask, Assess, Advise, Assist, Arrange); New Zealand – ABCD (Ask, Brief advice, Cessation support, Document) • Avoid passive smoking • Maintain non-smoking status (National Heart Foundation of Australia and Cardiac Society of Australia and New Zealand, 2012; National Heart Foundation of Australia, 2015; NZMOH, 2018; Royal Australian College of General Practitioners, 2011; Stroke Foundation, 2017)
Nutrition	• Reduced saturated fat • Healthy fat choices (i.e. polyunsaturated, monounsaturated) • Fruit, wholegrains • Reduce sugar and salt (use herbs and spices) • Water as a choice of drink (Heart Foundation, n.d.; National Heart Foundation of Australia and Cardiac Society of Australia and New Zealand, 2012; NZMOH, 2018)

Table 8.2   (cont.)

Risk factor	Management
Physical activity	• Thirty minutes on most days of the week (National Heart Foundation of Australia, 2015; National Heart Foundation of Australia and Cardiac Society of Australia and New Zealand, 2012; Royal Australian College of General Practitioners, 2011)
Body mass index (BMI), waist to hip ratio (WHR)	• BMI >18.5 to <25 kg/m^2 • WHR: women <80 cm • WHR: men <94 cm (National Heart Foundation of Australia and Cardiac Society of Australia and New Zealand, 2012)
Blood pressure (BP)/ diabetes/serum lipids	• Maintain healthy weight range through diet and exercise • Monitor – optimal BP <120/80 mmHg • Medications as prescribed (National Heart Foundation of Australia, 2010; 2106; National Vascular Disease Prevention Alliance, 2012)
Alcohol	• No more than two standard drinks per day; one standard drink if female and on antihypertensive medication (National Heart Foundation of Australia, 2010; National Heart Foundation of Australia and Cardiac Society of Australia and New Zealand, 2012; Stroke Foundation, 2017)
Signs and symptoms of CVD	• Awareness of signs of chest pain • Stroke awareness: FAST (Face, Arms, Speech, Time) (National Heart Foundation of Australia, 2010; National Stroke Foundation, 2017)

REFLECTION

Consider how cardiac rehabilitation, in conjunction with public health resources such as the National Heart Foundations in both Australia and New Zealand, have contributed to cardiovascular health promotion and prevention on a national scale. What impact do you think these programs and resources have had in reducing the prevalence of chronic CVD in these countries?

Person-centred care

Best practice in the management of chronic cardiovascular conditions is multidisciplinary in nature. Care should be evidence-based, individualised and patient-centred.

Person-centred care considers and responds to an individual's values, needs and preferences, while maintaining their respect and dignity (Atherton et al., 2018). The multidisciplinary team involved in the person-centred care of the chronic cardiovascular patient includes not only the patient and their family or carer, but extends to encompass informal supports, physicians, nurses, occupational therapists, pharmacists, social workers, dieticians and other allied health care professionals (Johansson & Harkey, 2014). Person-centred care includes the provision of emotional support, physical comfort, information, communication and care coordination. The key features of person-centred care is to access advice and support along with the consideration of family and carers. This approach provides continuity of care through care coordination and can improve quality of life for those with chronic CVD (Atherton et al., 2018).

When developing care plans for people who have experienced either a stroke or chronic heart failure, the generic principles of person-centred care need to be incorporated to suit the specific needs of the individuals and their families. Improving partnerships between clients and health care professionals so that they focus on communication, meaningfulness, relevance and quality are important because they encourage clients to be as active as possible in their care while in the acute care setting (Kessler & Liddy, 2017; Ulin, Malm & Nygardh, 2015). This also aligns with the ICCCF at the micro level where decision making and **self-care management** are major components. Kessler and Liddy (2017), and Ulin and colleagues (2015) demonstrated that such involvement in self-care management following a person's discharge resulted in a reduced length of stay, the maintenance of functional ability and an improved quality of life.

Self-care management – a process whereby the patient is able to independently function on a daily basis, with a sense of control and empowerment.

Care coordination

Care coordination is an essential component of person-centred care. The importance of care coordination can be seen throughout the management of chronic cardiovascular conditions. A common goal is the assurance of optimisation of management for the individual's condition by providing a seamless system of care for the entire health care journey, including community or hospital care. Atherton and colleagues (2018) discuss this goal in regard to heart failure management, indicating that to achieve care coordination, integration of other services such as cardiac rehabilitation and palliative management is essential. Multidisciplinary management programs are fundamental to the delivery of a complete package of care, including such services as follow-up with education, psychosocial support, optimisation of medical treatment using collaborative care models with general practitioners and improved access to care (Atherton et al., 2018). Coordination of care, along the continuum of chronic CVD and throughout the delivery of various services such as nurses, cardiologists and allied health, is the key to optimal management of every person. The stroke management guidelines from the National Stroke Foundation (2017) also emphasise care coordination and the continuum of care for people who have had a stroke with similar principles to those of CVD management, focusing on rehabilitation commencing in the acute phase. Evidence shows that the earlier rehabilitation is commenced, the better the outcome for the stroke survivor. Rehabilitation is a person-centred and goal-orientated process

Care coordination – a method of organising care between several participants to ensure that care delivery is appropriate to the individual.

aimed at reintegrating the stroke survivor into the community; therefore, the transition between hospital and community, with care coordination throughout, is of utmost importance (National Stroke Foundation, 2017).

The complex nature of chronic cardiovascular conditions indicates that an individualised approach to management needs to be adopted and person-centred programs developed to help promote self-care management. Self-care management should focus on content that is specific to the needs and preferences of the individual, so that the person develops skills like:

- decision-making
- problem-solving
- awareness of emotional and role management
- confidence building in management of their own condition
- understanding their role in the doctor/client relationship.

Education for chronic cardiovascular conditions is an important part of self-care management in person-centred care. By educating and empowering individuals with the knowledge necessary for them to help themselves, this can translate into a reduction of the need for hospital admissions, medical interventions and even specialist involvement in management (Atherton et al., 2018; National Stroke Foundation, 2017).

The nurse's role in the management of chronic cardiovascular conditions

Wilkes and colleagues (2013) discuss the nurse's role within the multidisciplinary team in regard to prevention and management of chronic cardiovascular conditions. They identify six main domains:

1. advocate
2. supporter
3. coordinator
4. educator
5. team member
6. assessor.

Person-centred care can only be achieved by gaining the cooperation of individuals and their active participation in all aspects of their care. The development of a therapeutic relationship between the nurse and the individual facilitates person-centredness for those with chronic conditions, and is a crucial element in health care provision. This is an essential component of the nurse's role in both acute care and community settings. Doherty and Thompson (2014) describe the process of establishing a therapeutic relationship, which is developed when a nurse is assessing, planning and delivering care. Doherty and Thompson (2014) also indicate that the therapeutic relationship is fostered by the nurse employing:

- listening and questioning techniques such as motivational interviewing and active listening
- information sharing

- support strategies
- person-centred care
- empathy and compassion.

Family and carers should not be excluded from the therapeutic relationship, as they provide a significant amount of support to the individual (Doherty & Thompson, 2014). Of utmost importance, the nurse must have skills in effective communication to support the development of a therapeutic relationship; this creates positive outcomes, increases engagement and enables self-care management of people with chronic cardiovascular conditions (Wilkes et al., 2013).

Advocating self-care management

Self-care management refers to 'the strategies, decisions and activities individuals take to manage a long-term health condition' (Boger, Demain & Latter, 2015, p. 175). This concept focuses on individuals effectively managing their treatment, symptoms, lifestyle, physical and psychological consequences of their chronic condition and own health within their own homes (Reynolds et al., 2018). To engage in self-care management, individuals and their families need to acquire skills and knowledge specific to their health problem from nurses, other services and health professionals (Boger et al., 2015). The nurse has a major role in providing support, follow up and education to enable and empower the person to self-manage their condition. Table 8.3 describes specific key points that need to be addressed by the nurse in the process of enabling self-care management for people with chronic cardiovascular conditions. This process begins in the acute setting and continues through the individual's health care journey in the community.

REFLECTION

Research indicates that for individuals who suffer from a chronic illness, a level of self-care management must be incorporated into their care to achieve the desired clinical outcomes. Consider the physical, psychological and social barriers that could impact on an individual's ability to self-manage their chronic cardiovascular condition. What interventions might be implemented to overcome these potential obstacles?

Advanced nursing practice and cardiovascular conditions

Advanced nursing practice in the management of cardiovascular conditions has addressed shortages in access to specialty health care, providing timely provision to appropriate services (Chang et al., 2012). The field of cardiovascular nursing encompasses a broad range of skills and knowledge. At an advanced level, the cardiovascular nurse has the skills and theoretical knowledge to interpret electrocardiograms (ECGs) and cardiac rhythms, monitor and maintain a person's haemodynamic status in stable

Table 8.3   The nurse's role in education and enabling self-care management for chronic cardiovascular conditions

Chronic cardiovascular condition	The nurse's role in educating and enabling self-care management
Coronary heart disease/acute myocardial infarction	• Medication management – antiplatelet agent(s), beta-blocker, ACE inhibitor, statin • Psychosocial factors – depression and social isolation • Cardiac rehabilitation programs • Lifestyle advice • Ongoing prevention • Chest pain management (Amsterdam et al., 2014; Chew et al., 2016)
Heart failure/cardiomyopathy	• Pharmacological treatment – beta-blocker, ACE inhibitor, diuretics • Non-pharmacological treatments • Monitoring of condition and adjustment of treatment – fluid management • Signs and symptoms of deterioration and when to seek health care • Lifestyle changes • Psychosocial factors (Atherton et al., 2018)
Hypertension	• Medication management – ACE inhibitor, calcium channel blockers, thiazide diuretics • Blood pressure monitoring • Lifestyle advice for modifications – physical activity, weight control, diet, smoking cessation and alcohol intake (National Heart Foundation of Australia, 2016)
Peripheral vascular disease	• Cardiovascular risk factor management • Lifestyle modification – smoking cessation, weight loss, exercise and healthy diet • Medication management – statin, antiplatelet, antithrombotic and antihypertensive • Optimal glucose level control in people with diabetes (Aboyans et al., 2018)
Stroke	• Focus on secondary prevention • Lifestyle modification • Medication management – antiplatelet, statin • Diabetes management • Rehabilitation • Support to access specific stroke self-care management programs (National Stroke Foundation, 2017)

and unstable environments, and an extensive understanding of the pharmacological and non-pharmacological management of CVD (Krum & Driscoll, 2013).

Nurses practising at an advanced level have a solid educational foundation in the context of chronic illness prevention and health promotion. Examples of these types of nurses include educators who have the ability to use their well-developed communication skills to provide high-quality care (Bishop & Jackson, 2013), or a heart failure nurse practitioner who supports patients to self-manage their chronic heart failure through comprehensive assessment, education and monitoring of their fluid status (Krum & Driscoll, 2013). In order to ensure that the needs of the person are met, nurses may take on roles with greater levels of responsibility and accountability. These situations mean that nurses who are practising at an advanced level are the first point of contact in the primary health setting, thus providing them with the autonomy to care for clients independently (Haidar, 2014).

Nurses with higher-level cardiovascular management skills are in a position to assist in the development of care models for chronic conditions which enable individuals to successfully engage in self-care activities (Haidar, 2014). It is also important to recognise that all nurses act as advocates. This encourages trust between nurses and individuals, and nurses and the individuals' families, thereby increasing the likelihood that self-care behaviours and lifestyle modifications will be accepted (Bishop & Jackson, 2013).

SKILLS IN PRACTICE

Swollen ankles

Joan is a 75-year-old lady who lives with her husband and two cats in an apartment block on the second floor. Joan has a history of hypertension, hypercholesterolaemia, osteoarthritis, type 2 diabetes mellitus and chronic heart failure. Her current medications are perindopril, carvedilol and frusemide. She is currently the carer for her husband Joe, who suffers from chronic obstructive pulmonary disease. Joan likes to smoke the occasional cigarette. Due to her husband's home oxygen, she does not smoke in the apartment, but finds it difficult to navigate the stairs because of her arthritis in her knees. Joan and Joe receive home help twice weekly with showering, and once weekly with a grocery shop. Their daughter, Jacinta, is only able to visit on weekends as she lives in the neighbouring town.

As the community nurse, you have been tasked with following up with Joan in her home as she has had a recent admissions to hospital because of shortness of breath, chest pain and swelling in her ankles. Joan admits to you that she continues to suffer from swelling in her feet and ankles, which limits her mobility and her ability to care for Joe. Due to her limited mobility, she has been having difficulty getting to the toilet in time after taking her frusemide, so has been reluctant to take this medication and admits to often skipping doses. When you ask Joan about her weight management, Joan reports that she has noticed that she has put on quite a significant amount of weight in the past few weeks, but she is unaware that she needs to monitor this.

QUESTION

Consider the impact that medication non-adherence and cigarette smoking has on Joan's ability to self-manage her chronic cardiovascular condition. How could nurses support Joan to improve on how she currently manages her chronic health condition?

SUMMARY

Learning objective 1: Demonstrate knowledge of the underlying pathogenesis of cardiovascular conditions and their associated risk factors.

Chronic CVD is an umbrella term used to identify a group of disease processes that involve the heart and blood vessels. It includes coronary artery disease, acute myocardial infarction, stroke, cardiomyopathy, heart failure, hypertension and peripheral vascular disease. These conditions are differentiated by their underlying pathophysiology. Chronic CVD is associated with a range of risk factors that are classified as either modifiable or non-modifiable.

Learning objective 2: Discuss the importance of promoting health and reducing risk in the management of chronic cardiovascular conditions.

Health promotion and prevention in the context of CVD must include early detection and lifestyle modification, with the aim to reduce the required number of hospitalisations. The prevention framework that should be followed is the micro, meso and macro system as outlined by the ICCCF. It is important that both primary and secondary prevention strategies are implemented to improve patient outcomes while reducing international health care expenditure on CVDs.

Learning objective 3: Understand the concepts of person-centred care and care coordination in relation to chronic cardiovascular conditions.

Person-centred care should be applied to the management of any chronic condition. It is important that nurses recognise that this care strategy includes not only the individual, but extends to encompass their family and the multidisciplinary health care team. Through well-developed and seamlessly executed care coordination, the individualised needs of the person can be met.

Learning objective 4: Identify the nurse's role in the care of chronic cardiovascular conditions.

To successfully engage the individual with chronic CVD, the nurse must assume several important care roles to facilitate the establishment of a strong therapeutic relationship. Families and carers should be considered in this process. The formation of these relationships will also assist in enabling self-care abilities in the individual suffering from CVD.

Learning objective 5: Identify the characteristics of the role of a nurse who practises at an advanced level in cardiovascular health.

Nurses working at an advanced level play a significant role in the management of chronic CVD. Advanced cardiovascular nursing practice is focused on the provision of education, leadership and consultancy. Advanced nursing practice has the potential to promote self-care behaviours in individuals, thereby enhancing quality health outcomes.

REVIEW QUESTIONS

1. Cardiovascular disease is differentiated by its underlying pathophysiology. What is the main pathological contributor to CVD and how does it contribute to differing chronic cardiovascular conditions?

2. Explain the purpose of both primary and secondary prevention in the management of CVD.
3. Discuss why individualised care coordination is important when discussing the concept of person-centred care in the management of CVD.
4. Nurses encompass six roles in the care of individuals with CVD. Identify these and explain how each enables the individual with CVD to self-manage their condition.
5. Nurses practising at an advanced level are integral in the management of CVD. Identify and discuss the key responsibilities that these skilled nurses have.

RESEARCH TOPIC

Atherosclerosis is a process that commences in adolescence and continues across a person's lifespan. Consider how this pathophysiological process is linked to the increasing obesity epidemic and the future impact this will have on global health care expenditure and resource allocation.

FURTHER READING

Atherton, J., Sindone, A., Pasquale, C., Driscoll, A., McDonald, P., Hopper, I., . . . & Connell, C. (2018). National Heart Foundation of Australia and Cardiac Society of Australia and New Zealand: Guidelines for the prevention, detection, and management of heart failure in Australia 2018. *Heart and Lung Circulation*, 27(10), 1123–208.

Mann, D. L., Zipes, D. P., Libby, P. & Bonow, R. O. (2014). *Braunwald's Heart Disease: A Textbook of Cardiovascular Medicine*. Philadelphia, PA: Elsevier Health Sciences.

National Rural Health Alliance. (2015). Cardiovascular disease in rural Australia. Deakin West, ACT: National Rural Health Alliance. Retrieved from http://ruralhealth.org.au/sites/default/files/publications/cardiovascular-disease-fact-sheet-may-2015.pdf

National Stroke Foundation. (2017). Clinical guidelines for stroke management 2017. Melbourne: National Stroke Foundation. Retrieved from https://informme.org.au/Guidelines/Clinical-Guidelines-for-Stroke-Management-2017

Perk, J., De Backer, G., Gohlke, H., Graham, I., Reiner, Ž., Verschuren, M., . . . & Wolpert, C. (2012). European guidelines on cardiovascular disease prevention in clinical practice (version 2012). *The Fifth Joint Task Force of the European Society of Cardiology and Other Societies on Cardiovascular Disease Prevention in Clinical Practice*, 33(13), 1635–1701. doi: http://10.1093/eurheartj/ehs092

REFERENCES

Aboyans, V., Ricco, J. B., Bartelink, M. L. E., Bjorck, M., Brodmann, M., Cohnert, T., . . . & Czerny, M. (2018). 2017 ESC Guidelines on the diagnosis and treatment of peripheral arterial diseases, in collaboration with European Society for Vascular Surgery (ESVS). *European Heart Journal*, 39(9), 763–816. doi: http://10.1093/eurheartj/ehx095

Amsterdam, E. A., Wenger, N. K., Brindis, R. G., Casey, D. E., Ganiats, T. G., Holmes, D. R., . . . & Zieman, S. J. (2014). 2014 AHA/ACC Guideline for the management of patients with non-ST-elevation acute coronary syndromes. *Circulation*, 130, e344–e426. doi: http://10.1161/CIR.0000000000000134

Atherton, J., Sindone, A., Pasquale, C., Driscoll, A., McDonald, P., Hopper, I., ... & Connell, C. (2018). National Heart Foundation of Australia and Cardiac Society of Australia and New Zealand: Guidelines for the prevention, detection, and management of heart failure in Australia 2018. *Heart and Lung Circulation*, 27(10), 1123–208.

Bishop, C. J. & Jackson, J. (2013). Motivational interviewing: How advanced practice nurses can impact the rise of chronic diseases. *Journal for Nurse Practitioners*, 9(2), 105–9. doi: http://10.1016/j.nurpra.2012.12.010

Boger, E. J., Demain, S. H. & Latter, S. M. (2015). Stroke self-management: A focus group study to identify the factors influencing self-management following stroke. *International Journal of Nursing Studies*, 52, 175–87.

Chang, A. M., Gardner, G. E., Duffield, C. & Ramis, M. A. (2012). Advanced practice nursing role development: Factor analysis of a modified role delineation tool. *Journal of Advanced Nursing*, 68(6), 1369–79.

Chew, D. P., Scott, I. A., Cullen, L., French, J. K., Briffa, T. G., Tideman, P. A., ... & Aylward, P. E. (2016). National Heart Foundation of Australia & Cardiac Society of Australia and New Zealand: Australian clinical guidelines for the management of acute coronary syndromes 2016. *Heart, Lung and Circulation*, 25(9), 895–951. doi: http://10.1016/j.hlc.2016.06.789

Dalal, H. M., Doherty, P. & Taylor, R. S. (2015). Cardiac rehabilitation. *British Medical Journal*, 351, h5000. doi: http://10.1136/bmj.h5000

Davidson, P. M. & Ferguson, C. (2014). Management of patients with complications for heart disease. In M. Farrell & J. Dempsey (eds), *Smeltzer and Bare's Textbook of Medical-Surgical Nursing* (3rd Australian and New Zealand edn, pp. 686–710). Sydney: Lippincott Williams & Wilkins.

Department of Health. (2015). Cardiovascular disease. Retrieved from www.health.gov.au/internet/main/publishing.nsf/Content/chronic-cardio

Doherty, M. & Thompson, H. (2014). Enhancing person-centred care through the development of a therapeutic relationship. *British Journal of Community Nursing*, 19(10), 502–7.

Farrell, M. (ed.). (2017). *Smeltzer & Bare's Textbook of Medical and Surgical Nursing* (4th edn). Sydney: Lippincott Williams & Wilkins.

Haidar, E. (2014). The reality of introducing advanced nurse practitioners into practice. *Journal of Community Nursing*, 28(1), 68–72.

Heart Foundation. (n.d.). Eating for heart health. Heart Foundation position statement. Retrieved from www.heartfoundation.org.au/images/uploads/main/Eating_for_Heart_Health_-_Position_Statement.pdf

Johansson, B. & Harkey, J. (2014). Care coordination in long term home and community-based care. *Home Healthcare Nurse*, 32(8), 470–5.

Kessler, D. & Liddy, C. (2017). An integrative literature review to examine the provision of self-management support following transient ischaemic attack. *Journal of Clinical Nursing*, 26(21–2), 3256–70.

Krishna, S., Moxon, J. & Golledge, J. (2015). A review of the pathophysiology and potential biomarkers for peripheral artery disease. *International Journal of Molecular Sciences*, 16(5), 11294–322.

Krum, H. & Driscoll, D. (2013). Management of heart failure. *Medical Journal of Australia*, 199 (5), 334–9.

Loades, J. M. (2017). Cardiovascular disease prevention: Where are we now? *Practice Nurse*, 47(9), 16–20.

Massaro, L. (2013). Ischemic stroke. In S. Alexander (ed.), *Evidence-Based Nursing Care for Stroke and Neurovascular Conditions* (pp. 36–67). Oxford: Wiley-Blackwell.

McCartan, C., Mason, R., Jayasinghe, S. & Griffiths, L. (2012). Cardiomyopathy classification: Ongoing debate in the genomics era. *Biochemistry Research International*, 1–10. doi: http://10.1155/2012/796926

National Heart Foundation of Australia. (2010). *Secondary Prevention of Cardiovascular Disease*. Retrieved from www.heartfoundation.org.au/SiteCollectionDocuments/ Secondary-Prevention-of-cardiovascular-disease.pdf

—— (2015). Know the risks. Retrieved from www.heartfoundation.org.au/your-heart/know-the-risks/Pages/default.aspx

—— (2016). *Guideline for the Diagnosis and Management of Hypertension in Adults*. Retrieved from www.heartfoundation.org.au/images/uploads/publications/PRO-167_Hypertension-guideline-2016_WEB.pdf

National Heart Foundation of Australia and Cardiac Society of Australia and New Zealand. (2012). *Reducing Risk in Heart Disease: An Expert Guide to Clinical Practice for Secondary Prevention of Coronary Heart Disease*. Melbourne: National Heart Foundation of Australia.

National Heart Foundation of New Zealand. (2015). Know the facts: Statistics. Retrieved from www.heartfoundation.org.nz/know-the-facts/statistics

National Stroke Foundation. (2017). Clinical guidelines for stroke management 2017. Melbourne: National Stroke Foundation. Retrieved from https://informme.org.au/ Guidelines/Clinical-Guidelines-for-Stroke-Management-2017

National Vascular Disease Prevention Alliance. (2012). Guidelines for the management of absolute cardiovascular disease risk. *National Health and Medical Research Council*. Retrieved from https://strokefoundation.com.au/~/media/strokewebsite/ resources/treatment/absolutecvd_gl_webready.ashx?la=en

New Zealand Ministry of Health (NZMOH). (2018). *Cardiovascular Disease Risk Assessment and Management for Primary Care*. Wellington: Ministry of Health. Retrieved from www.health.govt.nz/publication/cardiovascular-disease-risk-assessment-and-management-primary-care

Nuño, R., Coleman, K., Bengoa, R. & Sauto, R. (2012). Integrated care for chronic conditions: The contribution of the ICCC Framework. *Health Policy*, 105, 55–64.

Price, K. P., Gordon, B. A., Bird, S. R. & Benson, A. C. (2016). A review of guidelines for cardiac rehabilitation exercise programmes: Is there an international consensus? *European Journal of Preventive Cardiology*, 23(16) 1715–33.

Reynolds, N. A., Ski, C. F., Mcevedy, S. M., Thompson, D. R. & Cameron, J. (2018). Construct validity of the heart failure screening tool (Heart-FaST) to identify heart failure patients at risk of poor self-care: Rasch analysis. *Journal of Advanced Nursing*, 74(6), 1412–22.

Royal Australian College of General Practitioners. (2011). *Supporting Smoking Cessation: A Guide for Health Professionals*. Melbourne: The Royal Australian College of General Practitioners. Retrieved from www.racgp.org.au/your-ractice/guidelines/ smoking-cessation

Stroke Foundation. (2017). *Clinical Guidelines for Stroke Management 2017*. Melbourne: National Stroke Foundation. Retrieved from https://informme.org.au/Guidelines/ Clinical-Guidelines-for-Stroke-Management-2017

——(2018). Haemorrhagic stroke. Retrieved from https://strokefoundation.org.au/About-Stroke/Types-of-stroke/Haemorrhagic-stroke-bleed-in-the-brain

Ulin, K., Malm, D. & Nygardh, A. (2015). What is known about the benefits of patient-centred care in patients with heart failure. *Current Heart Failure Reports*, 12(6), 350–9.

Wilkes, L., Cioffi, J., Cummings, J., Warne, B. & Harrison, K. (2013). Clients with chronic conditions: Community nurse role in a multidisciplinary team. *Journal of Clinical Nursing*, 23, 844–55.

Williams, H. (2015). Hypertension: Pathophysiology and diagnosis. *Clinical Pharmacist*, 7(1).

World Health Organization (WHO). (2013). *Global Action Plan for the Prevention and Control of Noncommunicable Diseases (NCDs): 2013–2020*. Geneva: WHO. Retrieved from www.who.int/nmh/events/ncd_action_plan/en/

World Heart Federation. (2015). Cardiovascular disease risk factors. Retrieved from www.world-heart-federation.org/cardiovascular-health/cardiovascular-disease-risk-factors

9

Injury prevention

Linda Deravin, Sally-Anne Wherry
and Judith Anderson

With acknowledgement to Simone Brown

LEARNING OBJECTIVES

After studying this chapter, you should be able to:

1. understand the impact of injuries on the health and wellbeing of communities
2. identify the potential risk factors for falls
3. describe the main causes of transportation injuries
4. describe the signs, pathophysiology and long-term effects of an acquired brain injury (ABI)
5. outline the effects of interpersonal violence, including assault, and the effects of self-harm
6. consider the impact of chronic pain on an individual that occurs as a result of injury
7. understand the role of the nurse in injury prevention.

Introduction

Injury prevention has been identified as one of Australia's targeted national health priorities (Australian Institute of Health and Welfare (AIHW), 2015a). In New Zealand, injuries are the fifth most important cause of health loss (New Zealand Ministry of Health (NZMOH) and Accident Compensation Corporation, 2013). There is a significantly increasing trend in chronic illness and disability because of **falls**, transportation injuries, sporting and workplace accidents, and interpersonal violence. Many of these injuries result in hospitalisation. After receiving immediate treatment and stabilisation in the acute care setting, a person may require long-term physical rehabilitation or ongoing psychological support and counselling resulting from the injury sustained.

Falls – slips, trips or losses of balance that result in people coming to rest inadvertently on the ground or other lower level.

Health promotion and prevention programs are critical to raising awareness and reducing the incidence of injuries that occur. In Australia, falls account for 39.4 per cent of injuries; transportation 12 per cent; interpersonal violence, including **self-harm**, 5.9 per cent; assault 5.2 per cent; and other unintentional injuries 32.1 per cent. These alarming statistics have a significant impact on the cost to both people and health systems (AIHW, 2015b). A multi-layered approach is required to reduce the incidence of injuries. This includes government-led awareness programs such as driver safety campaigns (Proffitt & Beacham, 2012; Transport for NSW, 2015), domestic violence awareness (Parliament of Australia, 2011; Proffitt & Beacham, 2012), workplaces improving their safety systems, and individuals taking responsibility for their own safety. Falls, transportation injuries, ABIs, interpersonal violence as a result of assault, self-harm and the chronic pain that often results from injury will be the focus of this chapter.

Self-harm – when a person intentionally hurts themself without dying.

Falls

A fall is 'an event, which results in a person coming to rest inadvertently on the ground or other lower level' (World Health Organization (WHO), 2007). This definition includes slips, trips and a loss of balance. However, it does not cover near-miss events, which are key to identifying the person at risk. In 2012–13, there were 98 704 serious injuries due to falls in the over 65s, which is an increase of 3 per cent per year since 2002 (AIHW and Flinders University, 2017). Approximately one-third of people aged 65 or over fall each year, with 66–76 per cent requiring transportation to hospital (Paul et al., 2017). The risk of falls directly correlates with fragility and age, with those living in nursing homes being more likely to fall than those living independently (Bradley, 2013). Falls are the leading cause of injury in hospital and are recognised as a priority in the 10 Australian *National Safety and Quality Health Service Standards* (Australian Commission on Safety and Quality in Health Care (ACSQHC), 2012). They cause longer hospital stays and adverse outcomes. Falls are more likely in wards such as neurology, elderly care or rehabilitation. For example, in 2009–10, the number of falls in the in-patient population aged 65 or over was 83 800 in Australia (Bradley, 2013). Worldwide, the cost of falls is estimated at $648.2 million US and they account for 40 per cent of all injury death (WHO, 2007).

Risk factors

Effective prevention of falls is key to the prevention of more serious injuries, hospital admission or placement in a nursing home (Kenny et al., 2011; WHO, 2015). Risk factors for falls can be categorised by behavioural, environmental, biological and socioeconomic factors. Addressing these risk factors is part of the nurse's role in providing effective care.

Behavioural risk factors

Behavioural risk factors include actions, emotions or choices (WHO, 2007) that are potentially modifiable, such as lack of exercise or excessive alcohol use. The introduction of exercise programs, such as tai chi, can increase muscle strength as well as improve emotional wellbeing.

Environmental risk factors

Reducing the environmental hazards is a recommended part of any falls' reduction program. Introduction of safety devices such as hand rails, grab bars, ramps and appropriate lighting can reduce falls in the community (WHO, 2015). Multidisciplinary teams that target medical and environmental factors, for those with a history of falling or at high risk, are effective in reducing falls for the community-dwelling older person.

Biological risk factors

Polypharmacy – when a person is on four or more medications.

There are many medical conditions that can be targeted for falls reduction and multiple comorbidities. Some chronic diseases also increase the risk of falling (Rodrigues, Fraga & Barros, 2014). For example, 60–80 per cent of people with dementia fall within a year, which is double the amount of other people their age (Booth et al., 2015). **Polypharmacy** is also a large risk factor for falls, particularly psychotropic medication. A thorough medication review is therefore vital, with discontinuation of high-risk medications if possible (Slomski, 2012).

Socioeconomic risk factors

Low income, poor education, inadequate housing, limited social interactions, limited access to health care and lack of community resources all contribute to the risk of falling (Kiadaliri, Turkiewicz & Englund, 2018; Lee et al., 2018; Ryu et al., 2017; WHO, 2015). Encouraging people who are older and at risk of falling to participate in social gatherings can mitigate the risk of falling and build networks that can assist to reduce delays in seeking assistance if a fall occurs in the home. The role of the nurse would be to understand what services are available and recommend these services to the individual to provide socioeconomic support; for example, community transport, government-funded home modification programs, community-supported housing and diversional activity groups.

Promoting health and reducing risk

Multifactorial intervention — a customised approach often used in community situations — includes exercise, medical management, medication adjustments, environmental changes and education (Slomski, 2012; WHO, 2007). Lifestyle changes require a person to accept that change is necessary. The person also needs to have the resources to make the changes (WHO, 2007). Educating the health consumer is a vital part of the nursing role in preventing falls, as is working in collaboration with the person and the multidisciplinary team to reduce any risk and promote wellness. This information should be based on the frequency and outcomes of falls, causes of falls, consideration of individual risk, identification of problem areas, and prevention strategies and behaviours (Haines et al., 2011). Development of this education should be evidence-informed practice with a person-centred model. Haines and colleagues (2011) developed their program based on the health belief model, and covered the topics mentioned here in video and written information. Their positive results demonstrate that multidisciplinary work that includes an educational component produces positive results. This is supported by the work in other studies, including one by Hill and colleagues, which demonstrated that individual patient education reduced falls significantly (Hill et al., 2015). Working with the local health care team to develop these resources, if they are not already in place, would contribute to the care of at-risk people.

REFLECTION

What are some ways to reduce the risk of falls within your local community?

Transportation injuries

Transportation injuries are a major but preventable cause of death and injury. Males, and people in rural and remote areas have greater rates of death and disability related to transport injuries. Transport injuries include car occupants, motorcyclists, bicycle riders and pedestrians (AIHW and Flinders University, 2015; Ministry of Transport, 2014). Fifty to sixty per cent of major trauma hospitalisations are due to transport injuries, and these are most commonly head, neck and chest injuries (Ruseckaite et al., 2012).

Motorcyclists, bicycle riders and pedestrians are particularly vulnerable road users, and face significant injury if involved in accidents (NSW Government, 2012). Substantial success in reducing road trauma has been achieved with the mandated use of seat belts, random breath and drug testing, and speed enforcement programs (Stevenson & Thompson, 2014). These types of strategies sit within the macro level of the Innovative Care for Chronic Conditions Framework (ICCCF). Education programs for adolescents to reduce risk and subsequent injury from motor vehicle injuries have reduced the number of injuries (Layba et al., 2017), and road safety programs have had similar success when targeting children (Daniels & Risser, 2014). These achievements are significant as transport injuries can have ongoing ramifications – even non-serious transport injuries can lead to significant loss of earnings (Berecki-Gisolf, Collie & McClure, 2013).

In Australia, Indigenous Australians are more likely to die or sustain injury from transport injuries. This is likely to be related to a greater proportion of Indigenous

Australians living in rural and remote areas, where the majority of such injuries occur, and the risk factors related to these areas such as: speeding, unlicensed driving, lack of seat belt use, alcohol and drug use, driver fatigue, overcrowding of cars and poor-quality roads (Falster et al., 2013).

Due to the health benefits associated with riding bicycles, campaigns have been instigated to increase people's participation in this form of exercise. The benefit of increased physical activity is possibly well-known to nurses, but other benefits include reduced greenhouse gases, improved air quality and noise reduction. However, if the cycling campaigns are successful, there is the possibility that injuries in this area may increase. Safety equipment is mandated in several areas and offers some protection, but New Zealand bicycle riders indicate a greater use of such equipment than Australian bicycle riders (Poulos et al., 2015a; 2015b).

REFLECTION

There are a number of transport injury awareness programs promoted within the media. Identify a current program that targets injury prevention and discuss its main objectives. Consider the effectiveness of such programs when injuries continue to increase.

Acquired brain injury

Acquired brain injury includes both ischaemic stroke and traumatic brain injury (TBI), and is one of the common causes of disability and death in adults. Acquired brain injury results in deterioration in cognitive, physical, emotional or independent functioning. This injury can be a result of trauma, hypoxia, substance abuse, degenerative neurological diseases, infection, tumours or stroke. The deterioration can affect a person's cognitive ability or physical functioning; it can be temporary or permanent, and can lead to a partial or total disability, or psychosocial issues (Galgano et al., 2017). Traumatic brain injury is defined by the WHO Collaborating Centre Task Force as 'an acute brain injury resulting from mechanical energy to the head from external forces' (Cancelliere et al., 2012). This section will focus on TBI.

Diagnosis and treatment

A TBI can be identified by the following symptoms:

- confusion or disorientation
- loss of consciousness
- post-traumatic amnesia (PTA)
- focal neurological signs and seizures.

Glasgow Coma Scale (GCS) – a tool to measure neurological response that can be used to assess an ABI.

The severity of a TBI is classified as mild, moderate or severe and is based on scores from the **Glasgow Coma Scale (GCS)**. The GCS evaluates the person's ability to open their eyes, their verbal response and movement response (Green, Haukoos & Schriger, 2017).The risk factors for a TBI include age, alcohol intake, gender, ethnicity, socio-economic status and education level (Feigin et al., 2010).

X-rays, computed tomography (CT) and magnetic resonance imaging (MRI) scans may be performed to determine the nature and extent of the brain injury sustained. A CT scan can determine if the patient requires surgery. Brain swelling can occur after a significant brain injury, which can cause further damage (Galgano et al., 2017). Surgery may be needed to remove blood clots, foreign objects or bone fragments from the brain. The bone of a fractured skull may be temporarily lifted away from the brain to limit further damage, and a tube may be connected to a pressure monitor to measure brain swelling and indicate if further intervention is required. At times, an intracranial pressure monitor may be medically indicated and this may be inserted without the necessity of surgery (Galgano et al., 2017).

Post-traumatic amnesia is a symptom that is apparent when the patient regains consciousness; it may occur after an injury or surgery and last for hours or weeks. Post-traumatic amnesia is part of the recovery process of the brain; during this time the patient is unable to store new information, is confused and disorientated, and may be behaviourally disturbed (Vos et al., 2012). The length of time in PTA can be used as a guide to determine the severity of the brain injury (Agency for Clinical Innovation, 2011).

Health promotion and education

A brain injury is a devastating disability due to its wide range of effects. The number and severity of problems resulting from a brain injury will differ for each person affected. This is because the extent and location of the damage will differ in each person (Agency for Clinical Innovation, 2011). Cognitive changes can result in memory problems, poor concentration, depression, lack of initiative, poor planning and problem-solving abilities, changes in communication, lack of insight, slowed responses, inflexibility, impulsivity, irritability, **emotional lability** and socially inappropriate behaviour. Physical changes can result in loss of taste and smell, dizziness and balance issues, seizures, fatigue, headaches, chronic pain, paralysis and visual problems (Agency for Clinical Innovation, 2011).

Emotional lability – characterised by frequent and exaggerated changes in emotional displays or mood.

It is important for the person with a brain injury to resume an independent lifestyle safely, and this is approached in stages and based on the person's physical and cognitive abilities. In the home setting, the focus is on those issues related to everyday living, and the return to previous activities such as work, study and leisure. The ability of the brain-injured person to recognise their own strengths and limitations is important in order for specialised support to be made available (Agency for Clinical Innovation, 2011).

Nursing staff play a vital role in communicating with the rest of the multidisciplinary team with respect to the patient's progress. As ABI patients relearn activities through repetition, continuity of care is vital. When patients are confused, they may display aggressive behaviour. This may be due to the patient not understanding why the nursing staff act as they do and why they are having therapy. Naturally, people will often try to avoid activities that cause them discomfort or pain. Developing a relationship with the patient allows the nursing staff to work towards appropriate behaviours. The development of the relationship is dependent on a number of factors,

Empathy – understanding another person's experience from that person's perspective.

not least the nurse's ability to respect the patient, be sensitive to their changed circumstances, and have **empathy** with the patient and their situation (Valente & Fisher, 2011).

SKILLS IN PRACTICE

Living with an acquired brain injury

John is a 35-year-old male who lives with his wife, Sarah, and their three daughters aged ten, eight and six years old. John's parents live interstate; Sarah's father died many years ago and her mother lives locally. John is employed full time as a teacher and Sarah works part time in a bank. The children all attend the local private school.

John was involved in a motor vehicle accident. He was the driver and the sole person in the car. John sustained a TBI due to the accident and was transported to the local hospital. Once John's condition was stabilised and he was ready for rehabilitation, he was transferred to the nearest brain injury unit.

John had PTA for several weeks, during which time he displayed memory and behavioural changes, including aggression. Once John recovered from the PTA and before his discharge home, a family meeting was held where the therapists informed John and Sarah of a number of issues related to John's reintegration into the community. John had suffered significant changes to his memory, displayed poor concentration, poor planning, poor problem solving and a lack of insight into these changes, which would impact on his return into the community.

QUESTION

Using the knowledge that you have of John, his family and his role in the family before the accident, what are the key issues that could impact on family life once John is discharged home?

Interpersonal violence

Domestic violence – abusive behaviour in a relationship that is used by one person to gain or maintain power and control over another. It can include physical, sexual, emotional, economic or psychological actions or threats of actions.

Interpersonal violence includes both domestic and community violence. **Domestic violence** frequently takes place between family members or intimate partners. Community violence is usually between people who are not related, and who may or may not know each other. Alcohol and use of illicit drugs (such as ice) are major contributing factors in interpersonal violence. For this reason, health promotion to prevent interpersonal violence often targets alcohol and drug intake. Alcohol and other drugs also create other issues that can increase the severity of the injury, complicate treatment and rehabilitation, and worsen the patient's prognosis (Alcohol Healthwatch, 2012).

Community violence usually targets younger males, while intimate partner violence usually targets females (AIHW, Pointer & Kreisfeld, 2012; Alcohol Healthwatch, 2012). Violence may result in immediate, acute injuries, and, in the long term, can increase the risk of substance use, eating disorders, depression and post-traumatic stress disorder (Alcohol Healthwatch, 2012).

Approximately one in four women in Australia and one in three women in New Zealand have experienced physical violence (AIHW, 2018; New Zealand Family Violence Clearinghouse, 2017). Intimate partner violence and non-partner sexual violence can also have long-term effects, which may lead to sexually transmitted infections, substance abuse, anxiety and depression (WHO, Department of Reproductive Health and Research, London School of Hygiene and Tropical Medicine, South African Medical Research Council, 2013). Barriers to screening for intimate partner violence include inadequate training, time constraints, feelings of powerlessness and a lack of resources to refer victims to. Screening for this type of violence is more likely when nurses take a comprehensive health history and it should be perceived as preventative health care (Day et al., 2015). Women are unlikely to disclose intimate partner violence unless asked, so the role of the nurse can be essential. Women who have experienced intimate partner violence have advised that: nurses provide a rationale for their enquiry (to reduce feelings of shame and apprehension), ask the woman when she is alone in a safe and supportive environment, and offer information, support and access to relevant resources even if they are not disclosing at the time (Beynon et al., 2012). Nurses may have a legal mandate to report abuse against vulnerable populations (it varies by country and state or region) (Australian Nursing and Midwifery Federation (ANMF), 2016). Vulnerable populations are discussed to a greater extent in Chapter 5.

Neglect is most common among vulnerable populations such as children, people with disabilities and the elderly (Alcohol Healthwatch, 2012). Elder abuse is a term that covers physical, psychological, social and financial abuse, and neglect is often committed by family members. **Assault** across all ages is under-reported, but particularly so with the elderly, who often fear retaliation, feel ashamed when the act was committed by a family member, or fear institutionalisation (AIHW et al., 2012).

Neglect – to pay little attention to or disregard another person, leading to ill health. People who are not able to attend to all their own care are particularly vulnerable to abuse in this manner.

Assault – an intentional act that causes emotional, psychological or physical injury.

SKILLS IN PRACTICE

Holistic assessment: Nicky

Nicky presents to the emergency department (ED) with a fractured left wrist, which she says she sustained from falling over at home. Nicky is accompanied by her partner who insists on being present when you examine her, and answers many questions on Nicky's behalf. When you read Nicky's notes, you notice that she has had multiple presentations to the ED for a range of injuries; including bruising to the chest, abdomen and face; over the previous 12 months.

QUESTIONS
1. What strategies can you use to ensure that you have an unbiased assessment of Nicky (how would you separate Nicky from her partner without causing any further distress)?
2. What considerations do you need to implement to ensure that Nicky will be safe after discharge from the ED?
3. What safety measures are in place for staff when dealing with aggressive and potentially abusive people?

Self-harm

In New Zealand, self-harm accounts for approximately 33 per cent of injury-related health loss (measured by disability-adjusted life years) (NZMOH, 2013). Self-harm includes poisoning, cutting, burning, shooting and other self-inflicted injuries. Hospitalisation due to self-harm is more likely in females than males, and Indigenous Australians than non-Indigenous Australians (AIHW and Flinders University, 2015). It is important to remember that people who present with self-harm are experiencing stress, emotional pain and personal crisis (Callaghan & Waldock, 2012). It is particularly important to avoid appearing judgemental or negative towards the person who is self-harming, as this could increase the risk for further self-harm (Youd, 2013).

Chronic pain

Pain is a subjective experience. Every individual will experience pain differently and it is important that health professionals recognise that pain is what the person experiencing the pain says that it is. Chronic pain is pain that either lasts constantly or returns intermittently beyond the time of normal healing. Chronic pain is acknowledged as pain being present for longer than three months (NSW Agency For Clinical Innovations, 2015). The significant economic and social burdens of chronic pain are now being recognised as phenomena within chronic conditions that need to be addressed to improve the health of individuals. Having chronic pain affects people's ability to participate in normal activities of daily living. It may impact on a variety of aspects within a person's life, such as social relationships, or result in a loss of employment. People experiencing chronic pain have reported feelings of isolation, emotional distress and the stigma associated with having this chronic condition (Newton, et al., 2013).

Chronic pain may occur as a secondary disability linked to other chronic conditions, such as arthritis and multiple sclerosis, or mechanical physiological injuries. Even though it may be a secondary condition, pain is now recognised as being a chronic condition. Typically, within chronic pain, a person may present with a complex mixture of nociceptive and neuropathic pain. There are a range of treatment options available to people with chronic pain, including pharmacological interventions, surgical intervention and psychological support (Barrie & Loughlin, 2014). Nurses should encourage self-management strategies (Kawi, 2014) that support individuals to manage this chronic condition; they will need to have the knowledge and skills to provide person-centred care in line with best practice in the management of chronic pain (Barrie & Loughlin, 2014). Pain treatment and management is further explored in Chapter 21.

The nurse's role in injury prevention and care

As can be seen from the above discussion, the nurse will have multiple roles in injury prevention and rehabilitation, including care coordination, case management, counselling and complex nursing assessments. A holistic approach is therefore necessary, and a person-centred approach is vital. For example, the falls risk and ABI nurse works within the multidisciplinary team, and alongside allied health and medical teams, to improve the outcomes for patients. Health promotion is a significant role for nurses who need to educate clients and empower them to make informed choices to prevent injury (Stevenson & Thompson, 2014).The nurse also has a role to report abuse to authorities that protect children and the elderly. This is mandated in some countries so nurses need to be aware of their legal and ethical obligations in this area (ANMF, 2016).

Advanced nursing practice

Management of complex patients requires a teamwork approach, and nurses working as advanced practitioners in these areas must be able to operate in a teamwork environment. Due the extended hours that nurses spend working with clients, they are in an ideal position to advocate on their clients' behalf and to lead multidisciplinary teams. They also are often in management positions in rehabilitation units, aged-care facilities and community services. Nurse-led services, including health promotion and awareness programs that encourage and support empowerment of people with chronic conditions such as those who have had a brain injury or are in chronic pain, have demonstrated effectiveness in reducing adverse health outcomes such as falls and further hospitalisations (Imhof et al., 2012; Shiu, Lee & Chau, 2012).

SUMMARY

Learning objective 1: Understand the impact of injuries on the health and wellbeing of communities.

There is an increasing trend in injury-related chronic illness and disability from: falls, transportation injuries, sporting and workplace accidents, and interpersonal violence. These can have long-term, lasting effects both economically and socially on individuals and communities. Many injuries can be prevented.

Learning objective 2: Identify the potential risk factors for falls.

Falls are a multifactorial risk including biological, behavioural, environmental and socio-economic factors. Risk reduction requires a holistic, multidisciplinary team approach in both community and in-patient scenarios.

Learning objective 3: Describe the main causes of transportation injuries.

Transportation injuries occur to car occupants, motorcyclists, bicycle riders and pedestrians. Many of these injuries result from speeding, fatigue, lack of seat belts and substance abuse where people do not adhere to safety recommendations.

Learning objective 4: Describe the signs, pathophysiology and long-term effects of an ABI.

An ABI is an injury to the brain due to a stroke, TBI, tumours or degenerative neurological diseases. Acquired brain injury affects every person differently and can result in physical and cognitive changes. The injured person's ability to recognise their own strengths and limitations is important so that nurses are able to provide the appropriate specialised care required in the community setting.

Learning objective 5: Outline the effects of interpersonal violence, including assault, and the effects of self-harm.

Interpersonal violence may result in acute injuries, and in the long term can increase the risk of substance use, eating disorders, depression and post-traumatic stress disorder.

Learning objective 6: Consider the impact of chronic pain on an individual that occurs as a result of injury.

Having chronic pain affects people's abilities to participate in normal activities of daily living. It may impact on a variety of aspects within a person's life, such as social relationships, or result in a loss of employment. People experiencing chronic pain have reported feelings of isolation, emotional distress and the stigma associated with having this chronic condition.

Learning objective 7: Understand the role of the nurse in injury prevention.

The nurse may have multiple roles, including health promotion, care coordination, case management, counselling and complex nursing assessments.

REVIEW QUESTIONS

1. What are the categories of risk of falls?
2. What factors are involved in the prevention of falls?
3. List some risk-reducing programs that target transport injuries that you are aware of.
4. What are the impacts of ABI on family members?

5. Which vulnerable populations are more likely to be victims of interpersonal violence?

6. What is the nurse's role in assisting a person to manage a chronic pain condition?

RESEARCH TOPIC

How is your role in caring for a patient with ABI different in the acute setting, the rehabilitation setting and in the community? What important considerations would you consider for your nursing care in each of these areas?

FURTHER READING

Alcohol Healthwatch. (2017). Why we need to change our drinking culture. Auckland: Alcohol Healthwatch Trust. Retrieved from www.ahw.org.nz/Portals/5/Resources/Documents-other/2017/Our%20Drinking%20Culture.pdf

Australian Institute of Health and Welfare (AIHW). (2017). Injury. Canberra: AIHW. Retrieved from www.aihw.gov.au/reports-data/health-conditions-disability-deaths/injury/about

NSW Agency For Clinical Innovations. (2015). Chronic pain toolkit for clinicians. Retrieved from www.aci.health.nsw.gov.au/chronic-pain/health-professionals

World Health Organization (WHO). (2007). *WHO Global Report on Falls Prevention in Older Age*. Geneva: WHO.

REFERENCES

Agency for Clinical Innovation. (2011). *Adult Trauma Clinical Practice Guidelines: Initial Management of Closed Head Injury in Adults*. Sydney: NSW Ministry of Health. Retrieved from www.aci.health.nsw.gov.au/__data/assets/pdf_file/0003/195150/Closed_Head_Injury_CPG_2nd_Ed_Full_document.pdf

Alcohol Healthwatch. (2012). *Alcohol, Injuries and Violence*. Auckland: Alcohol Healthwatch.

Australian Commission on Safety and Quality in Health Care (ACSQHC). (2012). *National Safety and Quality Health Service Standards (September 2012)*. Sydney: ACSQHC. Retrieved from www.safetyandquality.gov.au/wp-content/uploads/2011/09/NSQHS-Standards-Sept-2012.pdf

Australian Institute of Health and Welfare (AIHW). (2015a). Injury. Canberra: AIHW. Retrieved from www.aihw.gov.au/injury.

—— (2015b). *Patterns and Trends in Hospitalised Injury*. Canberra: AIHW. Retrieved from www.aihw.gov.au/injury/patterns-and-trends

—— (2018). *Family, Domestic and Sexual Violence in Australia, 2018*. Canberra: AIHW Retrieved from www.aihw.gov.au/reports/domestic-violence/family-domestic-sexual-violence-in-australia-2018/contents/summary

Australian Institute of Health and Welfare (AIHW) and Flinders University. (2015). *Trends in Injury Deaths, Australia, 1999–00 to 2009–10. Injury Research and Statistics Series No. 74*. Cat no. INJCAT 150. Canberra: AIHW.

——(2017). *Trends in Hospitalisations Due to Falls by Older People, Australia 2002–03 to 2012–13, Injury Research and Statistics Series No. 106. Cat. no. INJCAT 182.* Canberra: AIHW. Retrieved from www.aihw.gov.au/reports/injury/hospitalisations-falls-older-people-2002-2013/contents/table-of-contents

Australian Institute of Health and Welfare (AIHW), Pointer, S. & Kreisfeld, R. (2012). *Hospitalised Interpersonal Violence and Perpetrator Coding, Australia 2002–05. Injury Research and Statistics Series No. 77.* Cat. no. INJCAT 153. Canberra: AIHW.

Australian Nursing and Midwifery Federation (ANMF). (2016). *Child abuse and neglect: ANMF Position Statement.* Kingston, ACT: ANMF.

Barrie, J. & Loughlin, D. (2014). Managing chronic pain in adults. *Nursing Standard,* 29(7), 50–8.

Berecki-Gisolf, J., Collie, A. & McClure, R. (2013). Work disability after road traffic injury in a mixed population with and without hospitalisation. *Accident Analysis & Prevention,* 51, 129–34. doi: http://dx.doi.org/10.1016/j.aap.2012.11.010

Beynon, C. E., Gutmanis, I. A., Tutty, L. M., Wathen, C. N. & MacMillan, H. L. (2012). Why physicians and nurses ask (or don't) about partner violence: A qualitative analysis. *BMC Public Health,* 12(473). doi: http://10.1186/1471-2458-12-473

Booth, V., Logan, P., Harwood, R. & Hood, V. (2015). Falls prevention interventions in older adults with cognitive impairment: A systematic review of reviews. *International Journal of Therapy and Rehabilitation,* 22(6), 289–96.

Bradley, C. (2013). *Trends in Hospitalisations Due to Falls by Older People, Australia.* Canberra: AIHW.

Callaghan, P. & Waldock, H. (2012). *Emergencies in Mental Health Nursing.* Oxford: Oxford University Press.

Cancelliere, C., Cassidy, J. D., Côté, P., Hincapié, C. A., Hartvigsen, J., Carroll, L. J., ... & Keightley, M. (2012). Protocol for a systematic review of prognosis after mild traumatic brain injury: An update of the WHO Collaborating Centre Task Force findings. *Systematic Reviews,* 1 (17). doi: http://10.1186/2046-4053-1-17

Daniels, S. & Risser, R. (2014). Road safety in a globalised and more sustainable world: Current issues and future challenges. *Accident Analysis & Prevention,* 62, 329–30. doi: http://dx.doi.org/10.1016/j.aap.2013.10.004

Day, S., Fox, J., Majercik, S., Redmond, F. K., Pugh, M. & Bledsoe, J. (2015). Implementing a domestic violence screening program. *Journal of Trauma Nursing,* 22(3), 176–81.

Falster, M. O., Randall, D. A., Lujic, S., Ivers, R., Leyland, A. H. & Jorm, L. R. (2013). Disentangling the impacts of geography and Aboriginality on serious road transport injuries in New South Wales. *Accident Analysis & Prevention,* 54, 32–8. doi: http://dx.doi.org/10.1016/j.aap.2013.01.015

Feigin, V. L., Barker-Collo, S., Krishnamurthi, R., Theadom, A. & Starkey, N. (2010). Epidemiology of ischaemic stroke and traumatic brain injury. *Best Practice & Research Clinical Anaesthesiology,* 24(4), 485–94. doi: http://10.1016/j.bpa.2010.10.006

Galgano, M., Toshkezi, G., Qiu, X., Russell, T., Chin, L. & Zhao, L.-R. (2017). Traumatic brain injury: Current treatment strategies and future endeavors. *Cell Transplantation,* 26(7), 1118–30. doi: http://10.1177/0963689717714102

Green, S. M., Haukoos, J. S. & Schriger, D. L. (2017). How to measure the Glasgow Coma Scale. *Annals of Emergency Medicine,* 70(2), 158–60. doi: http://10.1016/j.annemergmed.2016.12.016

Haines, T. P., Hill, A.-M., Hill, K. D., McPhail, S., Oliver, D., Brauer, S., . . . & Beer, C. (2011). Patient education to prevent falls among older hospital inpatients: A randomized controlled trial. *Archives of Internal Medicine*, 171(6), 516–24.

Hill, A.-M., McPhail, S. M., Waldron, N., Etherton-Beer, C., Ingram, K., Flicker, L., . . . & Haines, T. P. (2015). Fall rates in hospital rehabilitation units after individualised patient and staff education programmes: A pragmatic, stepped-wedge, cluster-randomised controlled trial. *The Lancet*, 385(9987), 2592–9.

Imhof, L., Naef, R., Wallhagen, M. I., Schwarz, J. & Mahrer-Imhof, R. (2012). Effects of an advanced practice nurse in-home health consultation program for community-dwelling persons aged 80 and older. *Journal of the American Geriatrics Society*, 60(12), 2223–31. doi: http://10.1111/jgs.12026

Kawi, J. (2014). Chronic low back pain patients' perceptions on self-management, self-management support, and functional ability. *Pain Management Nursing*, 15(1), 258–64. doi: http://10.1016/j.pmn.2012.09.003

Kenny, R. A. M., Rubenstein, L. Z., Tinetti, M. E., Brewer, K., Cameron, K. A., Capezuti, E. A., . . . & Rockey, P. H. (2011). Summary of the updated American Geriatrics Society/British Geriatrics Society clinical practice guideline for prevention of falls in older persons. *Journal of the American Geriatrics Society*, 59(1), 148–57.

Kiadaliri, A. A., Turkiewicz, A. & Englund, M. (2018). Educational inequalities in falls mortality among older adults: Population-based multiple cause of death data from Sweden. *Journal of Epidemiology and Community Health*, 72(1), 68–70.

Layba, C., Griffin, L. W., Jupiter, D., Mathers, C. & Mileski, W. (2017). Adolescent motor vehicle crash prevention through a trauma center-based intervention program. *Journal of Trauma and Acute Care Surgery*, 83(5), 850–3.

Lee, Y. G., Kim, S. C., Chang, M., Nam, E., Kim, S. G., Cho, S.-i., . . . & Park, S.-B. (2018). Complications and socioeconomic costs associated with falls in the elderly population. *Annals of Rehabilitation Medicine*, 42(1), 120–9.

Ministry of Transport. (2014). Motor vehicle crashes in New Zealand 2014. Retrieved from www.transport.govt.nz/research/roadcrashstatistics/motorvehiclecrashesinnewzealand/motor-vehicle-crashes-in-new-zealand-2014

New Zealand Family Violence Clearinghouse. (2017). *Data summaries 2017: Snapshot*. Wellington: New Zealand Family Violence Clearinghouse Retrieved from https://nzfvc.org.nz/sites/nzfvc.org.nz/files/Data-summaries-snapshot-2017.pdf

New Zealand Ministry of Health (NZMOH). (2013). *Health Loss: A Report from the New Zealand Burden of Diseases, Injuries and Risk Factors Study 2006–2016*. Wellington: Ministry of Health.

New Zealand Ministry of Health (NZMOH) and Accident Compensation Corporation. (2013). *Injury-Related Health Loss: A Report from the New Zealand Burden of Diseases, Injuries and Risk Factors Study 2006–2016*. Wellington: Ministry of Health.

Newton, B. J., Southall, J. L., Raphael, J. H., Ashford, R. L. & LeMarchand, K. (2013). A narrative review of the impact of disbelief in chronic pain. *Pain Management Nursing*, 14(3), 161–71. doi: http://10.1016/j.pmn.2010.09.001

NSW Agency For Clinical Innovations. (2015). Chronic pain toolkit for clinicians. Retrieved from www.aci.health.nsw.gov.au/chronic-pain/health-professionals

NSW Government. (2012). *NSW Road Safety Strategy 2012–2021*. Sydney: State of NSW.

Parliament of Australia. (2011). Domestic violence in Australia – An overview of the issues. Retrieved from www.aph.gov.au/About_Parliament/Parliamentary_Departments/Parliamentary_Library/pubs/BN/2011-2012/DVAustralia

Paul, S. S., Harvey, L., Carroll, T., Li, Q., Boufous, S., Priddis, A., … & Muecke, S. (2017). Trends in fall-related ambulance use and hospitalisation among older adults in NSW, 2006–2013: A retrospective, population-based study. *Public Health Research and Practice*, 27(4), e27341701.

Poulos, R. G., Hatfield, J., Rissel, C., Flack, L. K., Murphy, S., Grzebieta, R. & McIntosh, A. S. (2015a). Characteristics, cycling patterns, and crash and injury experiences at baseline of a cohort of transport and recreational cyclists in New South Wales, Australia. *Accident Analysis & Prevention*, 78, 155–64. doi: http://dx.doi.org/10.1016/j.aap.2015.02.008

—— (2015b). An exposure based study of crash and injury rates in a cohort of transport and recreational cyclists in New South Wales, Australia. *Accident Analysis & Prevention*, 78, 29–38. doi: http://dx.doi.org/10.1016/j.aap.2015.02.009

Proffitt, C. & Beacham, M. (2012). *The New Zealand Injury Prevention Outcomes Report – June 2012*. Wellington: Accident Compensation Corporation.

Rodrigues, I. G., Fraga, G. P. & Barros, M. B. d. A. (2014). Falls among the elderly: Risk factors in a population-based study. *Revista Brasileira de Epidemiologia*, 17, 705–18.

Ruseckaite, R., Gabbe, B., Vogel, A. P. & Collie, A. (2012). Health care utilisation following hospitalisation for transport-related injury. *Injury*, 43(9), 1600–5. doi: http://dx.doi.org/10.1016/j.injury.2011.03.011

Ryu, E., Juhn, Y. J., Wheeler, P. H., Hathcock, M. A., Wi, C.-I., Olson, J. E., … & Takahashi, P. Y. (2017). Individual housing-based socioeconomic status predicts risk of accidental falls among adults. *Annals of Epidemiology*, 27(7), 415–20. e2.

Shiu, A. T. Y., Lee, D. T. F. & Chau, J. P. C. (2012). Exploring the scope of expanding advanced nursing practice in nurse-led clinics: A multiple-case study. *Journal of Advanced Nursing*, 68(8), 1780–92. doi: http://10.1111/j.1365-2648.2011.05868.x

Slomski, A. (2012). Falls from taking multiple medications may be a risk for both young and old. *Journal of the American Medical Association*, 307(11), 1127–8. doi: http://10.1001/jama.2012.290

Stevenson, M. & Thompson, J. (2014). On the road to prevention: Road injury and health promotion. *Health Promotion Journal of Australia*, 25(1), 4–7. doi: http://dx.doi.org/10.1071/HE13075

Transport for NSW. (2015). NSW Centre for Road Safety – Campaigns. Retrieved from http://roadsafety.transport.nsw.gov.au/campaigns

Valente, S. M. & Fisher, D. (2011). Traumatic brain injury. *The Journal for Nurse Practitioners*, 7(10), 863–70. doi: http://10.1016/j.nurpra.2011.09.016

Vos, P. E., Alekseenko, Y., Battistin, L., Ehler, E., Gerstenbrand, F., Muresanu, D. F., … & von Wild, K. (2012). Mild traumatic brain injury. *European Journal of Neurology*, 19(2), 191–8. doi: http://10.1111/j.1468-1331.2011.03581.x

World Health Organization (WHO). (2007). *WHO Global Report on Falls Prevention in Older Age*. Geneva: WHO.

—— (2015). *Falls Prevention in Older Age*. Geneva: WHO.

World Health Organization (WHO), Department of Reproductive Health and Research, London School of Hygiene and Tropical Medicine, South African Medical Research Council. (2013). *Global and Regional Estimates of Violence Against Women: Prevalence and Health Effects of Intimate Partner Violence and Non-Partner Sexual Violence*. Geneva: WHO.

Youd, J. (2013). Self-harm. *Nursing Standard*, 28(3), 16. doi: http://10.7748/ns2013.09.28.3.16.s25

10

Living with mental health issues

Rhonda Brown, Denise McGarry,
Kathryn Kent, Maureen Miles
and Michelle Francis

LEARNING OBJECTIVES

After studying this chapter, you should be able to:

1. understand the prevalence of mental health conditions in Australia and New Zealand
2. understand the impact of living with mental health distress for individuals, families, communities and societies
3. discuss the significance of attitudes and beliefs, and the impact of stigma on individuals living with mental health conditions, as well as the impact on their carers
4. describe the nurse's capacity to engage with individuals, carers and families affected by mental health issues, and to guide them to reach optimal health through reflective practice
5. discuss the significant features of recovery principles and the nurse's role within mental health care settings.

Introduction

Nurses are at the forefront of health care profession, and have a vital role in supporting individuals and their family in recovery, as well as restoring the mental health of those in their care to optimal levels. Regardless of their practice, be it in a hospital or community setting, nurses have opportunities every day to promote mental health and provide interventions to assist recovery, improve mental health and wellbeing, reduce risk and prevent future episodes of illness. This can be achieved through meaningful connection with individuals and families, initiating health promotion and education, and facilitating connections with others.

Mental health is one of the major health priorities in Australia and New Zealand (Australian Institute of Health and Welfare (AIHW), 2014; New Zealand Ministry of Health (NZMOH), 2014a). Mental health is a state of wellbeing in which an individual can reach their own potential and cope with the normal stressors of life (World Health Organization (WHO) and the Calouste Gulbenkian Foundation, 2014a). Mental health and wellbeing are influenced by individual characteristics or attributes, socioeconomic circumstances and the broader environment in which people live.

The use of language in mental health is readily recognised as challenging. Language is acknowledged to be significantly entwined with the transmission of culture and cultural beliefs and values. In this field, language can therefore be a source for the transmission of stereotyping, discrimination and stigma in a way that is pervasive and can be poorly recognised. Terms with mental health heritage are frequently used as pejoratives ('psycho' or 'schizo', for example). Expressions which have general agreement as appropriate are changing and opinion is divided as to which terms are acceptable. In this chapter, we adopt expressions used by authors or documents cited when contextually appropriate, but in all other contexts we honour person-centred care principles and human rights in the selection of the terms we use. However, given the variation in acceptability and changeability of terms, our selections may be disputed.

This chapter provides an overview of common mental health issues (depression, anxiety, substance misuse and abuse), as well as those within a spectrum of psychosis. The role of nurses in supporting individuals and families affected by, and living with, mental health issues is also discussed. For more in-depth discussion of mental health issues and treatment, we recommend reading a comprehensive and dedicated mental health text. There is an expectation that this chapter provides basic information. We hope that it inspires you to take a journey of exploration, discovery and reflection, and learn how you can make a difference through your nursing practice for people experiencing mental health issues, alongside taking care of your own mental health.

Mental disorder – a temporary condition involving irrational behaviour that can vary in severity and duration, and requires temporary care, treatment or control to protect the person

Mental health in Australia and New Zealand

Almost half of all Australians aged 16–85 will experience **mental disorder** at some time in their lives and 1 in 5 will experience **mental illness** in any given year (AIHW, 2014). Anxiety disorders are the most commonly diagnosed mental illness affecting 1 in 7 (14.4 per cent) Australians aged between 16–85, followed by mood disorders,

Mental illness – a range of mental health conditions, which can be either temporary or permanent, that affect mood, thinking and behaviour; and cause serious impairment.

which affect 1 in 16 (6.2 per cent), and substance misuse and abuse disorders affecting 1 in 20 (5.1 per cent) (Slade et al., 2009). Similarly, in New Zealand, 1 in 6 people have a lifetime diagnosis of a common mental illness with high-prevalence conditions, including 1 in 6 experiencing depression (16.7 per cent), 1 in 8 experiencing anxiety (10.3 per cent) and 1 in 5 using hazardous alcohol consumption (19.5%) (NZMOH, 2018). Women are more likely to experience high-prevalence conditions in their mid-30–40s and men in their mid-40–50s (NZMOH, 2014b).

Less prevalent are psychotic disorders, which affect approximately 1 in 500 Australians (AIHW, 2018). Despite the lower prevalence, psychotic illness accounts for a third of individuals living with a severe mental illness (Morgan et al., 2011), and has one of the highest costs to the community including health care and lost productivity (Morgan et al., 2011; Tandon, Nasrallah & Keshavan, 2009).

Overall, mental disorders account for 13 per cent of the total disease burden (healthy life years lost) in Australia, which is fourth behind cancer (16 per cent), musculoskeletal disorders (15 per cent) and cardiovascular disease (14 per cent) (AIHW, 2012). In 2007, one-third of Australians (34.9 per cent) with a mental disorder had used services for a mental health problem in the previous 12 months, with women more likely than men to access services (40.7 per cent compared to 27.5 per cent) (AIHW, 2016). Those with depression were more likely to access services than those with anxiety or substance-use disorders (Slade et al., 2009). Individuals living with chronic mental illnesses are also more likely to experience physical comorbidities, with 1 in 9 Australians (13 per cent) having both a mental disorder and physical condition concurrently; the most common being anxiety with a physical condition (AIHW, 2012).

Childhood and adolescence are important formative times for mental health. Experiences of unsupported poor mental health may lead to disruptions in education, peer relationships, relationship development difficulties, loss of support networks, employment opportunities and an inability to participate in life opportunities. Australian parents, carers and young people reported that 13.9 per cent of those aged 4–17 years had experienced a mental health disorder in the 12 months prior to being surveyed (Lawrence et al., 2015). The most commonly experienced conditions in those aged 5–14 years were anxiety (10 per cent), depression (7 per cent) and conduct disorders (5.8 per cent). For those aged 15–24 years, the most commonly experienced conditions were suicide and self-inflicted injuries (8.4 per cent), anxiety (7.5 per cent) and depression (16.3 per cent), with males at a higher risk than females (16.3 versus 11.5 per cent) (Lawrence et al., 2015). In addition, 14.8 per cent of young people aged 4–17 years and 86.6 per cent of people who had experienced a severe disorder, had accessed health services in the previous 12 months (Lawrence et al., 2015).

In a New Zealand study of 1388 secondary school students, 19 per cent reported having experienced depression and 17 per cent reported having anxiety (Fernando et al. 2013). Young Māori and Pacific Islander peoples have an increased risk (Crengle et al., 2013), with 21 per cent having accessed mental health services (Malatest International, 2016). Young Māori peoples, aged 0–24 years, who had been hospitalised, were more likely to be diagnosed with disorders within the psychosis spectrum and mood disorders, while non-Māori young New Zealanders were more likely to be diagnosed with mood disorders, substance abuse and eating disorders (Simpson et al., 2017).

Both Australia and New Zealand have struggled to address the mental health gap between Indigenous and non-Indigenous populations. Limited access to affordable services is not a new problem and has often been cited as a major issue for Indigenous populations; however, it appears that more Māori people are accessing culturally sensitive services (NZMOH, 2014b). In Australia, mental health workers who identify as Aboriginal or as a Torres Strait Islander provide a vital role in addressing the specific mental health issues of their peoples, including culturally safe care (Jorm et al., 2009).

Understanding mental illness
Anxiety

Nurses are likely to encounter individuals exhibiting varying levels of anxiety and anxious responses to a variety of situations, including receiving care or during hospitalisation (Buchanan-Barker, 2009). A common experience of anxiety can be characterised by apprehension caused by fear from a threat, with nervous or anxious feelings stemming from being in new and unfamiliar situations. Symptoms of anxiety include rapid heart rate and breathing, muscle tension, a dry mouth, difficulty swallowing, sweating, nausea and diarrhoea, with symptoms ranging in intensity and frequency. Some people have sudden onsets of these feelings and sensations, resulting in severe and uncontrolled anxiety or panic attacks. During these episodes, palpitations, chest pain, sweating, shaking, a choking sensation, weakness and tingling of the hands and feet, fear of losing control, and/or fear of death can be experienced. Anxiety can also result in sleep disturbance, difficulty concentrating and a need for constant reassurance, especially when faced with change or going into new situations (Labott, 2019).

Depression

Depression can be a serious mental illness and can affect an individual at any stage of their life. Symptoms include: low and irritable mood; lack of energy; tiredness; sleep disturbance; loss of interest or pleasure; unexpected weight loss or weight gain; poor appetite; poor concentration; feelings of guilt, hopelessness and low self-esteem; and social withdrawal. It is important to note that having one or two of these symptoms does not necessarily mean that a person has depression disorder. Rather, depression disorder is characterised by the persistence of these feelings and symptoms over weeks, months or even years, and the symptoms significantly interfere with a person's ability to undertake day-to-day activities and responsibilities at home, school or work, and can lead to suicidal thoughts and behaviour (Lam, 2018).

Substance misuse and abuse

Substance misuse and abuse describes a person's use of legal and illegal substances at harmful levels, which affects their physical and mental health. It includes the

Hallucinations – sensory perceptions experienced in the absence of recognisable stimuli. Hallucinations may affect any sense and are experienced as real perceptions by the affected individual. Hallucinations are distinct from illusions and dreaming, which are associated with changes in an individual's level of consciousness.

Delusion – a false, fixed belief that is incongruent with the individual's education and cultural background. It is distinct from a belief that is based on incomplete or inaccurate knowledge.

Disorganised thinking (speech) – refers to the form in which thinking occurs that affects speech. The usual pattern of speech is disrupted in a variety of ways and in differing degrees of severity. Examples include poverty of speech, circumstantiality, tangentiality, clanging associations, blocking and echolalia.

Grossly disorganised or abnormal motor behaviour – seen in many psychotic disorders and includes, for example, slowing (lethargy) or accelerating (agitation) of motor activity, unusual poses (stereotypy), or tics or mutism.

Negative symptoms – a decrease in or loss of normal functioning such as reduced emotional expression and responsiveness, decreased ability to initiate activities, lowered motivation or drive, inability to feel pleasure, lack of spontaneity and reduced interest in other people.

misuse of prescribed and over-the-counter medications. A substance is a psychoactive material that is used to bring about a particular effect on the central nervous system. Psychoactive substances include licit (legal) substances, such as caffeine, nicotine and alcohol, and illicit (illegal) substances, such as cannabis, speed and heroin. These substances are categorised as stimulants, depressants or hallucinogens (see Table 10.1).

Table 10.1 Commonly misused substances

Stimulants	Depressants	Hallucinogens
• Amphetamine (e.g. speed) • Methamphetamine (e.g. ice) • Ecstasy • Cocaine • Nicotine • Caffeine • Ephedrine (Sudafed) • Cocaine	• Alcohol • Solvents • Barbiturates • Benzodiazepines • Opiates and opioids, including heroin, opium, morphine, codeine and methadone Cannabis – marijuana, hashish, hash oil • Sedatives and hypnotics, including Valium and Rohypnol • Some solvents and inhalants – petrol, glue, lighter fluids and paint thinners	• LSD (lysergic acid diethylamide) • Hallucinogenic (magic) mushrooms • Mescaline – naturally occurring psychedelic found in several cacti • Cannabis – may have hallucinogenic effects as well as depressant effects

The recurrent pattern of substance misuse and abuse causes significant impairment, including an inability to function, perform and attend to responsibilities at home, school or work. This inability to fully function can range from mild, moderate or severe, and can lead to substantial physical, emotional, psychological and interpersonal problems. The most commonly misused and abused substance in Australian and New Zealand is alcohol, with 78.2 per cent of people over the age of 14 years using alcohol and 17.2 per cent doing so at risky levels (that is, two or more standard drinks per day) (AIHW, 2014; Inter-Agency Committee on Drugs New Zealand, 2015).

Psychosis

Psychotic illnesses are conditions with varying symptoms, each with an individual clinical presentation, making diagnosis and treatment difficult. Psychotic illnesses are defined as abnormalities in one or more of five areas: **hallucinations, delusions, disorganised thinking (speech), grossly disorganised or abnormal motor behaviour** and **negative symptoms**. Negative symptoms, in particular, are often less evident than positive symptoms, making them more easily overlooked and more difficult to address. They may have a significant impact on a person's quality of life and capacity to recover (American Psychiatric Association, 2013, p. 87).

People experiencing psychotic illnesses may exhibit disturbances in thinking, perception, emotional responses and behaviour (Morgan et al., 2011). The DSM-5 (American Psychiatric Association, 2013) categorises a broad spectrum of psychotic illnesses, with the most common being **schizophrenia, bipolar disorder, schizo-affective disorder, schizotypal (personality) disorder, brief psychotic disorder** and **schizophreniform disorder.** Age of onset is in the late teens to early adulthood, with males (3.7 cases per 1000) experiencing earlier and more frequent episodes than females (2.4 cases per 1000). Early onset disrupts a person's development of critical life skills, education, employment and relationships (Morgan et al., 2011).

Contributing factors to mental illness

The variability and complexity of mental illness makes it difficult to be certain of the cause, which to a large extent is still unknown and requires further research. For example, while the cause of depression is unclear, some people are at higher risk because of genetic, psychological, personality, social or environmental stressors such as war, natural disasters and drought (Royal Australian and New Zealand College of Psychiatrists, 2018).

There have been no biomarkers established in psychotic disorders, and the role of neurotransmitters; such as dopamine, glutamate, gamma-amino buteric acid, serotonin and others; remains unclear with no causality yet shown (Keshavan, Nasrallah & Tandon, 2011). Genetic factors have been linked with the development of psychotic illness, but it is likely that the interaction between inherited risks and environmental factors triggers psychosis in adolescents and young people (Schlosser et al., 2012). Environmental factors such as the person's birth month being in late winter or early spring, pregnancy and birth complications, urban living, social determinants, stress, and migration have also been found to play important roles in the pathophysiology of psychotic illness (Schlosser et al., 2012).

Social determinants

Many factors are likely to play a part in the causation of mental health problems. Prominent factors are those referred to as social determinants such as the culture, social class and physical environment in which a person lives. Such risk factors can be present throughout a person's life and are especially significant in childhood and adolescence. Generally speaking, communities experiencing high social inequality have a high level of mental health risk factors (WHO and the Calouste Gulbenkian Foundation, 2014a). People living in rural and remote areas of Australia experience a higher level of mental ill health, especially depression (Johnson & Ragusa, 2014). Substance use, misuse and abuse may also lead to, or result from, depression. The role of illicit drug use in the development of psychotic disorders is contested, with studies of cannabis and amphetamine yet to clearly explain a causal link, in spite of well-established comorbidities (Miles et al., 2003; Proal et al., 2014). The implications of this are that treatment for those living with mental health conditions, which has in the past been focused on the individual, now also needs to be cognisant of

Schizophrenia – the experience of changes in thinking, social interactions, motivation and emotional expression that severely disrupts a person's life and may be long-lasting. Diagnosis is based on observation and self-reporting.

Bipolar disorder – an experience of a psychotic nature characterised by disturbances in mood. These take the form of alterations in emotional state unrelated to circumstances, which may switch from mania or euphoria to depression. At times neither may be experienced, and the individual will return to a normal emotional range between periods of mania or depression.

Schizoaffective disorder – characterised by features of both schizophrenia and mood disorders, with difficulties in thinking and emotional regulation.

Schizotypal (personality) disorder – refers to a way of interacting with the world that exhibits distortions in thinking resulting from misinterpretation of the world. It is frequently characterised by social anxiety, unusual behaviours and beliefs. Speech and dress may also show unusual properties.

Brief psychotic disorder – a short period of illness with psychotic symptoms such as delusions or hallucinations.

Schizophreniform disorder – refers to an experience that has the characteristics of schizophrenia but is distinguished from it by less severe symptoms and a duration typically of longer than a month but less than the six months required for a diagnosis of schizophrenia.

Social capital – a sociological concept that refers to the expected benefits, either collective or economic, that result from cooperative endeavours or preferential treatment between individuals and groups.

factors such as social capital, social isolation and social connection (WHO and the Calouste Gulbenkian Foundation, 2014b).

REFLECTION

The experiences of people diagnosed with psychotic mental health problems present multiple challenges, including complex, coexisting conditions. Consider how problems of a social nature contribute to the 'burden of disease' for people diagnosed with schizophrenia. What services are available in your local area to support people living with schizophrenia?

Traumatic experiences across the lifespan have also been recognised as contributing to the development of mental health issues. Abusive relationships in childhood or adulthood, including sexual, emotional, physical and/or psychological abuses, have all been implicated in the development of mental illness. Around 70 per cent of people seeking help from in-patient mental health services are recognised as having experienced trauma (Floen & Elklit, 2007). Experiences of social disruption, such as those witnessed in war or natural disasters, may also play a part. Trauma may be a single experience, or an ongoing trauma of significant duration such as in war (Bateman, Henderson & Kezelman, 2013).

Family, friendship and relationship difficulties can also contribute to anxiety and depression. Other factors are significant life events, such as a serious accident or work-related injury, or the development of a chronic health condition. Comorbidity of depression with a physical illness can make it difficult to recognise and diagnose depression, because some somatic symptoms of depression or anxiety may also be related to the physical illness (Olver & Hopwood, 2012). Physical illness is often associated with losses, resulting in feelings of sadness, worry and irritability which, while understandable (Olver & Hopwood, 2012), may mean depression is overlooked. It is therefore important for nurses to be particularly mindful of the presence of psychological symptoms that may be indicative of depression.

SKILLS IN PRACTICE

Comorbidity of depression with a physical illness

Joe is a 34-year-old man who lives at home with his wife Julia. They have one child, Ben, who is six months old. Joe is a successful sales representative and is often required to travel interstate. He works long hours and reports that he is missing out on important developmental milestones for Ben. Julia is an accountant and has not worked since the birth of their son. She is looking to return to work in the next few months and has asked Joe to spend more time at home. Joe and Julia are very supportive of each other in terms of their roles as parents and their careers. They live in an inner metropolitan area where housing prices and the cost of living are high.

While Joe can see the benefit in Julia returning to work both for herself and for the family, he is constantly worried about how he will be able to juggle his demands at work and at home.

Joe has no support from his parents and two siblings, and Julia's family live overseas. Due to his work and family commitments, he has limited interactions with his social supports. He has reported that his mother and father are heavy drinkers. His father has been treated for alcohol dependence in the past.

Since the birth of Ben, Joe has been experiencing low moods and anxiety about his ability to parent and provide for his family. Not long after the birth of Ben, Joe started to experience problems with sleeping, fatigue, sweating, loss of appetite and is complaining of stomach pains. He has been increasingly irritable and distressed, and has started to have the occasional drink after work to wind down after the day and cope with the new pressures of home life. This has increased, and he is now drinking eight to nine standard drinks per night. Joe reports that the only time during the day when he does not experience anxiety is when he is drinking. Julia is worried about Joe and has pointed out that he seems 'down', has less energy, and is starting to disconnect from her and Ben. Joe is insightful about this and is terrified that he is following in the same footsteps as his father.

QUESTIONS

1. What may be the contributing factors to Joe's anxiety and drinking? How do you think drinking and anxiety are related for Joe?
2. What are the protective factors and strengths for Joe and his supports?
3. What resources and support are available for Joe and Julia?

Impact of mental illness

Most people describe themselves as feeling stressed, anxious or depressed from time to time, but for some these feelings are persistent, impacting on their capacity to participate fully in life, and affecting their relationships and connections with others. Persistent anxiety or depression can result in a withdrawal from family and friends; being less productive in, or taking time away from, school and work; and generally impacting on a person's quality of life. Severe depression is also associated with self-harm and suicide. Some individuals resort to the use of alcohol and other drugs to deal with stressors and the symptoms of mental illness, which results in a high rate of comorbidity with substance abuse disorders (Lai et al., 2015; Miles et al., 2003). Substance misuse and abuse: interferes with the capacity to function effectively in daily activities; impacts on relationships with family, friends and social networks; and can lead to significant physical health problems, financial difficulties and legal problems or convictions. Substance misuse and abuse can also lead to dependency, where increasing levels of the substance are needed to achieve the same effect (Happell, Cowin & Roper, 2013).

Individuals living with a psychotic condition are at greater risk of experiencing poorer physical health than the general population and, as a result, have a reduced life expectancy of 15 to 25 years compared to the general population. Side effects from medication, chronic conditions such as heart disease, obesity and smoking, as well as drug and alcohol use, are among the leading risk factors for poorer physical health (Galletly et al., 2012; Morgan et al., 2011). Individuals living with a psychotic disorder are also at greater risk of suicide and self-harm (Morgan et al., 2011).

Mental health and stigma

Stigma is defined as negative attitudes and judgements that view an individual or group as having undesirable characteristics and personal traits, which need to be avoided (Clement et al., 2015). Labels such as 'mental disorders' and 'mental dysfunction' are common terms under the banner of mental illness, but have the potential to socially disempower rather than empower the individual (Hungerford & Kench, 2013). Misperceptions about mental ill health can result in stigmatisation, discrimination and prejudice (Corrigan, Druss & Perlick, 2014; Kopera et al., 2015). This is often challenging and has devastating consequences for those recovering from mental ill health. The most serious of these misrepresentations of people living with mental illness is that they are strange, dangerous and violent.

The experiences of stigma for individuals can include loss of self-esteem and distress, isolation from family and social supports, loss of employment or even homelessness. These negative attitudes towards mental ill health can be further internalised, leading to isolation and social exclusion, and dissuade people from seeking help (Clement et al., 2015).

Stigma can also come from health professionals with a poor understanding of mental health, and negative attitudes towards people experiencing mental health issues. Nurses need to be aware of their own attitudes, beliefs and understanding of mental health and challenge misunderstandings and assumptions in themselves and others. Understanding stigma and the effects of stigma is essential to improve the experience of care seeking and engagement in treatment (Corrigan et al. 2014).

> ## REFLECTION
>
> A friend discloses to you that they have recently been discharged from hospital where they were treated for severe depression. What do you think your friend might be experiencing at this time? How will you react and what will you say the next time you see them? Consider how the diagnosis of a mental illness might differ from a diagnosis of a physical illness.

Recovering from mental health distress

Historically, mental health care has been dominated by medical treatments including pharmacological interventions and a focus on curative interventions. Increasingly, however, there has been a shift to an emphasis on recovery in mental health policy and practice in both Australia and New Zealand (Commonwealth of Australia, 2013; O'Hagan, Reynolds & Smith, (2012). The notion of recovery is not new to mental health care (Buchanan-Barker, 2009), but recovery frameworks are now guiding practice and interventions from the first point of contact with the health system. Recovery is focused on living well whether or not in the presence or absence of a mental illness (Mental Health Advocacy Coalition, 2008). Recovery and living well is defined by the individual as being whatever gives meaning to their life. It is about individuals and families having strategies they can incorporate into their everyday lives to manage stress and anxiety. These strategies include having positive and supportive relationships with family, friends and work colleagues; and having a sense of inclusion and the ability to participate meaningfully in family, school, community and work. Recovery is also about having opportunities for personal growth, self-determination, finding new meaning and purpose, and being free to express one's culture, spiritual beliefs, gender and sexuality (Buchanan-Barker, 2009).

The goal of mental health care is to help individuals and families develop strategies for daily activities to deal with stress and manage symptoms. Interventions should be focused on factors important to mental health and wellbeing, including:

- social inclusion and connectedness
- feeling safe
- building resilience
- increasing sense of empowerment – self-determination/agency/responsibility
- sense of wellbeing
- self-esteem and self-worth
- optimism
- hope
- sense of wellness
- meaningful participation in life family/community/school/work – regaining meaning and purpose.

People experiencing mental health issues have individual needs. Nursing approaches should be collaborative, and build upon existing strengths and preferences of these individuals. It is difficult to be detailed and specific about such approaches simultaneously and recognise the individuality of those involved. However, there are a number of principles that can be helpful to bear in mind, and may ensure that nursing practice attains person-centred and strengths-based standards. This aligns with the micro level of the Innovative Care for Chronic Conditions Framework (ICCCF).

Promoting health and reducing risk

Promoting health and harm minimisation for people with substance-use disorder diagnoses can be achieved through supporting their healthy lifestyles to minimise the risk of them developing metabolic syndrome if prescribed psychotropic medications. This can mean a range of different approaches from formal to informal. Nurses' clinical practice may include group education sessions – perhaps for, or including, carers. Sessions might address distinct areas of concern, like mental health legislation or psychotropic medication. Sometimes it is more effective to support and empower the person to access their own knowledge or skills, and to help them recognise and address knowledge gaps. Peer-support workers can be an excellent guide and resource here as well as in other areas of nursing practice (Department of Health and Human Services, Victoria, 2016).

Collaborating care

Collaboration is an important nursing strategy – not only with the person experiencing mental health problems in a therapeutic relationship, but with a range of others, including carers. It is legally required in many jurisdictions that those identified as carers (not necessarily equivalent to next of kin) be consulted and informed about a person's treatment. Carers have much to contribute, given their experience of living with mental illness. Carers provide valuable insight and understanding of the pattern of symptoms and care needs (Olasoji, Maude & McCauley, 2017).

Collaboration with peers is an important strategy available for nurses to ensure that they achieve comprehensive person-centred care. Peers can make critical and unique contributions that are more attuned to support a person's care as they have shared, lived experiences of mental health problems and mental health service use.

Additionally, collaboration across a broad range of other disciplines and professions may be more prominent than in some other areas of nursing practice. The nurse is vital in enabling access to a range of allied health and multidisciplinary health workers; for example, speech pathologists may provide valuable support about swallowing difficulties arising as an adverse effect of psychotropic medications; exercise physiologists may help people individualise their approaches to minimise metabolic syndrome risk; dietitians may assist people with a range of challenges involved in eating disorders. Non-government organisations include groups providing housing services or job support. Non-government organisations also increasingly provide a range of services traditionally delivered as health clinical services, such as counselling or psychotherapy (Morgan et al., 2011).

Screening and assessment

Screening and assessment are central to all fields of nursing practice. They begin at the first point of engagement and continue throughout the care process. Individuals and their families can also learn to recognise and assess early warning signs and symptoms of mental health problems so that they are able to act, seek help early and implement strategies to manage symptoms.

Assessment is used, not only to identify needs and plan care, but also to evaluate the effectiveness of the care and strategies being implemented. Assessment should be a collaborative process where the individual and their family are engaged and involved in decisions about their care. In a comprehensive mental health assessment, the nurse is interested in what the client is doing (behaviour and actions), what is going on around them (at home and at work or school), what is going on inside (feelings and thoughts), the influence others are having (family, friends, social networks, work colleagues) and about their physical health. Learning about what strategies the client and their family have tried, what has worked in the past ('resilience'), their aspirations and goals, and their expectations of care, can also be useful. A comprehensive assessment should include:

- physical assessment
- risk assessment
- mental status examination
- substance use, misuse and abuse assessment

- family and relationship history
- social history
- developmental history
- psychiatric history
- medical history
- social history
- legal history
- review of major life events (for example, losses, transitions and changes) and responses, coping, recovery and resilience.

There are a number of screening and assessment tools specifically designed to assess depression, anxiety, and substance misuse and abuse, and these can be used in practice. The Depression and Anxiety Scale (DASS) and the Alcohol Use Disorders Identification Test (AUDIT) are two examples. Health of the Nation Outcome Scale (HoNOS) is a tool designed for use with people who have been diagnosed with severe mental illness; it measures health and social functioning. While the interpretation of these tools requires a degree of expertise and skill, they are useful for initial assessment, monitoring and evaluating progress. They can also be useful as self-assessment tools for individuals to use themselves.

More contentious, but critical, is the responsibility that nurses contribute to risk assessment. Risk is a broad concept and has a significant effect on the liberty of individuals because it commonly determines the application of legal sanctions, such as, for example, the NSW *Mental Health Act 2007*. The concept of risk is broad; its application in this context can sometimes be narrowed to the risk of suicide or homicide. Other aspects of risk that should be assessed by nurses are included in Table 10.2.

Table 10.2 Aspects of risk

Type of risk	Examples

Risk to self	• Self-harm and suicide, including repetitive self-injury
	• Self-neglect
	• Absconding and wandering (which may also be a risk to others)
	• Health, including:
	  – drug and alcohol use
	  – medical conditions; for example, alcohol withdrawal, unstable diabetes mellitus, delirium, organic brain injury and epilepsy
	• Quality of life including dignity, reputation, social and financial status

Risk to others	• Harassment • Stalking or predatory intent • Violence and aggression, including sexual assault or abuse • Property damage including arson • Public nuisance • Reckless behaviour that endangers others; for example, drink driving
Risk by others	• Physical, sexual or emotional harm or abuse by others • Social or financial abuse or neglect by others

Source: Mental Health Division, WA Department of Health (2008), p. 8

Risk can change rapidly in the nurse—client relationship and this characteristic limits the application of structured tools for assessing it (Large et al., 2016; Ribeiro et al., 2016; Singh et al., 2014). This feature reinforces the critical importance of establishing and maintaining a therapeutic relationship, both as an aid to assessment and as a measure to ameliorate against risk.

Resilience and protective factors refer to components of an individual's life circumstances that should also be assessed by nurses. These concepts refer to factors that enable individuals to withstand risk. They include factors such as social connectedness, a robust belief system (religious or other), strengths in emotion regulation, meaning-making and practising forgiveness (Banyard, Hamby & Grych, 2017). They can also be appreciated as being person-centred and supporting hope in recovery.

SKILLS IN PRACTICE

Revisiting Joe's story

Recall Joe, who you met earlier in the chapter: He presents to the emergency department accompanied by his partner, Julia, and their six-month-old son, Ben. Joe has a significant laceration to his head that he sustained at home after falling from a ladder and hitting his head (while trying to change a light bulb after having had a few drinks). Julia expresses how worried she had been about his moods lately and about his drinking. Joe's injury is assessed, his laceration is sutured and his wound dressed. He is medically cleared and is ready to go home. He appears distressed and tearful, and tells you that Julie and Ben would be better off without him. While Joe recognises something is wrong, he does not know what to do about it.

QUESTIONS

1. As the nurse caring for Joe, what would be your next step be before Joe goes home? What is your role and what are your responsibilities?

2. What are some of the factors that may get in the way of establishing a therapeutic relationship with Joe?

3. What personal attitudes, beliefs or experiences might affect or interfere with you developing a therapeutic relationship with Joe?

Recovery principles and the role of the nurse

Appreciating the diversity of needs and issues associated with mental health problems makes it clear that the skills required from a nurse in practice in this area may be different than in other clinical fields. Procedural approaches that have benefitted many people with health needs are perhaps less suited to meeting the requirements for those experiencing mental health problems. The advantages of generalising symptoms to guide practice and ensure a comprehensive coverage of health needs is less certain. This general model of nursing care is based on assumptions of uniformity and predictability that complex health experiences challenge. This is true also for mental health problems.

Mental health problems have been acknowledged in this chapter to range in complexity. Diagnosis may be contested, and the lived experience of mental health problems may be less responsive to medical model frameworks. The realisation that mental health problems both coexist with other health problems (for example, cardiac illness), including other mental health diagnoses (for example, anxiety, depression and substance use disorders), and may result in iatrogenic health problems (for example, metabolic syndrome and psychoses), challenges nurses to organise their strategies to meet the needs of people experiencing mental health problems in their clinical practice.

Insights from the 'recovery movement' provide some approaches. These have been adopted by both government and professional association standards of practice (Australian College of Mental Health Nurses, 2018). Essentially the recovery-orientated approach to clinical practice is based on person-centred care principles.

The Australian Health Ministers' Advisory Council and National Mental Health Strategy (2013) offer guidelines that are mandatory for clinical practice with people experiencing mental health problems. These are organised into what are termed 'Domains'. The principle domain, and the one which provides the underlying framework for the entire strategy, is 'Domain 1: Promoting a Culture and Language of Hope and Optimism' (Australian Health Ministers' Advisory Council and National Mental Health Strategy 2013, p. 12). This initial domain encompasses the four others, which are:

- Domain 2. Person first and holistic
- Domain 3. Supporting personal recovery
- Domain 4. Organisational commitment and workforce development
- Domain 5. Action on social inclusion and the social determinants of health, mental health and wellbeing.

Clearly, however, there are many challenges to implementing such practice guidelines in the field, especially when people may be experiencing extreme distress and disorganisation. The requirement that health care workers, like nurses, balance a range of other service and practice imperatives is recognised. These might include minimising risk and maintaining safety, and efficient delivery of services. The recovery guidelines (Australian Health Ministers' Advisory Council and National Mental Health Strategy 2013, p. 3) nominate the following as representing particular challenges:

- the offering of choice
- support of risk taking
- the dignity of risk
- medico-legal requirements
- duty of care
- promoting safety.

As Slade (2009, pp. 176–9) has clearly argued, the capacity to balance risk in a complex and changing environment that may regard risk as unacceptable to services is difficult to reconcile.

A further important understanding that is essential in guiding nursing practice is the recognition of the pervasiveness of the experience of trauma among those who have mental health problems. Previous experiences of trauma may not only be implicated in mental health problems, but may be further complicated by re-traumatising features of mental health practice (Floen & Elklit, 2007). Rather than indicating a necessity for establishing the detail of any pre-existing trauma experiences (which is addressed in focused therapy), these understandings about the prevalence of trauma necessitates nursing practice that does not re-traumatise. This practice, termed trauma-informed care and practice, is synergetic with recovery-orientated practice and emphasises the following features: safety, trustworthiness, choice, collaboration and empowerment (Kezelman & Stavropoulos, 2012).

Individuals working in mental health services are advised that their self-care strategies should therefore include addressing the high possibility of exposure to vicarious trauma or, on occasion, secondary trauma. The usual strategies for self-care − including attention to personal health, exercise, sleep, healthy eating, and vital social interests and relationships − has additional importance in this practice context. The additional benefits of a routine clinical supervision is also clear as a confidential forum to examine personal clinical practice. This allows space for reflection and feedback, and also for building resilience and gaining confidence in working with people with mental health issues (Rees et al., 2015).

Day-to-day the implications for clinical practice for nurses working with people experiencing mental health problems centres on the primacy of therapeutic communication aimed at establishing a therapeutic alliance. The point of this alliance is to support the person in understanding their recovery aims with or without continuing experience of mental health symptoms. Maintaining hope and optimism, while supporting the development of new paradigms for life that may incorporate mental health problems but also include a broad range of other elements (the person as friend, student and parent), is helpful. The challenge is to ensure that the support is flexible and responds to the changing capacity of the individual, resulting from their current experiences from distress.

Establishing a therapeutic relationship has been noted to be built on therapeutic communication. The features of this are not foreign to other fields of clinical practice. They incorporate respectful attention to the person's desires and preferences. This requires provision of time and giving value to developing circumstances to communicate. Privacy and confidentiality should be respected. A safety precaution would be to advise other team members of your physical location and expected time of return. This avoids any potential misunderstandings that may be compromising and reduces any risk to staff.

Listening is central to therapeutic communication. This can be challenging as it can seem similar but contrasts with the norms of ordinary social communication. The nurse−client relationship is not a friendship where equal exchange of confidences and knowledge of a personal nature occurs. Rather this is a professional relationship that is person-centred. Not only can this be tricky for a nurse to establish, at times the person experiencing mental health problems also expects the norms of ordinary social interactions to hold. The nurse needs to be skilful not to default to these familiar ways of communication, but runs the risk of offence as failure to share personal confidences sometimes limits the growth and closeness of a trusting relationship. However, genuine and authentic communication, which includes professional boundaries, is crucial (Dziopa & Ahern, 2009; Galon & Graor, 2012).

From time to time, nurses can feel overwhelmed when listening to the stress and distress of others; while it is important to learn to sit with this discomfort, nurses need support. This is a particular strength of clinical supervision of professional practice. While self-reflection is important, self-awareness is also enhanced through clinical supervision and debriefing where nurses not only have space to deal with their own personal issues, but also to learn new skills and address issues related to professional boundaries (Gerland & Gerland, 2012). This allows space for reflection and feedback, and also for building resilience and gaining confidence in working with people with mental illness (Rees et al., 2015). Reflective practice involves exploring and critiquing one's actions, thoughts and experiences as a process of continuous learning, developing practice and enhancing clinical knowledge (Caldwell & Grobbel, 2013).

SUMMARY

Learning objective 1: Understand the prevalence of mental health conditions in Australia and New Zealand.

An overview of the prevalence of the most common mental health conditions in Australia and New Zealand indicates that it affects a large percentage of the population. Both countries identify mental health as a health priority, with a range of initiatives being employed to reduce the impact of mental health issues on their populations. Nurses are identified as one the key agents for early detection, identification, mental health promotion and referral.

Learning objective 2: Understand the impact of living with mental health distress for individuals, families, communities and societies.

The impact of living with mental health distress are complex and can be socially isolating. The importance of the person's ability to engage with everyday activities; such as social inclusion and connectedness, feeling safe and building resilience; are important to their recovery. The impact to community and society is significant, given the high prevalence of mental health distress, including loss of productivity and high financial costs of providing ongoing support, care and services.

Learning objective 3: Discuss the significance of attitudes and beliefs, and the impact of stigma on individuals living with mental health conditions, as well as the impact on their carers.

Some of the challenges faced by individuals with mental health conditions include stigmatisation, discrimination and prejudice. The impact that negative attitudes and beliefs from the community, family, carers and health care providers can have on a person's recovery and maintenance can be significant in the care for the individual. Understanding and knowledge go a long way to improving the experience of individuals and families living with mental health distress.

Learning objective 4: Describe the nurse's capacity to engage with individuals, carers and families affected by mental issues, and to guide them to reach optimal health through reflective practice.

Person-centred care, reflective practice, therapeutic relationships and engagement are basic concepts for working with individuals experiencing mental health issues.

Learning objective 5: Discuss the significant features of recovery principles and the nurse's role within mental health care settings.

Caring and sensitive practice, based on trauma-informed and recovery principles, is an approach used by nurses when working with individuals and families affected by mental health distress. Nurses should also explore their own feelings and beliefs, and the impact that they can have on individuals and groups as an important professional benchmark.

REVIEW QUESTIONS

1. What are the determinants of mental health and wellbeing?
2. What is the impact of mental ill-health on individuals and communities?
3. How can nurses counter the stigma associated with mental illness?

4. How does trauma-informed care and practice, and recovery principles influence the delivery of nursing care to people living with mental health issues?

5. How do you prepare yourself to work with people who are living with mental health issues?

RESEARCH TOPIC

Identify two determinants of mental health and wellbeing, and describe their relevance to living with mental health issues. Critically analyse your role and responsibility as a nurse in enabling self-management and recovery for individuals with mental health issues.

FURTHER READING

Dudgeon, P., Milroy, H. & Walker, R. (eds). (2014). Working Together: Aboriginal and Torres Strait Islander Mental Health and Wellbeing Principles and Practice (2nd edn). Barton, ACT: Commonwealth of Australia.

Happell, B., Cowin, L. & Roper, C. (2013). *Introducing Mental Health Nursing: A Service User-Oriented Approach* (2nd edn). Sydney: Allen & Unwin.

Hungerford, C., Hodgson, D., Clancy, R., Monisse-Redman, M., Bostwick, R. & Jones, T. (2012). *Mental Health Care: An Introduction for Health Professionals* (2nd edn). Milton, QLD: John Wiley and Sons Australia Ltd.

New Zealand Ministry of Health (NZMOH). (2016). *Commissioning Framework for Mental Health and Addiction – A New Zealand Guide*. Wellington: Ministry of Health. Retrieved from www.health.govt.nz/system/files/documents/publications/commissioning-framework-mental-health-addiction-nz-guide-aug16.pdf

Nizette, D., McAllister, M. & Marks, P. (2013). *Stories in Mental Health: Reflection, Inquiry, Action*. Sydney: Elsevier.

Procter, N., Hamer, H., McGarry, D. E., Wilson, R. & Froggatt, T. (eds.). (2017). *Mental Health: A Person-Centred Approach* (2nd edn). Melbourne: Cambridge University Press.

REFERENCES

American Psychiatric Association. (2013). *Diagnostic and Statistical Manual of Mental Disorders* (vol. 5). Arlington, VA: American Psychiatric Association.

Australian College of Mental Health Nurses. (2018). *Mental Health Practice Standards for Nurses in Australian General Practice 2018*. Canberra: ACMHN.

Australian Health Ministers' Advisory Council and National Mental Health Strategy. (2013). *A National Framework for Recovery-Oriented Mental Health Services: Guide for Practitioners and Providers*. Canberra: Commonwealth of Australia.

Australian Institute of Health and Welfare (AIHW). (2012). *Comorbidity of Mental Disorders and Physical Conditions 2007*. Cat. no. PHE 155. Canberra: AIHW. Retrieved from www.aihw.gov.au/publication-detail/?id=10737421146

——(2014). *Australia's Health 2014. Australia's Health Series No. 14*. Cat. no. AUS 178. Canberra: AIHW.

——(2016). *Mental Health Services in Brief.* Cat. no. HSE 180. Canberra: AIHW. Retrieved from www.aihw.gov.au/getmedia/681f0689-8360-4116-b1cc-9d2276b65703/20299.pdf.aspx?inline=true

——(2018). *Australia's Health 2018. Australia's Health Series No. 16.* Canberra: AIHW.

Banyard, V., Hamby, S. & Grych, J. (2017). Health effects of adverse childhood events: Identifying promising protective factors at the intersection of mental and physical well-being. *Child Abuse & Neglect,* 65, 88–8.

Bateman, J., Henderson, C. & Kezelman, C. (2013). Trauma informed care and practice: Towards a cultural shift in policy reform across mental health and human services in Australia - *A national strategic direction.* Sydney: Mental Health Coordinating Council.

Buchanan-Barker, P. (2009). Reclamation: Beyond recovery. In P. J. Barker (ed.), *Psychiatric and Mental Health Nursing: The Craft of Caring* (2nd edn, pp. 661–89). London: Hodder Arnold.

Caldwell, L. & Grobbel, C. C. (2013). The importance of reflective practice in nursing. *International Journal of Caring Sciences,* 6(3), 319–26.

Clement, S., Schauman, O., Graham, T., Maggioni, F., Evans-lacko, S., Bezborodovs, N., . . . & Thornicroft, G. (2015). What is the impact of mental health-related stigma on help-seeking? A systematic review of quantitative and qualitative studies. *Psychological Medicine,* 45, 11–27. doi: http://10.1017/S0033291714000129

Commonwealth of Australia. (2013). *A National Framework for Recovery-Oriented Mental Health Services: Guide for Practitioners and Providers.* Retrieved from www.health.gov.au/internet/main/publishing.nsf/Content/mental-pubs-n-recovgde

Corrigan, P. W., Druss, B. G. & Perlick, D. A. (2014). The impact of mental illness stigma on seeking and participating in mental health care. *Psychological Science in the Public Interest,* 15(2), 37–70.

Crengle, S., Clark, T. C., Robinson, E., Bullen, P., Dyson, B., Denny, S., . . . & The Adolescent Health Research Group. (2013). *The Health and Wellbeing of Māori New Zealand Secondary School Students in 2012. Te Ara Whakapiki Taitamariki: Youth'12.* Auckland: The University of Auckland. Retrieved from www.fmhs.auckland.ac.nz/assets/fmhs/faculty/ahrg/docs/youth12-maori-report.pdf

Department of Health and Human Services, Victoria. (2016). *Preparing Your Organisation for the* Expanding Post-Discharge Support Initiative. Melbourne: Victorian Government.

Dziopa, F. & Ahern, F. (2009). What makes a quality therapeutic relationship in psychiatric/mental health nursing: A review of the research literature. *The Internet Journal of Advanced Nursing Practice,* 10(1), 1–9.

Fernando, A. T., Samaranayake, C. B., & Blank, C. J., Roberts, G. & Arroll, B. (2013). Sleep disorders among high school students in New Zealand. *Journal Primary Health Care,* 5(4), 276–82.

Floen, S. K. & Elklit, A. (2007). Psychiatric diagnoses, trauma, and suicidality. *Annals of General Psychiatry.* 6:12. doi: http://10.1186/1744-859X-6-12

Galletly, C. A., Foley, D. L., Waterreus, A., Watts, G. F., Castle, D. J., McGrath, J. J., . . . & Morgan, V. A. (2012). Cardiometabolic risk factors in people with psychotic disorders: The second Australian national survey of psychosis. *Australian and New Zealand Journal of Psychiatry,* 46(8), 753–61.

Galon, P. & Graor, C. H. (2012). Engagement in primary care treatment by persons with severe and persistent mental illness. *Archives of Psychiatric Nursing*, 26(4), 272–84. doi: http://10.1016/j.apnu.2011.12.001

Gerland, D. & Gerland, K. (2012). *Basic Personal Counselling: A Training Manual for Counsellors*. Sydney: Pearson.

Happell, B., Cowin, L. & Roper, C. (2013). *Introducing Mental Health Nursing: A Service User-Oriented Approach* (2nd edn). Sydney: Allen & Unwin.

Hungerford, C. & Kench, P. (2013). The perceptions of health professionals of the implementation of recovery-oriented health services: A case study analysis. *The Journal of Mental Health Training, Education and Practice*, 8(4), 208–18.

Inter-Agency Committee on Drugs New Zealand. (2015). *National Drug Policy 2015 to 2020*. Wellington: Ministry of Health. Retrieved from www.health.govt.nz/system/files/documents/publications/national-drug-policy-2015-2020-aug15.pdf

Johnson, S. J. & Ragusa, A. T. (2014). The impact of rurality on depression in rural Australia: Socio-cultural reflections for social change. In A. T. Ragusa (ed.), *Rural Lifestyles, Community Well-Being and Social Change: Lessons from Country Australia for Global Citizens* (pp. 206–52). Sharjah, UAE: Bentham Books.

Jorm, A., Allen, N., Morgan, A., Ryan, S. & Purcell, R. (2009). *A Guide to What Works for Depression* (2nd edn). Melbourne: beyondblue.

Keshavan, M. S., Nasrallah, H. A. & Tandon, R. (2011). Schizophrenia, "Just the Facts" 6. Moving ahead with the schizophrenia concept: From the elephant to the mouse. *Schizophrenia Research*, 127(1–3), 3–13.

Kezelman, C. A. & Stavropoulos, P. A. (2012). *Practice Guidelines for Treatment of Complex Trauma and Trauma Informed Care and Service Delivery*. Sydney: Adults Surviving Child Abuse.

Kopera, M., Suszek, H., Bonar, E., Myszka, M., Gmaj, B., Ilgen, M. & Wojnar, M. (2015). Evaluating explicit and implicit stigma of mental illness in mental health professionals and medical students. *Community Mental Health Journal*, 51(5), 628–34. doi: http://10.1007/s10597-014-9796-6

Labott, S. (2019) *Health Psychology Consultation in the Inpatient Medical Setting*. Washington, D.C.: American Psychological Association.

Lai, H. M. X., Cleary, M., Sitharthan, T. & Hunt, G. E. (2015). Prevalence of comorbid substance use, anxiety and mood disorders in epidemiological surveys, 1990–2014: A systematic review and meta-analysis. *Drug & Alcohol Dependence*, 154, 1–13. doi: http://10.1016/j.drugalcdep.2015.05.031

Lam, R. W. (2018). *Depression* (3rd edn). Oxford: Oxford University Press.

Large, M., Kaneson, M., Myles, N., Myles, H., Gunaratne, P. & Ryan, C. (2016). Meta-analysis of longitudinal cohort studies of suicide risk assessment among psychiatric patients: Heterogeneity in results and lack of improvement over time. *PLOS ONE*, 11(6), e0156322.

Lawrence, D., Johnson, S., Hafekost, J., Boterhoven de Haan, K., Sawyer, M., Ainley, J., & Zubrick, S. R. (2015). *The Mental Health of Children and Adolescents: Report on the Second Australian Child and Adolescent Survey of Mental Health and Wellbeing*. Canberra: Department of Health.

Malatest International. (2016). *Evaluation Report: The Youth Primary Mental Health Services*. Wellington: Ministry of Health.

Mental Health Advocacy Coalition. (2008). *Destination: Recovery: Te Unga ki Uta: Te Orangu*. Auckland: Mental Health Foundation of New Zealand.

Mental Health Division, WA Department of Health. (2008). *Clinical Risk Assessment and Management (CRAM) in Western Australian Mental Health Services: Policy and Standards*. Perth: Department of Health. Retrieved from www.health.wa.gov.au/CircularsNew/attachments/826.pdf

Miles, H., Johnson, S., Amponsah-Afuwape, S., Finch, E., Leese, M. & Thornicroft, G. (2003). Characteristics of subgroups of individuals with psychotic illness and a comorbid substance use disorder. *Psychiatric Services*, 54(4), 554–61. doi: http://10.1176/ appi.ps.54.4.554

Morgan, V. A., Waterreus, A., Jablensky, A., Mackinnon, A., McGrath, J. J., Carr, V., . . . & Saw, S. (2011). *People Living with Psychotic Illness 2010. Report on the Second Australian National Survey*. Canberra: Australian Government.

New Zealand Ministry of Health (NZMOH). (2014a). *Statement of Intent 2014 to 2018: Ministry of Health*. Wellington: Ministry of Health.

—— (2014b). *Annual Update of Key Results 2013/14: New Zealand Health Survey*. Wellington: Ministry of Health.

—— (2018). *Annual Update on Key Results 2016/17: New Zealand Health Survey*. Wellington: Ministry of Health. Retrieved from www.health.govt.nz/publication/annual-update-key-results-2016-17-new-zealand-health-survey

O'Hagan, M., Reynolds, P. & Smith, C. (2012). Recovery in New Zealand: An evolving concept? *International Review of Psychiatry*, 24(1), 56–63.

Olasoji, M., Maude, P. & McCauley, K. (2017). Not sick enough: Experiences of carers of people with mental illness negotiating care for their relatives with mental health services. *Journal of Psychiatric and Mental Health Nursing*, 24(6), 403–11.

Olver, J. & Hopwood, M. (2012). Depression and physical illness. *Medical Journal of Australia*, 199 (Suppl. 6), S9–12.

Proal, A. C., Fleming, J., Galvez-Buccollini, J. A. & DeLisi, L. E. (2014). A controlled family study of cannabis users with and without psychosis. *Schizophrenia Research*, 152(1), 283–8.

Rees, C. S., Breen, L. J., Cusack, L. & Hegney, D. (2015). Understanding individual resilience in the workplace: The International Collaboration of Workforce Resilience (ICWR) model. *Frontiers in Psychology*, 6, 1–7.

Ribeiro, J., Franklin, J., Fox, K. R., Bentley, K., Kleiman, E. M., Chang, B. & Nock, M. K. (2016). Self-injurious thoughts and behaviors as risk factors for future suicide ideation, attempts, and death: A meta-analysis of longitudinal studies. *Psychological Medicine*, 46(2), 225–36.

Royal Australian and New Zealand College of Psychiatrists. (2018). Depression. Retrieved from www.yourhealthinmind.org/mental-illnesses-disorders/depression

Schlosser D. A., Pearson R., Perez V. B. & Loewy R. L. (2012). Environmental risk and protective factors and their influence on the emergence of psychosis. *Adolescent Psychiatry*, 2(2),163–71. Retrieved from www.ncbi.nlm.nih.gov/pmc/articles/PMC3487693/

Simpson, J., Duncanson, M., Oben, G., Adams, J., Wicken, A., Pierson, M., . . . & Gallagher, S. (2017). *Te Ohonga Ake The Health of Māori Children and Young People in New Zealand Series Two*. Dunedin: New Zealand Child and Youth Epidemiology Service, University of Otago.

Singh, J. P., Desmarais, S. L., Hurducas, C., Arbach-Lucioni, K., Condemarin, C., Dean, K., . . . & Grann, M. (2014). International perspectives on the practical application of violence risk assessment: A global survey of 44 countries. *International Journal of Forensic Mental Health*, 13(3), 193–206.

Slade, M. (2009). *Personal Recovery and Mental Illness: A Guide for Mental Health Professionals*: Cambridge: Cambridge University Press.

Slade, T., Johnston, A., Teesson, M., Whiteford, H., Burgess, P., Pirkis, J. & Saw, S. (2009). *The Mental Health of Australians 2. Report on the 2007 National Survey of Mental Health and Wellbeing*. Canberra: Department of Health and Ageing.

Tandon, R., Nasrallah, H. A. & Keshavan, M. S. (2009). Schizophrenia, 'Just the Facts' 4. Clinical features and conceptualization. *Schizophrenia Research*, 110, 1–23.

World Health Organization (WHO) and the Calouste Gulbenkian Foundation. (2014a). Social determinants of mental health. Retrieved from www.who.int/mental_health/publications/gulbenkian_paper_social_determinants_of_mental_health/en

—— (2014b). Integrating the response to mental health disorders and other chronic diseases in health care systems. Retrieved from www.who.int/mental_health/publications/gulbenkian_paper_integrating_mental_disorders/en

11

Diabetes mellitus

Julia Gilbert
and Ysanne Chapman

With acknowledgement to Sharon Hooge

LEARNING OBJECTIVES

After studying this chapter, you should be able to:

1. gain an understanding of the global prevalence, risk factors and burden (complications and socioeconomic costs) that diabetes mellitus places on both individuals and the community
2. understand the pathophysiology, assessment and risk factors of diabetes mellitus
3. plan individualised care for people with diabetes mellitus, including health prevention and promotion
4. understand the nurse's role in supporting education and self-care management strategies.

Introduction

Diabetes mellitus is a serious chronic illness that alters the body's ability to metabolise carbohydrate, fat and protein; it is characterised by fasting plasma glucose levels above 7 mmol/L. The most common forms of diabetes mellitus, type 1 and type 2, are differentiated by unique pathophysiology, clinical presentation concerns, preventative efforts and treatments. Type 1 diabetes (T1D) accounts for 5–10 per cent of diabetes mellitus cases and is an autoimmune disorder with complete (or near complete) pancreatic cell dysfunction in producing insulin. Type 2 diabetes (T2D) accounts for 90–95 per cent of diabetes mellitus cases, and is associated with insulin resistance and some degree of insulin deficiency.

Prevalence of diabetes mellitus

Today, 9 per cent of the global adult population live with diabetes mellitus, with this figure projected to increase to approximately 366–439 million in 2030 (World Health Organization (WHO), 2015). Currently in Australia, over 787 500 people live with T2D and over 122 300 people live with T1D. However, the condition does not affect everyone equally, with 7 per 100 000 Aboriginal and Torres Strait Islander peoples being affected by diabetes, and 10 per 100 000 non-Indigenous people being affected (Australian Institute of Health and Welfare (AIHW), 2013). Type 1 diabetes is considered to be the most common chronic disease among children under the age of 14, affecting 1 in every 720 children (AIHW, 2015; Juvenile Diabetes Research Foundation (JDRF), 2015). In New Zealand, 257 000 people live with diabetes mellitus, with 40 new cases being diagnosed per day (New Zealand Ministry of Health (NZMOH), 2014). Currently, diabetes mellitus is the eighth leading cause of death globally and is expected to increase to the seventh leading cause of death by the year 2030 (WHO, 2015).

Diabetes mellitus is associated with microvascular and macrovascular damage because of prolonged hyperglycaemic exposure within the body. **Retinopathy**, **nephropathy** and **neuropathy** are potential microvascular complications (Moore, 2013). Cardiovascular disease (including stroke, peripheral vascular disease, myocardial infarction, angina and coronary vascular disease) is a major macrovascular complication, contributing to the leading cause of death due to diabetes (Royal Australian College of General Practitoners (RACGP) and Diabetes Australia, 2014). Research findings indicate **dyslipidaemia**, genetics and **hyperglycaemia** are key risk factors in cardiovascular disease prevalence (Chehade, Gladysz & Mooradian, 2013).

Global and community socioeconomic and personal costs associated with diabetes mellitus are staggering. Individual average costs reach $4669 annually for T1D alone (JDRF, Australia, 2015). Time that is consumed by seeking medical support; demands of daily self-monitoring (diet, activity, stress and lifestyle); and the expenses of recreational equipment, insulin, medication and testing equipment are but some of the personal burdens placed on individuals and communities (Rhee et al., 2016).

Retinopathy – damage to the eye due to blood vessels inside the retina at the back of the eye leaking fluid and resulting in vision loss.

Nephropathy – damage to the blood vessels in the glomerulus within the kidney, which reduces its function.

Neuropathy – dysfunction or damage to peripheral nerves that may result in tingling, numbness or weakness.

Dyslipidaemia – any disorder of lipoprotein metabolism; for example, overproduction or deficiency of lipoprotein.

Hyperglycaemia – an excess of glucose in the blood.

Pathophysiology, risk factors and assessment

There are various types of diabetes mellitus found in the global population. This chapter focuses on the most common types – T1D and T2D. The differences between T1D and T2D are shown in Figure 11.1.

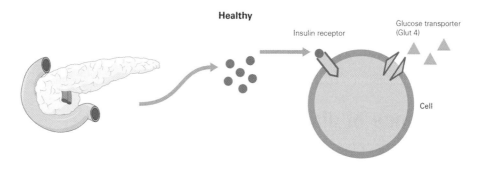

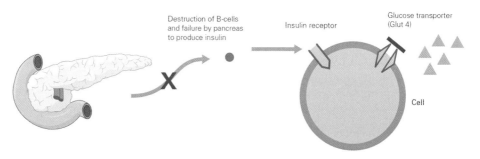

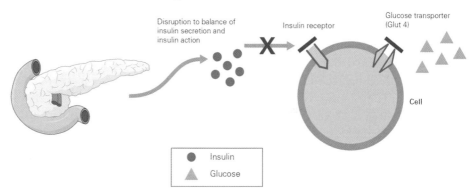

Figure 11.1   Differences between type 1 and type 2 diabetes

Type 1 diabetes

Type 1 diabetes results from the complete (or near complete) destruction of β cells (beta cells) of the pancreas through autoimmune-mediated cell destruction; it is characterised by hyperglycaemia, **hypoglycaemia**, **lipolysis** and **ketoacidosis** (Orchard et al., 2015; Oikawa & Shimada, 2015). The rate of destruction of β cells of the pancreas is variable, so diagnosis can occur at any age (Oikawa & Shimada, 2015). The aetiology of β-cell destruction is unknown, but research continues into the link between T1D and genetics, the environment and other autoimmune disorders (Diabetes Australia, 2018).

Individuals with T1D present in a variety of clinical scenarios from diabetic ketoacidosis (DKA), requiring hospitalisation at one end of the spectrum to the incidental discovery of elevated blood glucose values during routine screening at the other. Symptoms associated with T1D include polyuria, polydipsia, vomiting, hyperventilation, ketonuria and abdominal pain. There is no known cure and no known preventative actions for T1D. Insulin replacement is critical to the successful management of T1D, in conjunction with blood glucose self-monitoring, diet, increased physical activity and continual monitoring for complications (Lind et al., 2017).

Hypoglycaemia – low levels of glucose in the blood.

Lipolysis – the breakdown of lipids which involves hydrolysis of triglycerides creating glycerol and fatty acids.

Ketoacidosis – a serious complication of diabetes which involves an accumulation of ketones in the blood.

Type 2 diabetes

Type 2 diabetes involves disruption to the intrinsic balance of insulin secretion and insulin action, and occurs when β cells of the pancreas are unable to respond appropriately. Obesity body mass index (BMI) more than $30 \, kg/m^2$ and waist circumference more than 90 cm for adult males), increased levels of cholesterol or fats within the blood, and limited physical activity, increase insulin resistance and the development of T2D (Chehade et al., 2013; Moore, 2013). Genetic (that is, family history), environmental (that is, exposure during pregnancy) and a Westernised diet are factors being researched to determine links to T2D (DeFronzo et al., 2015). Type 2 diabetes is not age dependent (Moore, 2013). Children and adolescents who are overweight are at greater risk of insulin resistance. Insulin resistance is also increased during puberty, resulting in increased prevalence in this age group (Diabetes Australia, 2015).

Type 2 diabetes symptoms are often insidious and may be unnoticed by the individual for prolonged periods of time. These symptoms include fatigue, blurry vision, dysphagia, polyuria, polydipsia and weight changes, and a history of frequent illness, nausea, vomiting, irritability and paraesthesia (Diabetes New Zealand, 2014; Nichols, 2014). Type 2 diabetes treatment includes maintenance of a healthy weight through balanced energy intake, low saturated fat intake, low sodium, high fibre intake and low glycaemic index foods spread evenly through the day, low alcohol intake and avoidance of high protein diets. It also includes daily physical activity, healthy diet, blood glucose testing, healthy cholesterol levels, blood pressure management, and monitoring of renal excretion (Diabetes Australia, 2015). Oral hypoglycaemics and insulin may be required to achieve neuroglycaemic levels for some individuals (RACGP and Diabetes Australia, 2014).

Diabetes mellitus diagnostic criteria

The diagnosis of diabetes mellitus is determined through blood level analysis, with the following criteria (National Prescribing Service Medicinewise, 2011a; 2011b):

- fasting blood glucose ≥ 7.0 mmol/L
- random blood glucose ≥ 11.1 mmol/L on oral glucose tolerance test
- HbA1c ≥ 7.0% (53 mmol/mol).

Prediabetes

Adults, children and adolescents may experience impaired glucose tolerance (IGT) or impaired fasting glucose (IFG) prior to diagnosis. This is known as prediabetes and affects over 2 million Australians over the age of 25 (Shaw & Tanamas, 2012). Obesity is linked to prediabetes and accounts for 80–85 per cent risk of T2D development (Diabetes.co.uk, 2015). Diagnosis of prediabetes is made when:

- fasting blood glucose (FBG) is between 6.1 mmol/L, but under 7.0 mmol/L (known as IFG)
- oral glucose tolerance test is above 7.8, but less than 11.1 mmol/L (known as IGT) (Diabetes Australia, 2015).

Individuals with prediabetes may continue to function within the boundary of their pancreatic and metabolic needs without progression to a diagnosis of T2D. Monitoring and reduction of obesity is important as this factor contributes directly to insulin resistance (abdominal fat release of pro-inflammatory chemicals interferes with insulin responsiveness), disrupts body fat metabolism, and increases the risk of T2D development (DeFronzo et al., 2015). The RACGP Diabetes Australia (2014) suggests asymptomatic individuals with IFG and IGT (of any age) be tested with fasting blood glucose every three years. Treatment of prediabetes includes efforts aimed at prevention and delay. Diabetes Queensland (2012–13) suggests weight loss of 5–10 per cent body weight through moderate physical activity for at least 150 minutes per week for those with risk factors. Oral medication may be necessary for prediabetes.

Risk factors

Risk factors associated with T1D and T2D are presented in Table 11.1.

Table 11.1   Risk factors associated with type 1 and type 2 diabetes

Risk factor	T1D	T2D
Common age of diagnosis (but not exclusive)	In Australia, 44% of T1D found in children age 0–14 years, but can occur at any age (AIHW, 2015)	Typically more than 45 years of age (Garvan Institute of Medical Research, 2013), but rising in children and adolescents globally due to the obesity epidemic (DeFronzo et al., 2015)
Characteristics linked to diagnosis	Genetic, environmental, autoimmune and idiopathic (Nichols, 2014)	Lower social and economic status, obesity, central visceral adiposity, **acanthosis nigricans**, hypertension, hyperlipidaemia, genetic history of cardiovascular event, history of gestational diabetes mellitus (GDM)[*], sedentary lifestyle, poor diet, polycystic ovarian syndrome with obesity and prediabetes (Diabetes New Zealand, 2014; RACGP and Diabetes Australia, 2014)

Acanthosis nigricans – dark, velvet-like hyperpigmentation of the skin.

Risk factor	T1D	T2D
Populations with higher incidence	All populations (Nichols, 2014)	African-American, Southern European, Latino/Hispanic, Māori, Native American, Asian and Pacific Islander (RACGP and Diabetes Australia, 2014) and Australian Indigenous groups less than 14 years of age (Maple-Brown, Sinha & Davis, 2010)

* Gestational diabetes mellitus (GDM): diabetes mellitus with diagnosis during pregnancy and disappearance post pregnancy. Prevalent in 1 in 20 pregnancies, with 50 per cent progressing to T2D within 15 years (RACGP and Diabetes Australia, 2014).

REFLECTION

What are the important factors to be aware of when assessing the risk for developing diabetes mellitus?

Nursing assessment of diabetes mellitus

Nursing assessment of the individual with T2D is required throughout their lifetime. A patient-centred approach with a focus on the whole individual is required to identify, monitor, educate and support individuals. Assessment is focused on potential and actual physical, emotional, social, environmental and historical factors that may impact on the individual (Diabetes Queensland, 2012–13). A commonly used tool to assess risk is the Australian Type 2 Diabetes Risk Assessment Tool (Baker IDI Heart and Diabetes Institute, 2010).

It is important to gather a detailed history as part of the assessment of the person with diabetes. This should include: immunisation status; familial history of cardiac, endocrine, autoimmune, metabolic, neurological, renal and retinal disease; applicable economic history; occupational history; environmental exposures (including travel) and other social factors (access to community resources and social support systems). Physical assessment includes:

- general appearance – general health, present blood sugar and individual general care habits are assessed. Hypoglycaemia may cause dilated pupils, pallor, low energy, moodiness and inability to concentrate. Hyperglycaemia may cause states of over activity and excessive energy
- vital signs – a rapid pulse, elevated blood pressure and an elevated respiratory rate may be noted with cardiac or kidney dysfunction. Baseline readings are important to document and refer to at each health visit to aid the understanding of changes and the early identification of complications
- weight and height – the signs of polyphagia (severe hunger), polydipsia (severe thirst) and weight changes may go unnoticed during normal times of growth and development or stress. Height measurements require documentation and a

comparison to growth charts to assess the impact of disease on normal growth and development.

Body mass index of 18.5–24.9 is recommended (RACGP and Diabetes Australia, 2014). For adults with BMI more than $40\,kg/m^2$, weight loss strategies are suggested. Waist circumference measurements are made around the bare abdomen at the level of the pelvis. Waist measurements of $\geq$ 94 cm for men and $\geq$ 80 cm for women are indicative of visceral fat (RACGP and Diabetes Australia, 2014).

Dietary assessment of appetite, usual food intake patterns, likes and dislikes, food availability, food options, family or ethnic influences on food choices, developmental age and dependency on others are important components to understand. Carbohydrate amount, type and daily distribution are influenced by insulin, medication, activity level, age and individual personal response

- blood glucose and HbA1c values – routine self-monitoring of blood glucose (SMBG) levels is not recommended by the RACGP and Diabetes Australia (2014) for T2D individuals utilising oral glucose-lowering medications (excluding sulphonylureas). Self-monitoring of blood glucose is required during illness, pregnancy, insulin usage, unreliable HbA1c levels, and when glucose level data is desired. Consistent and frequent daily SMBG monitoring is recommended for individuals with T1D
- cardiovascular – includes examination for oedema (central and peripheral), peripheral and apical pulses, chest pain, skin colour, moisture, turgor, capillary refill, shortness of breath and presence of exertion. Heart sound and lung sounds auscultation, level of physical activity and tolerance of stair climbing may also be assessed. ECG and blood samples may be taken and assessed regularly
- neurological – reflexes, gait and balance, coordination, strength of muscles, pain sensation, and presence of paraesthesia are important indicators of potential neurological complications
- musculoskeletal – assessment of the individual's gait, reflexes, ambulatory status, posture, movement (independent) and symmetry of movements should be observed. Range of motion, alterations from prior injuries, surgical history, as well as present physical activity level and goals, should be discussed
- integumentary – skin integrity, sensation, ability to conduct personal daily assessment of extremities, pain sensation, redness, wound healing and presence of sustained pressure to extremities is necessary at each visit. Foot assessment is critical
- renal – individuals with prediabetes, T1D and T2D may experience polyuria with hyperglycaemia. Proteins and ketones may be passed. Women with diabetes mellitus are especially prone to asymptomatic urinary tract infections. Assessment of urine output and character (colour, odour, dysuria, frequency, bladder emptying and clarity) are necessary. Annual screening for albuminuria and estimation of glomerular filtration rate are needed to monitor kidney functioning.
- retinal – an ophthalmologist should be involved in the individual's care for annual review of potential retinal changes. Nursing assessment of vision, pupil dilation response and use of glasses should be conducted. Driving status may require further assessment with high incidences of hypoglycaemia
- reproductive – assessment of libido, sexual discomfort and ability to perform may indicate neurological involvement.

Promoting health and reducing risk

In line with the *National Strategic Framework for Chronic Conditions* (Australian Health Ministers' Advisory Council, 2017), a vital component of individualised, person-centred care is the active engagement of the individual with the condition in critical health care decisions. Establishing a partnership arrangement with individuals allows them to develop a better understanding of their chronic health conditions, and facilitates active management of risk factors and good health outcomes (Ceriello & Kilpatrick, 2013). In addition to the clinical need for individualised treatment, the diverse goals and preferences of the individual will require additional treatment regime adjustments by health care practitioners.

Traditionally, health care practitioners dictate treatment regimes with little variation, and minimal consideration and validation is given to individual preferences and decision making. A three-step health care model to facilitate shared decision making involves providing information on choices available to the individual, a description of options for treatment, and assisting people to identify and explore their preferences and make decisions in collaboration with their health care team members (Elwyn et al., 2012). Shared decision making between the clinician and the individual, in addition to the input of other health care team members, involves the sharing of information and discussion of the person's preferences and values, enhancing treatment adherence and engagement (Barry & Edgman-Levitan, 2012). Shared decision making validates the individual's preference for treatment, and respects their decisions and priorities in order to facilitate compliance with treatment programs (Elwyn et al., 2012). Individualised care involves assisting people with diabetes to access and interpret information for treatment of diabetes that empowers them and helps them to achieve their lifestyle goals (Denig et al., 2014). This collaborative model of caring for people with chronic conditions can form part of regular diabetes check-ups with health care providers, and involves identifying problems and formulating treatment plans (Ahmann et al., 2014; Denig et al., 2014). The importance of individualised care is often disregarded by health care providers who target specific test results as a measure of health and compliance. For example, some individuals living with diabetes will face daily challenges to control glucose levels, blood pressure and lipid levels within the confines of delineated clinical treatment – there may be little consideration given by their health care team to the support required for empowerment and decision making (Denig et al., 2014). Individualised care programs are designed to focus on meeting the health, cultural, knowledge, physical limitation and health literacy needs of the person.

A recent report by Sainsbury and colleagues (2018) has, however, revealed a deficit in the routine checks of people with diabetes. Up to 71 per cent of people with diabetes attend a health care professional for annual HbA1c estimation; in the Australian Indigenous population, up to 68 per cent complete this cycle (Sainsbury et al., 2018). These routine checks also include eye checks, foot care, and lipid and kidney monitoring. Sainsbury and colleagues (2018) conclude that the management of diabetes in Australia is sub-optimal and the time for action is imperative.

Integrated health care is defined as goal-directed and person-centred, and emphasises education and self-management. The change from a didactic and generic approach to an integrated and cohesive health care approach requires a shift towards mutual problem solving and open communication across the team to prevent and minimise both microvascular and macrovascular complications of living with diabetes. The use of web-based interventions to encourage self-management of an individual's diabetes is a powerful strategy that has been successful in facilitating information access and exchange between the individual and health care team members (Ramadas et al., 2012). Web-based education programs have also been successfully utilised for the prevention and management of chronic diseases such as diabetes mellitus in a variety of settings (Ramadas et al., 2012). In addition, Diabetes Australia and state-run diabetes associations have concentrated their efforts in the promotion of risk aversion, partnerships in the health care of diabetics, and education programs that inform the person with diabetes of balancing their medication, exercise and diet (Australian Government Department of Health, 2015).

Education and management of diabetes mellitus is complex and challenging for the newly diagnosed individual, and includes making a multitude of daily choices and complex care decisions to manage the disease. These choices include dietary intake, whether to increase or decrease physical activity, and the use of medications such as oral hypoglycaemics and insulin (Jarvis et al., 2010).

SKILLS IN PRACTICE

Assessing the person with type 2 diabetes

Sandu is a 43-year-old male of Indian descent. He and his wife have one child. He presents at the community health centre with complaints of frequent nocturnal urination, blurred vision and fatigue. Sandu claims he is restless and has had trouble sleeping over the past three months.

On examination, the following observations are recorded: height is 182 cm, weight is 95 kg, but was 105 kg three months ago. Sandu's waist circumference is 106 cm. Blood tests and urinalysis show the presence of elevated HbgA1c, ketones and glucose. No other abnormalities are detected.

QUESTION

As the nurse, what education would you provide to Sandu and his family on the preliminary diagnosis of T2D? In your response include lifestyle modifications, and the need for ongoing self-care management and assessment of this condition.

The future of diabetes education and management

Some research has explored the potential of combining traditional patient–provider education strategies and electronic resources designed to support diabetes self-management (Harrison et al., 2014; Vuong et al., 2012). Studies found that many individuals with diabetes preferred face-to-face contact and education sessions with their health care team members, but also utilised technology as a tool to support their self-management decisions and to receive individualised information from health care providers (Holtz & Lauckner, 2012). The desire to receive real-time assistance with their daily behavioural decision making and the ability to share information with their health care team were considered to be beneficial in self-management (Lyles et al., 2011).

Continued advancements in smartphone technology have resulted in an increased interest in the use of mobile phone apps for diabetes self-management. Some mobile phone apps can support self-management via measuring and recording physical exercise duration, medication dosage and effectiveness, blood glucose testing results, and changes to an individual's diet. Other apps provide alerts when medication is due or appointments are required, as well as interfacing with medical practitioners' information systems and allowing data to be transferred directly between the individual and members of the health care team (Lyles et al., 2011). These advancements promote holistic and positive interactions between the individual living with diabetes and their health care team, and enhance health outcomes.

In addition, technological advancements have been made in the delivery of insulin through insulin pumps, and continuous glucose monitoring can be established in conjunction with these pumps which can vary the delivery of insulin in the event of hypoglycaemia. Recently, continuous glucose monitoring has been made available regardless of the insulin delivery system, and interstitial glucose can be monitored 24 hours a day via a small transducer that is attached to the outer aspect of the arm. The hardware of these technological systems can be costly (transducers, software of delivery systems and pumps themselves), but the improvements in health outcomes outweigh these costs. Some members of the population (for example, children) can receive these advancements free of charge. The reduction in the development of complications and an improved quality of life are testament to the value of this technology (Alsaleh, Smith & Taylor, 2012).

The issue of lower socioeconomic status can impact on the ability of the individual with diabetes to manage their condition successfully. Diabetes self-management strategies for these individuals need to engage them and facilitate behaviour change where possible, while addressing barriers to self-care. Health literacy and the ability to problem solve are common barriers to diabetes self-care, and intensive, condensed education programs and community support can form the basis for self-management for these individuals (Hill-Briggs et al., 2011). Peer support can be an effective strategy to promote diabetic self-management for individuals struggling to overcome barriers. Effective peer support involves connecting individuals who have diabetes with non-professionals who themselves have diabetes or are familiar with diabetes management. Peers can provide daily management advice and assistance in addition to social and emotional support, leading to improvements in dietary choices, blood glucose levels and symptom management. By emphasising the importance of peer support to newly diagnosed diabetics, diabetes management programs can be successfully implemented across a variety of community settings.

In addition to peer support, frequent contact with friends, partners and family members has been associated with increased self-management behaviours for individuals with diabetes, such as increased exercise and dietary choices. Conversely, social support barriers, such as a poor social network, have been associated with decreased self-care, poor diet and increased emotional distress (Schiotz et al., 2012). Health care team members need to include social support networks in assessment for the newly diagnosed person with T2D to facilitate optimum care outcomes.

REFLECTION

How will the continued use and acceptance of technology in everyday life impact on the self-care management of diabetes?

The nurse's role in the management of diabetes mellitus

Nurses often engage regularly with the individual living with diabetes by acting as a conduit for information to and from other health care team members, promoting flexibility within the team, and promoting optimum health outcomes (Inzucchi et al., 2015). The nurse's role can include the provision of diabetic education such as insulin administration, education on problem-solving skills and promoting self-management (Barry & Edgman-Levitan, 2012).

The following ongoing assessments are required by the nurse:

- growth and development
- cognitive function
- psychological coping
- blood glucose management
- insulin administration technique and effectiveness
- medication adherence and routine
- nutritional pattern and daily intake
- foot integrity
- lifestyle choices (diet, exercise, alcohol intake, stress management)
- immunisation status
- management of hypoglycaemic episodes (Chung et al., 2015; RACGP and Diabetes Australia, 2018).

Individual lifestyle choices, including smoking, sedentary lifestyle and alcohol use, can result in cardiovascular, renal and eye diseases, diabetic neuropathy, and premature death (Weaver et al., 2014; Wilkinson, Whitehead & Ritchie, 2014).

Individualised assessment and person-centred strategies at the time of diagnosis, such as promoting good blood glucose control, cessation of smoking and the adoption of healthy lifestyle habits, have been proven to overcome perceived barriers to self-management and improve health outcomes (Inzucchi et al., 2015). The focus on integrated care and promotion of self-management have been identified in the Innovative Care for Chronic Conditions Framework (ICCCF), which promotes a multidimensional approach to the management of chronic conditions to achieve optimum health outcomes (Nuño, et al., 2012).

Issues influencing the ability of adults with diabetes to self-care include day-to-day management, vulnerability to social pressure, bias from others in the community and wider situational, and cultural and social issues such as low socioeconomic status and literacy levels (Wilkinson et al., 2014). For individuals living with diabetes, lifestyle modifications, such as eating a healthy diet, regular exercise and frequent monitoring of blood glucose levels, are vital. However, for some people, a healthy diet and exercise is insufficient to keep blood glucose levels within the normal range, so they require the addition of oral hypoglycaemic medications or insulin.

Advanced nursing practice

Diabetes nurse educators are an integral part of the diabetes management team; they work closely with medical staff to educate individuals living with diabetes about their condition and how to manage it. Their primary role is to facilitate diabetes self-management by working with the individual and other members of the health care team to improve self-care ability, health and quality of life (Packer et al., 2012). Nurses working at an advanced level can provide counselling and support, and information regarding what diabetes is and how it develops. They can also address the practical aspects of day-to-day diabetes management, including medication management, the need for regular blood glucose checking and the identification of complications (Rodriguez, 2013).

Treatment involves individualised person-centred care (RACGP and Diabetes Australia, 2014).Weight loss, increased physical activity, a balanced diet that is healthy and adequate, smoking cessation and a limited alcohol intake are the basis for care of diabetic individuals. Techniques to enhance problem solving, decision making, education and skill development should be tailored to individual learning needs, culture, roles, language, literacy, age, and social and financial environments. Reduction of complications includes interventions aimed at screening, monitoring, treatment (including pharmacology), awareness training, self-care management, counselling and ongoing education (Canadian Diabetes Association Clinical Practice Guidelines Expert Committee et al., 2013). National standards for diabetes self-management education provide evidence-based educational and supportive curricula for diabetes nurse educators and health care professionals (Haas et al., 2013).

As this is so, diabetes impacts on all personal areas of an individual's life. Coping styles, living situation, social support systems (formal and informal), health care provider relationships and experience within the health care system will all affect a person's participation in their health care. A knowledge of ethnic descent, religious customs, social values, cultural norms and primary language are critical to providing effective care. An awareness of professional values, reactions and feelings associated with caring for other populations is also necessary. Professional, respectful nursing care is demanded for all individuals.

Diagnoses of depression have been connected to people experiencing diabetes, so affect, mood, coping and thoughts regarding the experience of living with the disease are crucial to assess. Individual effort, motivation, reality and outcomes are important aspects to understand from the individual's point of view (Holt, 2009). Therefore, the involvement of a health care team should address the physical, emotional and spiritual needs of the individual.

SKILLS IN PRACTICE

Type 1 diabetes mellitus

Kandy Smith is a 14-year-old student at Oakreach High School. She plays touch football three nights a week and referees netball on the weekends. She lives with her parents and younger brother, Keith, who is nine years old. They are all in excellent health.

Kandy has an uneventful medical history with no significant illnesses until recently. Over the past two weeks, she has complained of polydipsia, polyuria, polyphagia, 5 kg weight loss and increasing fatigue. She states that she has to go to the toilet five to six times a night and that it makes her even more tired by morning.

Kandy's mother has brought her to the family's general practitioner (GP), as she is concerned about Kandy. On examination, the GP notes that Kandy looks tired, has a BMI of 16.8, has all general observations within the normal range, and a blood glucose Level of 21.8 mmol/l. He organises for Kandy to be admitted to hospital for further testing and diabetic education.

The goals of treatment are as follows.

- Achieve glycaemic control.
- Monitor blood glucose levels.
- Initiate self-management education for Kandy and her family on insulin administration, dietary choices, signs and symptoms of hyper and hypoglycaemic episodes, and exercise.

Kandy was discharged from hospital two days later and was invited to a party Saturday night. She tested her blood glucose level prior to leaving home and it measured 8.9 mmol/L, so she administered 10 units of NovoRapid insulin. On arrival at the party she had two full strength beers, began to feel lightheaded and woke up in the emergency department.

QUESTION

Discuss how Kandy might have avoided being taken to the emergency department. What advice would you give to Kandy to help her manage her diabetes, yet retain her social life?

SUMMARY

Learning objective 1: Gain an understanding of global prevalence, risk factors and burden (complications and socioeconomic costs) that diabetes mellitus places on both individuals and the community.

The number of individuals living with diabetes mellitus is increasing worldwide. Diabetes mellitus is a serious chronic illness that alters the body's ability to metabolise carbohydrate, fat and protein, and is characterised by fasting plasma glucose levels above 7 mmol/L. The most common forms of diabetes mellitus, type 1 and type 2, are differentiated by unique pathophysiology, clinical presentation concerns, preventative efforts and treatments.

Learning objective 2: Understand the pathophysiology, assessment and risk factors of diabetes mellitus.

The diagnosis of diabetes mellitus is based in the presence of a fasting blood sugar $\geq$ 7.0 mmol/L, or HbA1c $\geq$ 7.0% (53 mmol/mol). While it is currently not possible to prevent the development of T1D, strategies to reduce the incidence of developing T2D centre on maintaining a healthy weight, healthy lifestyle choices and increased physical activity. Populations at increased risk of developing T2D include Pacific Islanders, southern Europeans, native Americans and Indigenous Australians.

Learning objective 3: Plan individualised care for people with diabetes mellitus, including health prevention and promotion.

A vital component of individualised, person-centred care is the active partnership with the individual with the condition, and involving that person in critical health care decisions. In addition to the clinical need for individualised treatment, the diverse goals and preferences of the person requiring treatment undergo regime adjustments by health care practitioners.

Learning objective 4: Understand the nurse's role in supporting education and self-care management strategies.

The education and self-management of individuals living with diabetes mellitus is complex and challenging, involving a myriad of daily complex care decisions. Effective self-management is based on individualised assessment, education, and ongoing support of the individual and their family/carers.

REVIEW QUESTIONS

1. Describe the signs and symptoms of diabetes mellitus.
2. Diabetes mellitus is a predisposing risk factor for other chronic conditions. Identify some of these conditions.
3. Identify five risk factors for diabetes.
4. What advice would you give a client to reduce the risk of developing diabetes?
5. Identify three issues that would inhibit a person with diabetes from effectively implementing a self-care management strategy.
6. Identify the latest technological advancements in insulin delivery systems and continuous glucose monitoring. How would you manage a person in your care with these systems in place?

RESEARCH TOPIC

One of the most significant complications of diabetes is diabetic ketoacidosis (DKA). Find out what signs and symptoms you would notice upon clinical presentation. What are the treatment options for this life-threatening condition?

FURTHER READING

Abouzeid, M., Philpot, B., Janus, E. D., Coates, M. J. & Dunbar, J. A. (2013). Type 2 diabetes prevalence varies by socioeconomic status within and between migrant groups: Analysis and implications for Australia. *BMC Public Health*, 13, 252–61.

D'Adamo, E. & Caprio, S. (2011). Type 2 diabetes in youth: Epidemiology and pathophysiology. *Diabetes Care*, 34(Suppl. 2), S161–5.

Inzucchi, S. E., Bergenstal, R. M., Buse, J. B., Diamant, M., Ferrannini, E., Nauck, M., ... & Matthews, D. R. (2015). Management of hyperglycaemia in type 2 diabetes: A patient-centered approach. Position statement of the American Diabetes Association (ADA) and the European Association for the Study of Diabetes (EASD). *Diabetes Care*, 35(6), 1364–79.

Kalea, A. Z., Harrison, S. C., Stephens, J. W. & Talmud, P. J. (2012). Genetic susceptibility for coronary heart disease and type 2 diabetes complications. *Clinical Chemistry*, 58(5), 818–20.

Lind, M., Polonsky, W., Hirsch, I. B., Heise, T., Bolinder, J., Dahlqvist, S., ... & Ahlén, E. (2017). Continuous glucose monitoring vs conventional therapy for glycemic control in adults with type 1 diabetes treated with multiple daily insulin injections: The GOLD randomized clinical trial. *Journal of the American Medical Association*, 317(4), 379–87.

REFERENCES

Ahmann, A., Szeinbach, S. L., Gill, J., Traylor, L. & Garg, S. K. (2014). Comparing patient preferences and healthcare provider recommendations with the pen versus vial and syringe insulin delivery in patients with type 2 diabetes. *Diabetes Technology & Therapeutics*, 16(2), 76–83.

Alsaleh, F. M., Smith, F. J. & Taylor, K. M. (2012) Experience of children/young people and their parents, using pump therapy for the management of type 1 diabetes: Qualitative review. *Journal of Clinical Pharmacy*, 37, 140–7.

Australian Government Department of Health. (2015). Australian National Diabetes Strategy 2016–2025. Canberra: Australian Government Department of Health. Retrieved from www.health.gov.au/internet/main/publishing.nsf/Content/nds-2016-2020

Australian Health Ministers' Advisory Council. (2017). *National Strategic Framework for Chronic Conditions*. Canberra: Australian Government.

Australian Institute of Health and Welfare (AIHW). (2013). *AIHW Analysis of 2013 National (Insulin-Treated) Diabetes Register (NDR)*. Canberra: AIHW.

—— (2015). *Prevalence of Type 1 Diabetes among Children aged 0–14 in Australia 2013. Diabetes Series No. 24*. Cat no. CVD 70. Canberra: AIHW.

Baker IDI Heart and Diabetes Institute. (2010). *Australian Type 2 Diabetes Risk Assessment Tool*. Canberra: Australian Government Department of Health and Ageing.

Barry, M. J. & Edgman-Levitan, S. (2012). Shared decision making – the pinnacle of patient-centered care. *New England Journal of Medicine*, 366(9), 780–1. doi: http://10.1056/NEJMp1109283

Canadian Diabetes Association Clinical Practice Guidelines Expert Committee, Ransom, T., Goldenberg, R., Mikalachki, A., Prebtani, A. P. & Punthakee, Z. (2013). Reducing the risk of developing diabetes. *Canadian Journal of Diabetes*, 37(Suppl. 1), S16–19. doi: http://10.1016/j.jcjd.2013.01.013

Ceriello, A. & Kilpatrick, E. S. (2013). Glycemic variability: Both sides of the story. *Diabetes Care*, 36(Suppl. 2), S272–5. doi: http://10.2337/dcS13-2030.

Chehade, J. M., Gladysz, M. & Mooradian, A. D. (2013). Dyslipidemia in type 2 diabetes: Prevalence, pathophysiology, and management. *Drugs*, 73, 327–39.

Chung, C.-C., Pimentel, D., Jor'dan, A., Hao, Y., Milberg, W. & Novak, V. (2015). Inflammation-associated declines in cerebral vasoreactivity and cognition in type 2 diabetes. *Neurology*, 85(5), 450–8.

DeFronzo, R. A., Ferrannini, E., Groop, L., Henry, R. R., Herman, W. H., Holst, J. J., ... & Simonson, D. C. (2015). Type 2 diabetes mellitus. *Nature Reviews Disease Primers*, 1, 15019.

Denig, P., Schuling, J., Haaijer-Ruskamp, F. & Voorham, J. (2014). Effects of a patient orientated decision aid for prioritising treatment goals in diabetes: Pragmatic randomised controlled trial. *British Medical Journal*. doi: http://dx.doi.org/10.1136/bmj.g5651

Diabetes Australia. (2015). About diabetes – Pre-diabetes. Canberra: Diabetes Australia. Retrieved from www.diabetesaustralia.com.au/pre-diabetes

—— (2018). About diabetes – Prevention. Retrieved from www.diabetesaustralia.com.au/prevention

Diabetes New Zealand. (2014). About type 2 diabetes. Retrieved from www.diabetes.org.nz/home

Diabetes Queensland. (2012–13). Diabetes management. In *General Practice: Guidelines for Type 2 Diabetes*. Melbourne: Royal Australian College of General Practitioners.

Diabetes.co.uk. (2015). Diabetes risk factors. Retrieved from www.diabetes.co.uk

Elwyn, G., Frosch, D. Thomson, R., Joseph-Williams, N., Lloyd, A., Kinnersley, P., ... & Showless, M. B. (2012). Shared decision making: A model for clinical practice. *Journal of General Internal Medicine*, 27(10), 1361–7.

Garvan Institute of Medical Research. (2013). Diseases we research: Diabetes – type 2. Retrieved from www.garvan.org.au/research/diseases-we-research/diabetes-type-2

Haas, L., Marynuik, M., Beck, J., Cox, C., Ducker, P., Edwards, L., ... & 2012 Standards Revision Task Force (2013). *National Standards for Diabetes Self-Management Education and Support. Diabetes Care*, 36(Suppl. 1), S100-8. Retrieved from www.diabetesjournals.org

Harrison, S., Stradler, M., Ismail, K., Amiel, S. & Herrmann-Werner, A. (2014). Are patients with diabetes mellitus satisfied with technologies used to assist with diabetes management and coping? A structured review. *Diabetes Technology & Therapeutics*, 16(11), 771–83.

Hill-Briggs, F., Lazo, M., Peyrot, M., Doswell, A., Chang, Y.-T., Hill, M.N., . . . & Brancati, F. L., (2011). Effect of problem-solving-based diabetes self-management training on diabetes control in a low income patient sample. *Journal of General Internal Medicine,* 26(9), 972-8. doi: http://10.1007/s11606-011-1689-6

Holt, P. (2009). *Diabetes in Hospital: A Practical Approach for Healthcare Professionals* (pp. 1-23). Oxford: Wiley-Blackwell.

Holtz, B. & Lauckner, C. (2012). Diabetes management via mobile phones: A systematic review. *Telemedicine and e-Health*, 18(3), 175–84.

Inzucchi, S. E., Bergenstal, R. M., Buse, J. B., Diamant, M., Ferrannini, E., Nauck, M., . . . & Matthews, D. R. (2015). Management of hyperglycaemia in type 2 diabetes: A patient-centered approach. Position statement of the American Diabetes Association (ADA) and the European Association for the Study of Diabetes (EASD). *Diabetes Care*, 35(6), 1364–79.

Jarvis, J., Skinner, T. C., Carey, M. E. & Davies, M. J. (2010). How can structured self-management patient education improve outcomes in people with type 2 diabetes? *Diabetes, Obesity and Metabolism*, 12(1), 12–19. doi: http://10.1111/ j.1463-1326 .2009.01098.x

Juvenile Diabetes Research Foundation (JDRF). (2015). About type 1 diabetes. Juvenile Diabetes Research Foundation (Australia). Retrieved from www.jdrf.org.au

Lind, M., Polonsky, W., Hirsch, I. B., Heise, T., Bolinder, J., Dahlqvist, S., . . . & Ahlén, E. (2017). Continuous glucose monitoring vs conventional therapy for glycemic control in adults with type 1 diabetes treated with multiple daily insulin injections: The GOLD randomized clinical trial. *Journal of the American Medical Association*, 317(4), 379–87.

Lyles, C. R., Harris, L. T., Le, T., Flowers, J., Tufano, J., Britt, D., . . . & Ralston, J. D. (2011). Qualitative evaluation of a mobile phone and web based collaborative care intervention for patients with type 2 diabetes. *Diabetes Technology & Therapeutics*, 13(5), 563–9.

Maple-Brown, L. J., Sinha, A. K. & Davis, E. A. (2010). Type 2 diabetes in Indigenous Australian children and adolescents. *Journal of Paediatrics and Child Health*, 46, 487–90.

Moore, P. (2013). Improving glycaemic control in people with type 2 diabetes: Expanding the primary care toolbox. *Best Practice Journal*, 53, 6–15.

National Prescribing Service Medicinewise. (2011a). Tests to diagnose type 1 diabetes. Retrieved from www.nps.org.au/conditions/hormones-metabolism-nutritional-problem/diabetes-type-1/for-individuals/diagnosis

——(2011b). Tests to diagnose type 2 diabetes. Retrieved from www.nps.org.au/ conditions/hormones-metabolism-nutritional-problem/diabetes-type-2/for-individuals/diagnosis

New Zealand Ministry of Health (NZMOH). (2014). About diabetes. Wellington: Ministry of Health. Retrieved from www.health.govt.nz/our-work/diseases-and-conditions/ diabetes/about-diabetes

Nichols, H. (2014). What is the difference between diabetes type 1 and diabetes type 2? *Medical News Today*. Retrieved from www.medicalnewstoday.com/articles/75-4 .php

Nuño, R., Coleman, K., Bengoa, R. & Sauto, R. (2012). Integrated care for chronic conditions: The contribution of the ICCC Framework. *Health Policy*, 105(1), 55–64. doi: http://dx.doi.org/10.1016/j.healthpol.2011.10.006

Oikawa, Y. & Shimada, A. (2015). Type 1 diabetes. *Nihon Rinsho. Japanese Journal of Clinical Medicine*, 73(12), 1997–2002.

Orchard, T. J., Nathan, D. M., Zinman, B., Cleary, P., Brillon, D., Backlund, J. Y. C. & Lachin, J. M. (2015). Association between 7 years of intensive treatment of type 1 diabetes and long-term mortality. *Journal of the American Medical Association*, 313(1), 45–53.

Packer, T. L., Boldy, D., Ghahari, S., Melling, L., Parsons, R. & Osborne, R. H. (2012). Self-management programs conducted within a practice setting: who participates, who benefits and what can be learned? *Patient Education and Counseling*, 87(1), 93–100. doi: http://10.1016/j.pec.2011.09.007

Ramadas, A., Quek, K. F., Oldenburg, B., Chan, C. K. Y. & Zanariah, H. (2012). Improvement in dietary knowledge, attitude and behavior of patients with type 2 diabetes mellitus: Results from a tailored web-based dietary education program (myDIDeA). *International Journal of Behavioral Medicine*, 19(Suppl. 1), 1–341.

Rhee, S. Y., Hong, S. M., Chon, S., Ahn, K. J., Kim, S. H., Baik, S. H., . . . & Kim, Y. S. (2016). Hypoglycemia and medical expenses in patients with type 2 diabetes mellitus: An analysis based on the Korea National Diabetes Program Cohort. *PLOS ONE*, 11(2), e0148630.

Rodriguez, K. M. (2013). Intrinsic and extrinsic factors affecting patient engagement in diabetes self-management: perspectives of a certified diabetes educator. *Clinical Therapeutics*, 35(2), 170–8. doi: http://10.1016/j.clinthera.2013.01.002

Royal Australian College of General Practitioners (RACGP) and Diabetes Australia. (2014). *General Practice Management of Type 2 Diabetes – 2014–15*. Melbourne: RACGP and Diabetes Australia.

Sainsbury, E., Shi, Y., Flack, J. & Colagiuri, S. (2018). *Burden of Diabetes in Australia: It's time for a change*. Baulkham Hills, NSW: Nordisk Pharmaceuticals Pty Ltd.

Schiotz, M. L., Bogelund, M., Almdal, T., Jensen, B. B. & Willaing, I. (2012). Social support and self-management behaviour among patients with type 2 diabetes. *Diabetic Medicine*, 29(5), 654–61. doi: http://10.1111/j.1464-5491.2011.03485.x

Shaw, J. & Tanamas, S. (2012). *Diabetes: The Silent Pandemic and its Impact on Australia*. Melbourne: Baker IDI Heart and Diabetes Institute.

Vuong, A. M., Huber, J. C., Bolin, J. N., Ory, M. G., Moudouni, D. M., Helduser, . . . & Forjuoh, S. N. (2012). Factors affecting acceptability and usability of technological approaches to diabetes self management: A case study. *Diabetes Technology and Therapeutics*, 14(12), 1178–82.

Weaver, R. R., Lemonde, M., Payman, N. & Goodman, W. M. (2014). Health capabilities and diabetes self management: The impact of economic, social and cultural resources. *Social Science & Medicine*, 102, 58–68.

Wilkinson, A., Whitehead, L. & Ritchie, L. (2014). Factors influencing the ability to self-manage diabetes for adults living with type 1 or 2 diabetes. *International Journal of Nursing Studies*, 51(1), 111–22.

World Health Organization (WHO). (2015). Diabetes. Retrieved from www.who.int/diabetes/en

12

Chronic respiratory conditions

Michelle Baird, Amanda Moses
and Maria Davies

With acknowledgement to Elizabeth Forbes, Jody Hook and Heather Latham

LEARNING OBJECTIVES

After studying this chapter, you should be able to:

1. define asthma, chronic obstructive pulmonary disease (COPD) and bronchiectasis; identify the pathophysiological differences, risk factors and presentations of these chronic conditions, and explain the principles of their nursing care
2. provide education to patients and their families on health promotion and prevention strategies regarding asthma, COPD and bronchiectasis
3. discuss the nurse's role in a variety of health care settings
4. describe the benefits of advanced nursing practice in the management of patients with asthma, COPD and bronchiectasis.

Introduction

The three chronic conditions affecting the respiratory system discussed in this chapter are asthma, COPD and bronchiectasis. These conditions are serious chronic health problems in Australia and New Zealand, and while the symptoms experienced by clients can be similar, the aetiology, pathophysiology and treatments vary between the conditions. The important role that nurses have in the management of these conditions is discussed in this chapter.

Asthma is Australia's most widespread chronic health problem, contributing to 29 per cent of the overall burden of respiratory disease, with one in nine Australians identifying as a person with asthma in 2014–15 (Australian Institute of Health and Welfare (AIHW), 2017; 2018). In children aged 5–14, asthma is the leading contributor to the burden of disease for males and the second-leading cause for females (AIHW, 2018). As females reach adolescence, the prevalence is likely to increase (AIHW, 2018). Asthma has a 9.9 per cent prevalence rate in Australia, which is high by international standards. The rate of asthma among Indigenous Australians is almost twice as high as the rate for non-Indigenous Australians. This difference in prevalence is common in all age groups but particularly so for older Indigenous peoples (AIHW, 2018). For men, the prevalence of asthma secondary to remoteness and socioeconomic status is not significant, but for women living in remote and rural areas, the prevalence of asthma is increased at 15 per cent compared to women living in metropolitan areas at 11 per cent (AIHW, 2018). Since the year 2000, New Zealand has experienced an increase of 16.4 hospitalisations per year for respiratory disease (Telfar Barnard & Zhang, 2016). Pacific Islander peoples are the most affected across all respiratory disease, with a hospitalisation rate 3.1 times greater than non-Pacific Islander and non-Asian peoples (Telfar Barnard & Zhang, 2016). New Zealand has the second-highest prevalence of asthma in the world, with one in seven children aged 2–14 years (14 per cent) requiring asthma medication, and with one in nine adults (11 per cent) diagnosed with asthma. Although the mortality rate of asthmatics has declined, lower socioeconomic groups, and Māori and Pacific Islander peoples are disproportionately affected by asthma (Telfar Barnard & Zhang, 2016).

In Australia, COPD is the fifth-leading cause of death (AIHW, 2015). Chronic obstructive pulmonary disease is the fourth-leading cause of death in New Zealand, ranked second in men and seventh in women for years lost to disability (Lawes et al., 2012). It is currently ranked third in New Zealand and fifth in Australia for the burden of disease manifested in disability-adjusted life years (Institute for Health Metrics and Evaluation, 2016). Disability-adjusted life years is defined as the 'measurement of the gap between current health status and an ideal health situation where the entire population lives to an advanced age, free of disease and disability' (World Health Organization (WHO), 2015). The hospitalisation of Australian patients with COPD accounted for an estimated $929 million for 2008–09 (AIHW, 2012). As with asthma, the disparity of the disease burden for Indigenous Australians and for Indigenous New Zealanders is higher, with a mortality rate 2.6 times greater for COPD then for non-Indigenous peoples (AIHW, 2014; Telfar Barnard & Zhang, 2016).

Bronchiectasis is estimated to affect up to 50 per cent of people diagnosed with COPD in Australia, although exact figures are hard to determine due to a lack of available data (Bullock & Hales, 2012). In 2013, nearly 300 deaths were attributed to bronchiectasis. It is more commonly seen in people of lower socioeconomic backgrounds, particularly Indigenous peoples (AIHW, 2016). There is significantly more data available on the incidence in children, with the identified prevalence in Indigenous children anticipated to be more than 1400 in 100 000. New Zealand shows a similar trend, with a higher incidence in the Māori population – 33 in 100 000 children under 15 years of age are diagnosed with bronchiectasis, with variations depending on ethnicity. Overall, 17 in 100 000 children from Pacific descent and 4.8 in 100 000 Māori children are identified as having a diagnosis of bronchiectasis (Bullock & Hales 2012; Thoracic Society of Australia and New Zealand, 2018).

Common respiratory conditions

Asthma and COPD are common respiratory diseases that have similar characteristics, which are differentiated by their airflow response to bronchodilator therapy. They vary in their onset, presentation and demographics, and occur singularly or, in some cases, together when the illness is known as asthma-COPD overlap syndrome (ACOS) (Louie et al., 2013; Reddel et al., 2015). Bronchiectasis is predominantly caused by COPD and chronic bronchitis, and many of the predisposing factors align with those identified for these conditions. The presence of a systemic inflammatory condition is also identified as a predisposing factor (Thoracic Society of Australia and New Zealand, 2018). A comprehensive medical assessment, including history (smoking, frequency of lung infections, response to medical therapy), presentation, physical examination and diagnostic tests such as lung function testing, and CT scanning (if bronchiectasis is suspected), allows clinicians to determine if the condition is asthma, COPD or bronchiectasis. Furthermore, careful questioning to elicit exposure to an allergen or timing of symptoms (at night or with exercise) may be associated more with asthma (National Asthma Council Australia, 2015), whereas COPD may exhibit symptoms of fatigue, decreased exercise tolerance, waking at night short of breath, ankle swelling, poor appetite and weight loss; bronchiectasis may present with a history of persistent sputum production (National Institute for Clinical Excellence, 2018). Table 12.1 lists the characteristics of asthma, COPD and bronchiectasis.

Table 12.1 Characteristics of asthma, chronic obstructive pulmonary disease and bronchiectasis

Characteristic	Asthma	COPD	Bronchiectasis
Onset	Variable	Insidious	Insidious
Presentation	Variable	Chronic	Acute and chronic
Dyspnoea	Episodic	Persistent – increases with severity and exertion	Episodic
Cough	Episodic/variable	Chronic	Chronic

Characteristic	Asthma	COPD	Bronchiectasis
Sputum	Episodic/variable	Variable	Usually daily, copious, purulent, difficult to drain
Wheeze	Likely	Can be present	May be present
Chest tightness	Present	Can be present	May be present
Timing	Worse at night or early morning	Always present	Always present
Airflow reversibility	Reversible	Minimal/not fully reversible. FEV1 * < 0.7 (diagnostic of COPD post bronchodilator)	Variable
Spirometry	Obstructive	Obstructive	More commonly obstructive, may be mixed obstructive/restrictive, restrictive or normal
Airway modification	Narrowing	Fibrosis and narrowing	Permanent dilation of bronchial airway (small airway)
Disease progression	Acute flare ups	Progressive with acute flare ups	Progressive with frequent flare ups
Demographics	Children, although can be adults	Adults	Children or adults Disadvantaged groups

* FEV1 is the forced expiratory volume that can be forcibly exhaled over one second
   Sources: Adapted from Abramson et al. (2014); National Asthma Council Australia (2015); Stretton et al. (2013)

Asthma

The Global Initiative for Asthma (GINA) has described asthma as

> a heterogeneous disease, usually characterised by chronic airway inflammation. It is defined by the history of respiratory symptoms such as wheeze, shortness of breath, chest tightness and cough that vary over time and in intensity, together with variable expiratory airflow limitation. (GINA, 2018, p. 14)

During an attack of asthma, epithelial cells, which line the airway, initiate an inflammatory response that leads to excess mucus production and smooth muscle contraction of the airways (airway hyper-responsiveness; see Figure 12.1) (Doeing & Solway, 2013). These epithelial cells respond by releasing cytokines, which act upon mast cells, dendritic cells and innate lymphoid cells to release the T helper (Th) 2 cytokines that contribute to asthma symptomology (Erle & Sheppard, 2014). Airway remodelling occurs due to structural changes in the epithelium (bronchial thickening and oedema, mucous metaplasia and bronchoconstriction), which contributing to variable airflow obstruction (Doeing & Solway, 2013; Erle & Sheppard, 2014).

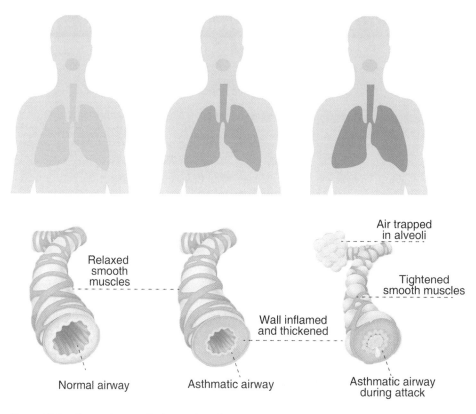

Figure 12.1 Airway changes that occur in asthma
Source: Emma Hammett, 2014

More recently, asthma pathogenesis has been described in terms of phenotyping, with each phenotype differing in its aetiology. A phenotype has been defined as 'the integration of different characteristics that are the product of the interaction of the patient's genes with the environment' (Wenzel, 2012, p. 650).

The Global Initiative for Asthma (2018) identifies common asthma phenotypes:

- allergic asthma
- non-allergic asthma
- late-onset asthma
- asthma with fixed-airflow limitation
- asthma with obesity.

Allergic (atopic) asthma is a cell-mediated response to an allergen, such as dust mites and respiratory infections. The correlation of atopy – IgE antibodies in response to an environmental allergen – and asthma is well documented in younger age groups but less so in adult-onset asthma (Al-Alawi, Hassan & Chotirmall, 2014) or as a result of exposure to hazardous substances, such as cigarettes (non-atopic asthma), which causes airway inflammation, increased sputum production and bronchoconstriction (Athanazio, 2012). Identifying the underlying aetiology of asthma is paramount to effective treatment. Phenotyping of asthma as defined by aetiology (for example, cough-variant asthma and aspirin-intolerant asthma) optimises the management and treatment of asthma since clinicians are able to prescribe pharmacological (reliever and preventer medications), and non-pharmacological treatments (such as avoidance of allergens, like dust, pets or other triggers, like aspirin) (Ko et al., 2014). Although asthma is an inflammatory response, a diagnosis of asthma should not be excluded if clients exhibit variable respiratory symptoms or airflow limitation (Reddel et al., 2015). Further testing may be needed, such as bronchial provocation testing or allergy testing (GINA, 2018), to confirm or refute a diagnosis of asthma.

Asthma is now described in terms of symptom control and future risk of adverse outcomes (GINA, 2018). Asthma severity may change over time and is defined as mild, moderate or severe. It is classified once a client has been on adequate controller therapy for a few months and their response to therapy is assessed (GINA, 2018). Initially, a patient may require high doses of controller therapy, but if they have reduced symptoms over a few months, their controller therapy may be stepped down (GINA, 2018).

Chronic obstructive pulmonary disease

Chronic obstructive pulmonary disease is characterised by airflow limitation that is usually progressive and not fully reversible (Global Initiative for Chronic Obstructive Lung Disease (GOLD), 2018). The initials 'COPD' are often used as an umbrella term to also encompass emphysema and chronic bronchitis. Frequently, clients with COPD will exhibit symptoms of both emphysema and chronic bronchitis, but the proportion of each will differ from patient to patient.

Irritation to the airways by the inhalation of noxious particles or gases initiates an inflammatory process in the airways. The inflammatory process seen in COPD is different to that of asthma, as the inflammation is characterised by the presence of neutrophils, whereas the inflammation in asthma is primarily driven by eosinophils. The difference in the type of inflammation impacts on the prognosis and pharmacological management of COPD. However, there may be an increase in eosinophils, especially in COPD and ACOS (GOLD 2018, p.13)

Repeated irritation to the airways by noxious particles or gases leads to a chronic inflammatory process. This process is not yet well understood (GOLD, 2018); however, the effect of the presence of inflammatory cells leads to fibrosis of the airways, epithelial metaplasia and increased mucus secretion. The ongoing cycles of injury and repair to the airway results in the airways becoming narrowed, ultimately leading to reduced airflow (chronic bronchitis).

In further response to irritation, the large and small airways (that is, the **bronchi and bronchioles**) try to protect themselves by increasing the amount and tenacity of the mucus lining the airways in order to reduce the damage done by the inhaled irritants. To increase the mucus production, the mucous glands increase in number and size. The excessive mucus production and its tenacity results in the destruction of the cilia that line the airways. A combination of the increased mucus production and the destruction of cilia mean that the lungs cannot remove mucus effectively, which can clog the airways (GOLD, 2018). Additionally, structural changes occur in the lung with repeated cycles of injury and repair.

The gradual destruction of **alveoli** (emphysema) is also due to inflammation and is often a result of cigarette smoking or other inhaled irritants. These irritants initiate an inflammatory response in the peripheral airways and lung tissue, leading to neutrophils and macrophages releasing multiple proteinases that break down and destroy

Bronchi and bronchioles – the trachea splits into two breathing tubes (bronchi) and the breathing tubes continue to divide into smaller and smaller breathing tubes (bronchioles).

Alveoli – the air sacs at the base of the bronchioles where gas exchange takes place.

alveoli and connective tissue (Barnes, 2000). The destruction of the alveoli walls means that individual alveoli sacs merge together and become one large sac. This decreased alveoli surface area for oxygen and carbon dioxide gas exchange results in impairment, which then leads to dyspnoea (breathlessness).

These damaged, larger alveoli sacs are inelastic and often unable to provide structure to the surrounding lung tissue and airways. As a result, the small airways can collapse during expiration, trapping air in the lung and leading to further poor gas exchange. In response to the increased levels of trapped carbon dioxide (**hypercapnia**), the client increases their respiratory rate, which leads to further air trapping and a feeling of dyspnoea. When a client has trapped air or hyperinflated lungs, the diaphragm becomes flattened. This changes the way the inspiratory muscles move, making them inefficient and easily fatigued. The client then has to use more energy to perform the normal task of breathing; it may take so long to breathe out that the client will not have enough time to empty their lungs before they need to breathe in again (see Figure 12.2).

Hypercapnia – abnormally high levels of carbon dioxide.

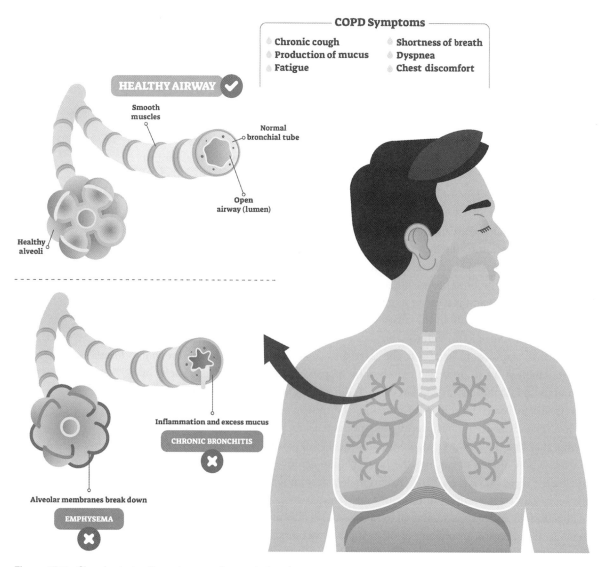

Figure 12.2   Chronic obstructive pulmonary disease in the airways

The disease trajectory of COPD can vary from client to client, but is commonly described as a slow physical decline with potentially serious exacerbations scattered throughout (Pinnock et al., 2011). Table 12.2 outlines the scale of severity and symptoms of COPD.

Table 12.2   Guide to the severity of chronic obstructive pulmonary disease

COPD severity	FEV % predicted*	Symptoms	History of exacerbations	Comorbid conditions**
Mild	60–80	• Breathlessness on moderate exertion • Recurrent chest infections • Little or no effect on daily activities	Frequency may increase with severity	Present across all severity groups
Moderate	40–59	• Increasing dyspnoea • Breathlessness walking on level ground • Increasing limitation of daily activities • Cough and sputum production • Exacerbations requiring corticosteroids and/or antibiotics		
Severe	< 40	• Dyspnoea on minimal exertion • Daily activities severely curtailed • Experiencing regular sputum production • Chronic cough		

* FEV = forced expiratory volume.
** Common comorbid conditions include cardiovascular disease, skeletal muscle dysfunction, metabolic syndrome, osteoporosis, anxiety or depression, lung cancer, peripheral vascular disease and sleep apnoea.

Source: Abramson et al. (2014)

Bronchiectasis

While bronchiectasis is associated with asthma and COPD, there is a difference in the pathophysiology of this condition. Changes in the airway musculature combined with damage to the elastin, secondary to inflammatory processes and oedema, leads to permanent dilation of the bronchial airway and decreased gas exchange (Bullock & Hales, 2012). This results in impaired drainage of secretions; a common feature of bronchiectasis is the presence of increased quantities of purulent sputum and chronic infection. If not well managed, this leads to permanent damage to the parenchyma of the lung. Bronchiectasis may be present in specific lobes of the lung or disseminated throughout the lungs. It may also be present in one or all three of the identified forms. These forms include:

- cylindrical, where bronchioles are dilated, smooth and cylindrical in shape
- varicose, where the bronchioles are irregular with areas that are constricted and dilated
- cystic, where dilated bronchioles occur in clusters, as most commonly seen in cystic fibrosis (Thoracic Society of Australia and New Zealand, 2018).

The person with bronchiectasis may present with symptoms similar to that of COPD; however, the differentiating aspect of bronchiectasis is the excessive sputum that is produced and the frequency of infective exacerbations, presenting with pneumonia-like symptoms.

A diagnosis of bronchiectasis includes completing a comprehensive medical history, with consideration of smoking, lung conditions, frequency of lung infections and duration of symptoms, and the presence of systemic inflammatory disorders. Clinical examination may identify increased sputum production, often purulent, **adventitious sounds** on chest auscultation, and peripheral changes such as **nail clubbing**, associated with chronic lung conditions. High-resolution CT scanning, which demonstrates the irregularity and dilation of the bronchial tubes, is considered the gold standard for diagnosis of bronchiectasis. (Bullock & Hales, 2012; Thoracic Society of Australia and New Zealand, 2018)

Adventitious sounds – abnormal breath sounds heard on lung auscultation. Examples of adventitious sounds are: crackles (discontinuous, popping sounds) , and wheezes (continuous musical sounds, either high or low (rhonchi) pitched).

Nail clubbing – widening and increased curvature of the nail bed. It can occur in both the fingers and toes. The angle between the nail and cuticle is more acute, with curvature of the nail like an upside-down spoon.

REFLECTION

Describe the differences and similarities between asthma, COPD and bronchiectasis. Think about the key characteristics, the effects on lung function and client presentation in each chronic condition.

Risk factors

Atopy – an allergic response to an environmental pathogen, contributing to disease symptomology such as asthma.

Risk factors identified in asthma are **atopy**, respiratory virus, allergen exposure and family history (Ko et al., 2014; National Asthma Council Australia, 2015). Avoidance of triggers such as dust and weather changes (for example, by staying inside) minimises flare ups, except in the case of exercise-induced asthma (EIA), which is an unavoidable trigger that can be managed with the use of reliever and preventer medications (National Asthma Council Australia, 2015).

Spirometry – a non-invasive test to detect obstruction or restriction in the lungs. Spirometry measures the maximum volume of air in litres that can be forcibly exhaled (forced vital capacity, or FVC) and the volume of air in litres that can be forcibly exhaled over one second (forced expiratory volume, or FEV1).

Smoking is the number one risk factor for the development of COPD; there is a close relationship between the amount of cigarettes smoked and the decline in the volume of air in litres that can be forcibly exhaled over one second as measured by **spirometry**. However, people who have not smoked can also develop COPD. Other risk factors for COPD can include:

- genetic factors including α1-antitrypsin deficiency
- second-hand smoke (or passive smoking)
- long-standing asthma

- outdoor air pollution from traffic or other sources
- biomass smoke (cooking with coal, wood, crop waste and animal dung)
- occupational exposure (working in coal and hard rock mines, tunnels, concrete manufacturing and non-mining industries)
- poor diet, and low intake of vitamin C and other antioxidants (Einser et al., 2010).

Bronchiectasis is predominantly caused by COPD and chronic bronchitis, and many of the predisposing factors align with those identified for these conditions. The presence of a systemic inflammatory condition is also identified as a predisposing factor (Thoracic Society of Australia and New Zealand, 2018).

Impact on activities of daily living

Living with asthma, COPD and bronchiectasis can socially isolate and decrease a client's self-efficacy. The impact on the client physically, mentally and socially varies with disease severity. The impact of these chronic conditions on activities of daily living (ADL) is greater among the young and the elderly. In 42.4 per cent of children aged 0–14 years with asthma, asthma contributed to school absenteeism. Similarly, 44 per cent of elderly people with asthma confirmed that asthma had impacted on their daily living (Australian Bureau of Statistics, 2013).

Chronic obstructive pulmonary disease is progressive, and in its mild stage has little impact on the client's ADL. As the disease progresses, the individual's ability to perform ADL is inhibited, and they will require support for such activities as showering and shopping, and they may also require modified dietary intake. This is similar for those diagnosed with bronchiectasis, with the frequent infective exacerbations limiting their activity and the ongoing need for the management of sputum production impacting on their daily life.

It is important for clients with these chronic conditions to conserve their energy and modify ADL. Clients with asthma may need to minimise exposure to allergens, such as cleaning products and dust, when they are unwell. For clients with COPD and bronchiectasis, vacuuming or showering can become difficult and produce fatigue and/or respiratory distress (Hinkle & Cheever, 2014). Nurses should work with the client to plan activities during the times of day that the client feels at their best and spread ADL out. According to MacLeod (2012), the introduction of SMART goals encourages robust discussion between the nurse and client to set client-centred goals that are:

- Specific
- Measurable
- Achievable
- Realistic
- Timely.

It is essential for the client to plan, pace and prevent avoidable stress associated with shortness of breath by taking regular breaks to focus on breathing during activities. It is common that, as COPD progresses, the client may need assistance at home with ADL. There are many government and non-government community organisations that can provide this assistance. Examples of services include transport, cleaning, shopping, cooking meals, and providing equipment to make activities easier (for example, a shower chair).

Respiratory assessment

The nurse needs to be able to perform and interpret a respiratory assessment of the asthma, COPD and bronchiectasis client. The nurse needs to focus on the following.

- Observe respiratory rate, work of breathing (use of accessory muscles), colour (central and peripheral) and mental acuity (anxiety, fatigue).
- Ask the client how they are feeling: Are they able to talk in full sentences or just single words?
- Assess the flow of air through the bronchioles and the presence of obstruction or fluid in the lungs by thoracic auscultation. Place the stethoscope firmly against the chest wall and compare one side with the other starting at the apices, instructing the patient to take slow, deep breaths through the mouth.
- Check for symmetrical chest movement by placing hands on the back of the chest and assess symmetry on inspiration.
- Monitor pulse oximetry (SpO_2 per cent) to assess the need for administration/response to prescribed bronchodilator therapy or supplemental oxygen.
- Assess sputum production and quality, including changes in quantity and colour.

Assessment should also include the use of spirometry to diagnose asthma or COPD (see Figure 12.3). Spirometry measures the maximum volume of air in litres that can be forcibly exhaled (forced vital capacity; that is, FVC) and the volume of air in litres that can be forcibly exhaled over one second (FEV1). It is the ratio of these two measures FEV1/FVC post bronchodilator (2–4 puffs of a short-acting beta$_2$ agonist (SABA)) via

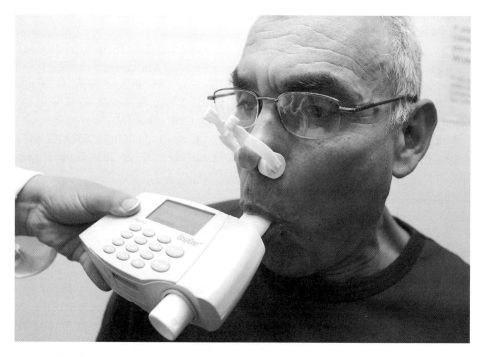

Figure 12.3 Spirometry

a spacer that indicates whether airflow obstruction is reversible. Chronic obstructive pulmonary disease should be considered in anyone over 35 years old with a history of more than a 15 pack-year history of smoking (1 pack-year history of smoking = 20 cigarettes per day for 1 year; for example, 35 cigarettes a day for 25 years = 35/20 × 25 years [number of years smoked] = 44 pack-year history of smoking) or with occupational exposure to dust or gas/fumes (Abramson et al., 2014). Bronchiectasis should be considered in patients who have a history of increased sputum production and a productive cough for more than 8 weeks duration (Chang et al., 2010).

Asthma is reversible with more than 12 per cent or 200 mL increase in FEV1 post bronchodilator (National Asthma Council Australia, 2015), whereas COPD is defined by its lack of reversibility post-bronchodilator and an FEV1/FVC (FEV1 per cent) of less than 0.70 (Abramson et al., 2014). Spirometry findings in bronchiectasis may show obstructive patterns, but restrictive patterns may also be present. Undertaking spirometry at diagnosis of bronchiectasis will assist in monitoring the decline in lung function (Chang et al., 2010).

There is much that can be done for the client to manage their asthma, COPD or bronchiectasis. Bronchiectasis and COPD clients live with the condition every single day, so it affects their physical, emotional and psychosocial wellbeing. The nurse has an opportunity to assist clients with respiratory disease to minimise disease progression and to help them effectively self-manage it, which, in turn, minimises exacerbations and maximises their quality of life. This approach aligns with the micro level of the Innovative Care for Chronic Conditions Framework (ICCCF), where interaction with the individual and their family encourages self-care management strategies and the development of empowerment to manage the condition; it is a focus of the partnership of care. (Further detail on this is provided in Chapter 4.) Clients should be encouraged to take an active participatory role in their care planning; it is important for nurses to respect the knowledge and experience a client has about their asthma, COPD or bronchiectasis.

Treatment options

Oxygen (O_2) therapy is used in an acute asthma attack to maintain O_2 saturations of 93–95 per cent (94–98 per cent in children aged 6–11 years) (Adams, Sutter & Albertson, 2012; Reddel et al., 2015) or in the management of bronchiectasis or COPD to maintain a SpO_2 of 88–92 per cent (Beasley et al., 2015) for those who have **hypoxemia**. Oxygen therapy can be used as short-term therapy (often in hospital to assist in recovery from an exacerbation), or for client long-term home therapy if hypoxemia is persistent, as diagnosed from arterial blood gases measuring $PaO_2 < 55$ mmHg (GOLD, 2018). Oxygen is generally not used in the delivery of inhaled bronchodilators unless prescribed by a medical officer. When caring for a client with O_2, it is essential to know what the O_2 prescription is in L/min. The correct delivery device for the flow rate of O_2 must be supplied to the client; for example, nasal prongs or a mask. The nurse must ensure that there is correct equipment set up or on standby to enable the client to move around, and that the person is educated on home O_2 safety considerations – this includes avoiding smoking and any naked flames, storing and travelling with O_2, as well as cleaning and replacing equipment and tubing.

Hypoxemia – abnormally low levels of oxygen in the blood.

The nurse can monitor the response to supplemental O_2 by using pulse oximetry, assessing vital signs and the level of consciousness. It is important to understand that providing more O_2 than necessary to maintain O_2 target saturations in some COPD patients is not beneficial to them. Hyperoxia leads to complex mechanisms of events, including a decrease in minute ventilation and an increase in carbon dioxide (CO_2) (Austin et al., 2010). Symptoms of high levels of CO_2 include drowsiness, somnolence, headache and disorientation (McDonald, Crocett & Young, 2005).

Correct device usage will ensure that an effective dose of the inhaled medication is provided. Nurses should take every opportunity to check a client's technique and educate any misconceptions on usage. Metered-dose inhalers (MDI) should be used with a spacer to enhance the deposition of the medications into the lungs. Inhalers containing corticosteroids have the potential side effects of oral thrush infection and hoarseness of the voice. After using these inhalers, the client should be instructed to rinse their mouth (gargle and spit) to prevent these side effects.

When breathing becomes difficult, clients with asthma will compensate by using a tripod position. It is important to minimise the client's anxiety to ensure effective breathing. Clients with COPD often have a shallow, rapid and inefficient breathing pattern, where the lungs become hyperinflated due to air trapping. The nurse can teach breathing exercises, such as pursed-lip breathing, to help slow and deepen expiration, prevent collapse of small airways and reduce feelings of panic (Hinkle & Cheever, 2014).

Surgical interventions can be beneficial in carefully selected COPD patients. Interventions may include:

- bullectomy (removing large bulla that do not contribute to gas exchange so that the adjunct lung parenchyma is decompressed)
- lung volume reduction surgery (LVRS), including bronchoscopic LVRS and endobronchial valve replacement (LVRS involves removing parts of the lung to reduce hyperinflation, enabling the respiratory muscles to be more effective by improving mechanical efficiency and overall gas exchange)
- lung transplantation (single or double) (Clini & Ambrosino, 2008).

Non-invasive positive pressure ventilation can also be used to improve inspiratory flow rate, correct hypoventilation, rest respiratory muscles and reset the central respiratory drive (Hanania et al., 2005). Nutritional status is very important, with studies consistently showing greater mortality rates in underweight compared to people who are overweight with COPD. This may be caused by an imbalance between low energy intake and high energy requirements. Muscle wasting and depletion is a common problem in people with COPD (Clini & Ambrosino, 2008). The nutritional status of clients should be evaluated by a professional, with supplements and support readily implemented.

Management of bronchiectasis can depend on the comorbidity with other respiratory conditions. It is aimed at improving quality of life, managing sputum production and early intervention to prevent infective exacerbations. Physiotherapy and airway clearance are useful interventions for the management of sputum production and maintenance of exercise capacity (Thoracic Society of Australia and New Zealand, 2018). Antibiotic therapy is essential early in the course of infective exacerbation, and the use of action plans assists in ensuring this is implemented (Chang et al., 2010). The use of long-term antibiotics is considered on an individual basis, but is not currently encouraged (Chang et al., 2010). Inhaled bronchodilators and corticosteroids are not recommended for bronchiectasis alone, but will support comorbid COPD or asthma, and will help management of acute exacerbations (Chang et al., 2010). Pulmonary rehabilitation with education and regular exercise, nutritional support and encouragement of annual vaccinations are all important components of appropriate management of bronchiectasis (Bullock & Hales, 2012).

SKILLS IN PRACTICE

Living with chronic obstructive pulmonary disease

John is a previously healthy 60-year-old man, who has presented to hospital after experiencing a productive cough (green sputum), fevers and increased shortness of breath over the last two days.

John reports that he smokes 15–20 cigarettes per day and has done so for the last 25 years. He works in the construction industry and volunteers with the local country fire authority. He has been feeling 'very tired' over the last six months but ascribes this to 'working too hard, and not doing any exercise'. His general practitioner (GP) had recently prescribed him Ventolin PRN via an inhaler for his shortness of breath.

On further questioning, John reports that he has had a 'bit of a cough' on and off for a year and has noted that he has been increasingly short of breath on exertion over the past six months. He reports that he does get the occasional 'chest infection' three to four times per year that requires antibiotics and he finds he experiences more shortness of breath when the local council undertakes hazard-reduction burns for bushfire management in his local area.

On physical examination, John's vital signs are as follows: heart rate 85 bpm, respiratory rate 18 bpm, blood pressure 142/70 mmHg, SpO_2 91 per cent on room air, and FEV1/FVC 56 per cent. Chest auscultation demonstrated reduced breath sounds bilaterally and crackles in the bases of his lungs. The GP has diagnosed John as having COPD.

QUESTION

Explain John's in-hospital management and discuss the important issues that you would like to educate John about regarding the management of COPD.

Promoting health and reducing risk

The principles of nursing care for clients with asthma, COPD or bronchiectasis include minimising the progression of the disease and ensuring that the client's quality of life is maintained. Nurses are an integral part of a client's journey across the continuum of care from acute to community care. Nurses should be equipped with the skills to provide education to clients to maximise their quality of life. It is essential that nurses have the knowledge and the ability to impart their knowledge, and can guide and counsel clients on their journey to a healthier lifestyle. Education needs to be culturally appropriate and may need to involve a translator, or in the case of Indigenous clients, an Indigenous health worker may need to be present.

Smoking cessation

Smoking cessation is a modifiable risk factor that can prevent or slow the progression of all three conditions outlined in this chapter (GOLD, 2018). Nurses are pivotal in promoting smoking cessation by providing opportunistic intervention, education and referral. The 5As strategy is currently accepted as best practice for brief intervention.

- **A**sk and identify smokers. Document smoking status in the medical record.
- **A**ssess the degree of nicotine dependence using the Fagerstrom Tolerance Scale (Mendelsohn, 2011) and motivation or readiness to quit.
- **A**dvise smokers about the risks of smoking and the benefits of quitting, and discuss options.
- **A**ssist cessation – this may include specific advice about pharmacological interventions or referral to a formal cessation program.
- **A**rrange follow up to reinforce messages (Mendelsohn, 2015).

Nicotine replacement therapy (NRT) – the substitution of nicotine to satisfy cravings by using skin patches, lozenges, mouth spray, chewing gum or dissolvable oral strips. These items do not contain the harmful toxins contained in inhaled smoke and aim to assist with the symptoms of nicotine withdrawal.

The ICCCF focus on health prevention at the meso level incorporates policies that ensure hospitals are smoke-free and provide patients admitted with the opportunity for **nicotine replacement therapy (NRT)**, which in some instances will be nurse-initiated. Checking of CO_2 levels via a Smokerlyzer provides the patient with a measurable variable to encourage smoking cessation (Mendelsohn, 2015). Although brief intervention during hospitalisation is effective, follow up post-hospitalisation with counselling for one month has been shown to increase quit rates (Mendelsohn, 2015). It is imperative the nurse be aware of decreased smoking and drug interactions such as theophylline, as dosages may need to be reduced (Mendelsohn, 2015).

Vaccinations

Immunisation is recommended in clients with asthma, COPD and bronchiectasis. Nurses should encourage individuals to have their annual influenza and pneumococcal vaccinations as prescribed by their GP. It is recommended that all Aboriginal and Torres Strait Islander peoples receive an annual influenza vaccination, and adults older than 50 years should receive the pneumococcal vaccination (*Australian Medicines Handbook 2018*). Aboriginal and Torres Strait Islander peoples who have a chronic condition and are 15–49 years old may be eligible for the pneumococcal vaccination (*Australian Medicines Handbook 2018*). Influenza immunisations reduce the risk of exacerbations, hospitalisations and death from asthma or COPD (Yang et al., 2018). Māori and Pacific Islander peoples are recommended to have the influenza vaccination annually and the pneumococcal vaccination every five years (Harwood, Martin & Reid, 2012).

Pulmonary rehabilitation

Pulmonary rehabilitation (PR) – a holistic program that helps to improve the wellbeing of patients with chronic lung issues.

According to the COPD-X guidelines, **pulmonary rehabilitation (PR)** 'reduces dyspnoea, fatigue, anxiety and depression, improves exercise capacity, strength, emotional function and heath related quality of life and enhances clients' sense of control over their condition' (Yang et al., 2018, p. 53). Pulmonary rehabilitation is a suitable program for anyone with a chronic lung condition experiencing breath-lessness while attending ADL. It is also recommended for those on O_2 therapy.

Pulmonary rehabilitation is a six-to-twelve-week exercise training and education program run by health professionals. It is often held at local hospitals or community centres two to three times per week and focuses on the following core components:

1. assessment
2. goal setting
3. exercise training
4. client education, behavioural change
5. program evaluation
6. maintenance.

These programs provide clients with a secure, controlled place to exercise and gain self-confidence in their ability to exercise, manage breathlessness and anxiety. Pulmonary rehabilitation is also a forum for clients to discuss their chronic condition and become more knowledgeable so as to enhance their ability to self-manage and feel in control of their lung disease. On completion of PR it is envisaged that clients will be equipped with the skills and confidence to be able to continue to exercise in local fitness centres or gentle exercise programs in their communities.

Education about recognising signs and symptoms

Recognising signs and symptoms is paramount in self-managing asthma, COPD and bronchiectasis. Understanding how each condition occurs, its triggers and risk factors, and how to treat it when well or unwell, are synonymous with good client outcomes. Prescribing and effectively using respiratory inhalers are essential to managing asthma and COPD.

Education regarding worsening of symptoms, including increased dyspnoea, fatigue and tightness of chest, and changes in sputum colour, consistency or amount, should be provided to the client. These changes may indicate an infection or exacerbation of asthma or COPD, which needs to be treated. An individual asthma or COPD action plan should be developed in conjunction with the client and a medical officer (Shah et al., 2011). People with bronchiectasis should be provided with a treatment plan, which is individualised and suitable for early intervention of infective exacerbation (Chang et al., 2010). It is important that at each visit the nurse educates the client on how to use their treatment plan.

The nurse's role in the management of asthma, chronic obstructive pulmonary disease and bronchiectasis

Nurses have a key role in the management of people with asthma, COPD and bronchiectasis in a variety of settings, including in-patient and outpatient settings in hospitals, GP clinics and in the community. Community-based multidisciplinary teams, which enable better integration of services and support for individuals and their carers, have resulted in improved health outcomes for individuals experiencing these chronic illnesses (Hefford & Ehrenberg, 2011, p. 2). Generalist community nurses are key members of these teams and operate in six main role domains: advocate, supporter, coordinator, educator, team member and assessor, as identified in research by Wilkes and colleagues (2013, p. 850).

Advance care planning and palliation of end-stage respiratory disease is essential for the client, and family and health professionals who care for these clients, to appropriately manage functional and cognitive decline (Patel, Janssen & Curtis, 2012). Although it is often a difficult conversation to initiate, nurses need the confidence and knowledge to discuss end of life with respiratory patients. Advance care planning is encouraged and should be discussed early in the disease trajectory (Curtis, 2008) so that the client and family are able to make informed decisions regarding their end-of-life management, such as whether they want to stay at home, or enter a hospital or hospice (Patel et al., 2012).

REFLECTION

Nurses are key members of multidisciplinary teams working with individuals experiencing asthma, COPD and bronchiectasis. Reflect on the role of various team members and explain how they apply to individuals with asthma, COPD and bronchiectasis in hospital and community settings.

Advanced nursing practice

Fletcher and Dahl (2013), and Zakrisson and Hagglund (2010) believe that nurses engaged in advanced nursing practice are in a key position to assume a leading role in the management of asthma, COPD and bronchiectasis, and have the potential to make a positive impact on the health of individuals. They argue that advanced nursing practice results in reduced fragmentation of services, better integration of evidence-based care, and a higher level of support for the individual and their family or carer (Fletcher & Dahl 2013; Zakrisson & Hagglund, 2010, p. 154). Watts and colleagues (2009, p. 167) report that nurse practitioners have unique strengths in leading multidisciplinary teams to provide evidence-based, patient-centred holistic care. Advanced nursing practice involves flexibility, depth of knowledge and skill in clinical decision making, application of clinical guidelines, coordination, case management, and the use of technology, education, research and leadership to implement change. Research by Kadu and Stolee (2015, p. 4) has identified facilitators and barriers to implementing change that nurses need to consider when leading this process. These relate to individuals, team members, the organisation and the wider health system.

SKILLS IN PRACTICE

Multidisciplinary approaches to treatment

Mary, who is 67 years old, has a history of chronic bronchitis, obesity and osteoarthritis. Recently she has experienced several severe exacerbations of her lung condition, characterised by significant increase in sputum production and acute shortness of breath. Mary has required numerous hospitalisations over the past four months for intravenous antibiotics and nebulised bronchodilators, as she was not able to adequately utilise non-nebulised inhaled medications. Her respiratory physician has today advised her that the microscopy, culture and sensitivity (MC&S) of her sputum shows that she has a pseudomonas infection in her lungs, and her CT scan indicates she has developed disseminated varicose bronchiectasis. Mary lives with her husband, Jim, in rural NSW. Jim has a diagnosis of COPD, type 2 diabetes and reduced mobility due to a farming injury where he sustained damage to his thoracic spine. They receive some support with housework and, until recently, Mary had been doing most of the cooking.

QUESTIONS

1. Considering the change in diagnosis that has now occurred for Mary, what additional measures need to be put in place for her to appropriately manage her condition?

2. What multidisciplinary team members may be useful in assisting with this?

SUMMARY

Learning objective 1: Define asthma, COPD and bronchiectasis; identify the pathophysiological differences, risk factors and presentations of these chronic conditions, and explain the principles of their nursing care.

Asthma and COPD are common respiratory diseases that have similar characteristics, but are differentiated by their airflow response to bronchodilator therapy. They vary in their onset, presentation and demographics, and occur singularly or together (ACOS). Bronchiectasis is linked to these conditions, but may exist alone, and is characterised by significant increased sputum production. The nurse has an important role in assisting clients with asthma, COPD and bronchiectasis to minimise disease progression and to help them to effectively self-manage, which, in turn, minimises exacerbations of the disease and maximises the clients' quality of life.

Learning objective 2: Provide education to patients and their families on health promotion and prevention strategies regarding asthma, COPD and bronchiectasis.

Nurses are an integral part of a client's journey across the continuum of care from acute to community care. Nurses should be equipped with the skills to provide education to clients to maximise their quality of life. It is essential that nurses have the knowledge and ability to impart their knowledge, and can guide and counsel clients on their journey to a healthier lifestyle. Education needs to be culturally appropriate.

Learning objective 3: Discuss the nurse's role in a variety of health care settings.

Nurses have been identified as key members of multidisciplinary teams who work with clients experiencing asthma, COPD and bronchiectasis in a variety of settings. The definition of the nurse's role is key to the provision of more integrated care.

Learning objective 4: Describe the benefits of advanced nursing practice in the management of patients with asthma, COPD and bronchiectasis.

Advanced nursing practice results in reduced fragmentation of services, better integration of evidence-based care and a higher level of support for the client and their family or carer. Nurses with advanced skills are able to identify and manage changes in symptoms within their scope of practice.

REVIEW QUESTIONS

1. As a nurse working in a multidisciplinary team, how would you ensure integration of services and continuity of care for clients experiencing asthma, bronchiectasis or COPD?
2. Nurses involved in leading change in care practices will experience facilitators and barriers during the process. Discuss how these factors will impact on the implementation of change.
3. Discuss how smoking is a contributing factor to COPD, and the role that the nurse can play in educating and supporting clients with smoking cessation.
4. What are some of the issues and supports you need to consider when discharging a client with a chronic respiratory condition from your care?
5. How could you assist a client to attend PR? Discuss the benefits with them of the PR program.

RESEARCH TOPIC

Investigate the role that the nurse has in advance care planning with clients who have a chronic respiratory condition. Examine the legislative requirements in both Australia and New Zealand related to advance care planning. Explore the variations in terminology used in jurisdictions across Australia and New Zealand.

FURTHER READING

Alison, J. A., McKeough, Z. J., Johnston, K., McNamara, R., J., Spencer, L. M.,
    Jenkins, S. C., . . . & The Thoracic Society of Australia & New Zealand. (2017).
    *Australian and New Zealand-Pulmonary Rehabilitation Clinical Practice
    Guidelines. Respirology,* 22(4), 800–19. Retrieved from https://
    onlinelibrary.wiley.com/doi/full/10.1111/resp.13025

Bunker, J., Reddel, H., Dennis, S., Middleton, S., Van Schayck, C., Crockett, A., . . . & Zwar,
    N. (2012). A pragmatic cluster randomized controlled trial of early intervention for
    chronic obstructive pulmonary disease by practice nurse–general practitioner
    teams: Study protocol. *Implementation Science,* 7(83), 1–10.

Kadu, M. & Stolee, P. (2015). Facilitators and barriers of implementing the chronic care
    model in primary care: A systematic review. *BMC Family Practice,* 16(12), 1–14.

Wang, K. Y., Chu, N.-F., Lin, S.-H., Chiang, I. C., Perng, W.-C. & Lai, H.-R. (2014). Examining
    the causal model linking health literacy to health outcomes of asthma patients.
    Journal of Clinical Nursing, 23(13/14), 2031–42.

Zakrisson, A. B., Engfeldt, P. & Hagglund, D. (2012). Nurse-led multidisciplinary programme
    for patients with COPD in primary health care: A controlled trial. *Primary Care
    Respiratory Journal,* 20(4), 427–33.

REFERENCES

Abramson, M., Frith, P., Yang, I., McDonald, C., Hancock, K., Jenkins, S., . . . & Scowcroft, C.
    (2014). COPD-X concise guide for primary care. Brisbane: Lung Foundation
    Australia

Adams, Y. A., Sutter, M. E. & Albertson., T. E. (2012). The patient with asthma in the
    emergency department. *Clinical Reviews in Allergy & Immunology,* 43, 14–29.

Al-Alawi, M., Hassan, T. & Chotirmall, S. H. (2014). Advances in the diagnosis and
    management of asthma in older adults. *The American Journal of Medicine,* 127,
    370–8.

Athanazio, R. (2012). Airway disease: Similarities and differences between asthma, COPD
    and bronchiectasis. *Clinics (Sao Paulo),* 67(11), 1335–43.

Austin, M. A., Wills, K. E., Blizzard, L., Walters, E. & Wood-Baker, R. (2010). Effect of
    high flow oxygen on mortality in chronic obstructive pulmonary disease patients
    in prehospital setting: Randomized control trial. *British Medical Journal,* 341,
    c5462.

Australian Bureau of Statistics. (2013). *Australian Health Survey: Health Service Usage and
    Health Related Actions, 2011–12.* ABS cat no. 4727.055.001. Canberra: Australian
    Bureau of Statistics.

Australian Institute of Health and Welfare (AIHW). (2012). *Risk Factors Contributing to Chronic Disease*. Cat. no. PHE 157. Canberra: AIHW.

—— (2014). *Mortality from Asthma and COPD in Australia*. Cat. no. ACM 30. Canberra: AIHW.

—— (2015). COPD – chronic obstructive pulmonary disease. Retrieved from www.aihw .gov.au.copd.

—— (2016) *Chronic Respiratory Conditions*. Cat. no. AUS119. Canberra: AIHW.

—— (2017). *The Burden of Chronic Respiratory Conditions in Australia: A Detailed Analysis of the Australian Burden of Disease Study 2011*. Australian Burden of Disease Study series no. 14. BOD 15. Canberra: AIHW.

—— (2018). Asthma snapshot. Retrieved from www.aihw.gov.au/reports/chronic-respiratory-conditions/asthma/contents/asthma

Australian Medicines Handbook (2018). Adelaide: Australian Medicines Handbook Pty Ltd.

Barnes, P. J. (2000). Chronic obstructive pulmonary disease. *New England Journal of Medicine*, 343, 269–80.

Beasley, R., Chien, J., Douglas, J., Eastlake, L., Farah, C., King, G., . . . & Walters, H. C. (2015). Thoracic Society of Australia and New Zealand oxygen guidelines for acute oxygen use in adults: 'Swimming between the flags'. *Respirology*, 20, 1182–91.

Bullock, S. & Hales, M. (2012). *Principles of Pathophysiology*. Sydney: Pearson.

Chang, A. B., Bell, S. C., Byrnes, C. A., Grimwood, K., Holmes, P. W., King, P. T., . . . & Torzillo, P. J. (2010). Chronic suppurative lung disease and bronchiectasis in children and adults in Australia and New Zealand: A position statement from the Thoracic Society of Australia and New Zealand and the Australian Lung Foundation. *Medical Journal of Australia*, 193, 356–65.

Clini, E. M. & Ambrosino, N. (2008). Nonpharmacological treatment and relief of symptoms in COPD. *European Respiratory Journal*, 32, 218–28.

Curtis, R. (2008). Communication and palliative care in ICU. *Journal Compilation, Asian Specific Society of Respirology*, 13(5), A80.

Doeing, D. C. & Solway, J. (2013). Airway smooth muscle in the pathophysiology and treatment of asthma. *Journal of Applied Physiology*, 114, 834–43.

Einser, M. D., Anthonisen, N., Coultas, D., Kuenzli, N., Perez-Padilla, R., Postma, D., . . . & Balmes, J. R. (2010). An official American Thoracic Society public policy statement: Novel risk factors and the global burden of chronic obstructive pulmonary disease. *American Journal of Respiratory and Critical Care Medicine*, 182, 693–718.

Erle, D. J. & Sheppard, D. (2014). The cell biology of asthma. *Journal of Cell Biology*, 205(5), 621–31.

Fletcher, M. & Dahl, B. (2013). Expanding nursing practice in COPD: Is it key to providing high quality, effective and safe patient care? *Primary Care Respiratory Journal*, 22(2), 230–3.

Global Initiative for Asthma (GINA). (2018). *Global Strategy for Asthma Management and Prevention, 2018*. Retrieved from www.ginasthma.org

Global Initiative for Chronic Obstructive Lung Disease (GOLD). (2018). *Global Strategy for the Diagnosis, Management and Prevention of COPD*. Retrieved from www.goldcopd.org

Hanania, N. A., Ambrosino, N., Calverley, P., Cazzola, M., Donner, C. F. & Make, B. (2005). Treatments for COPD. *Respiratory Medicine*, 99, S28–40. doi: http://10.1016/ j.rmed.2005.09.013

Harwood, M., Martin, P. & Reid, J. (2012). Diagnosis and management of COPD in Māori and Pacific peoples. *Best Practice Journal*, 43, 14–25. Retrieved from www.bpac .org.nz/BPJ/2012/April/copd.aspx

Hefford, M. & Ehrenberg, N. (2011). *Telehealth Support for Patients with Long Term Conditions. Evaluation of a Rural Pilot*. Retrieved from www.srgexpert.com/ Telehealth_Evaluation_Final_Report_18_Feb_11.pdf

Hinkle, J. L. & Cheever, K. H. (2014). *Brunner & Suddarth's Textbook of Medical-Surgical Nursing* (13th edn, vol. 1). Sydney: Lippincott Williams & Wilkins.

Institute for Health Metrics and Evaluation. (2016). Country profiles. Retrieved from www.healthdata.org/results/country-profiles

Kadu, M. & Stolee, P. (2015). Facilitators and barriers of implementing the chronic care model in primary care: A systematic review. *BMC Family Practice*, 16(12), 1–14.

Ko, F. W. S., Lim, T. K., Hancox, J. & Yang, I. A. (2014). Year in review: Chronic obstructive pulmonary disease, asthma and airway biology. *Respirology*, 19, 438–47.

Lawes, C., Thronley, S., Young, R., Hopkins, R., Marshall, R., Cheuk Chan, W. & Jackson, G. (2012). Statin use in COPD patients is associated with a reduction in mortality: A national cohort study. *Primary Care Respiratory Journal*, 21, 35–40.

Louie, S., Zeki, A. A., Schivo, M., Chan, A. L., Yoneda, K. Y., Avdalovic, M, ... & Albertson, T. E. (2013). The asthma-chronic obstructive pulmonary disease overlap syndrome: Pharmacotherapeutic considerations. Expert review. *Clinical Pharmacology*, 6(2), 197–219.

MacLeod, L. (2012). Making SMART goals smarter. *Physician Executive*, 38(2).

McDonald, C. F., Crocett, A. J. & Young, I. H. (2005). Adult domiciliary oxygen therapy. *Position tatement of the TSANZ. Medical Journal of Australia*, 182, 612–16.

Mendelsohn, C. (2011). Nicotine dependence: Why is it so hard to quit? *Medicine Today*, 12(10), 35–44.

—— (2015). Managing nicotine dependence in NSW hospitals under the Smoke-Free Health Care Policy. *Public Health Research and Practice*, 25(3), e2531533. doi: http://dx.doi.org/10.17061/phrp2531533

National Asthma Council Australia. (2015). *Australian Asthma Handbook, Version 1.1.* Melbourne: National Asthma Council Australia.

National Institute for Clinical Excellence. (2018). *Chronic Obstructive Pulmonary Disease in Over 16s: Diagnosis and Management*. London: National Institute for Clinical Excellence. Retrieved from www.nice.org.uk/guidance/NG115

Patel, K., Janssen, J. A. & Curtis, J. R. (2012). Advanced care planning in COPD. *Respirology*, 17(1), 72–8.

Pinnock, H., Kendall, M., Murray, S. A., Worth, A., Levack, P., Porter, M., ... & Sheikh, A. (2011). Living and dying with severe chronic obstructive pulmonary disease: Multi-perspective longitudinal qualitative study. *British Medical Journal*, 342, d142.

Reddel, H. K., Bateman, E. D., Becker, A., Boulet, L. P., Cruz, A. A., Drazen, J. M. & FitzGerald, J.M. (2015). A summary of the new GINA strategy: A roadmap to asthma control. *European Respiratory Journal*, 46(3), 622–39.

Shah, S., Sawyer, S. M., Toelle, B. G., Mellis, C. M., Peat, J. K., Lagleva, M., ... & Jenkins, C. R. (2011). Improving paediatric asthma outcomes in primary health care: A randomised controlled trial. *Medical Journal of Australia*, 195, 405–9.

Stretton, R., Schembri, S., Short, P., Poppelwell, L., Singnayagam, A., Akram, A., ... & Williamson, P. (2013). The impact of bronchiectasis on outcomes in a large cohort of patients hospitalised with exacerbations of COPD. *European Respiratory Journal,* 42(Suppl. 57), 4647. Retrieved from http://erj.ersjournals.com/content/42/Suppl_57/4647

Telfar Barnard, L. & Zhang, J. (2016). *The Impact of Respiratory Disease in New Zealand: 2016 Update.* Wellington: Asthma and Respiratory Foundation NZ.

Thoracic Society of Australia and New Zealand. (2018). *Bronchiectasis Toolbox.* Melbourne: Digital Agency. Retrieved from http://bronchiectasis.com.au/

Watts, S., Gee, J., O'Day, M., Schaub, K., Lawrence, R., Aron, D. & Kirsh, S. (2009). Nurse practitioner-led multidisciplinary team to improve chronic illness care: The unique strengths of nurse practitioners applied to shared medical appointments/group visits. *Journal of the American Academy of Nurse Practitioners*, 21, 167–72.

Wenzel, S. (2012). Severe asthma: From characteristics to phenotypes to endotypes. *Clinical & Experimental Allergy*, 42, 650–8.

Wilkes, L., Cioffi, J., Cummings, J., Warne, B. & Harrison, K. (2013). Clients with chronic conditions: Community nurse role in a multidisciplinary team. *Journal of Clinical Nursing*, 23, 844–55.

World Health Organization (WHO). (2015). Health statistics and information systems, metrics: disability-adjusted life year (DALY). Retrieved from www.who.int/healthinfo/global_burden_disease/metrics_daly/en

Yang I. A., Brown J. L., George J., Jenkins S., McDonald C. F., McDonald V., . . . & Dabscheck E. (2018). *The COPD-X Plan: Australian and New Zealand Guidelines for the Management of Chronic Obstructive Pulmonary Disease 2018. Version 2.55.* Brisbane: Lung Foundation Australia.

Zakrisson, A. & Hagglund, D. (2010). The asthma/COPD nurses' experience of educating patients with chronic obstructive pulmonary disease in primary health care. *Scandinavian Journal of Caring Sciences*, 24, 147–55.

13

Arthritis and musculoskeletal conditions

Amanda Stott
and Louise Wells

LEARNING OBJECTIVES

After studying this chapter, you should be able to:

1. recognise the biopsychosocial impact arthritis has on the individual as well as the community
2. understand the underlying pathophysiology, and associated modifiable and non-modifiable risk factors relating to osteoarthritis (OA), rheumatoid arthritis (RA) and osteoporosis
3. identify and discuss health prevention, and promote strategies relevant to these conditions
4. highlight the nurse's role in the collaborative management of these conditions
5. discuss opportunities for advanced nursing practice in relation to arthritis and osteoporosis.

Introduction

In Australia and New Zealand, arthritis and other musculoskeletal conditions affect a significant proportion of the general population. For example, in Australia, 15.3 per cent of the population was affected by at least one form of the condition during 2014–15. This figure is slightly higher in New Zealand where 17 per cent of adults have been diagnosed with some form arthritis (Ackerman et al., 2016; New Zealand Ministry of Health (NZMOH), 2018). People tend to view arthritis as a single-disease entity when, in fact, it may be more accurately described as an umbrella term for more than 100 conditions that affect the musculoskeletal system (Arthritis and Osteoporosis Victoria, 2013). The word 'arthritis' originates from the Greek words for joint – 'arthron' –and inflammation – 'itis' – with the hallmarks of the condition being pain, swelling and stiffness (Australian Institute of Health and Welfare (AIHW), 2014). Arthritis is a significant contributor to disability in that it limits physical activity subsequently affecting the quality of life of those affected (Ackerman et al., 2016)

The way these conditions affect individuals is highly variable. However, despite their diversity in relation to functional changes, these conditions are linked anatomically in terms of their association with pain and impaired physical functioning (Ackerman et al., 2016; AIHW, 2014). The burden of this group of diseases on the Australian and New Zealand health systems is considerable. The health care costs of arthritis in Australia are estimated to have exceeded $5.5 billion in 2015, with these costs predicted to exceed $7.6 billion by 2030 (Ackerman et al., 2016). The latest figures available from New Zealand report an annual cost of $12.2 billion in 2018 (Deloitte Access Economics, 2018).

In view of these facts, it is imperative that nurses are well educated in relation to this group of conditions. Nurses make a significant contribution to the health care team, and play a pivotal role in the care of clients with arthritis and musculoskeletal conditions. On completion of this chapter, greater knowledge and expertise will be gained in relation to the coordination and provision of care to those patients experiencing OA, RA and osteoporosis in a variety of contexts. Particular focus is given to discussing the underlying pathophysiology and associated risk factors of these conditions. In addition, health promotion and prevention strategies, as well as the role of the nurse in relation to education and self-care management, are discussed.

Osteoarthritis, rheumatoid arthritis and osteoporosis

Osteoarthritis and RA are the two most common forms of arthritis. Other forms of arthritis include **gout**, **ankylosing spondylitis**, juvenile arthritis, **systemic lupus erythematosus** and **scleroderma** (Arthritis Australia, 2015a). Osteoarthritis currently affects approximately 2.2 million people in Australia and 305 000 people in New Zealand (Ackerman et al., 2016; Arthritis New Zealand, 2015). It is estimated that half of all adults over the age of 50 have radiological changes consistent with OA, although

Gout – a condition where uric acid is poorly metabolised and causes arthritis through the deposition of chalk stones. Affected areas include the smaller bones of the feet.

Ankylosing spondylitis – arthritis of the spine that is more common in young males and can lead to fusion of joints resulting in the spine becoming less flexible and a hunched posture.

Systemic lupus erythematosus – an autoimmune disease affecting the body's immune system. In this condition the immune system mistakenly attacks healthy tissue affecting the skin, joints, kidneys, brain and other organs.

Scleroderma – a chronic condition that affects the connective tissue, and hardens and contracts the skin.

many of these will be asymptomatic. Rheumatoid arthritis is the second-most common form of arthritis, affecting approximately 400 000 people in Australia and 40 000 in New Zealand (Ackerman et al., 2016; Arthritis New Zealand, 2015). Both conditions can affect people of all ages, but are more common in older people, with RA being more common in women (AIHW, 2014). While these two conditions share certain clinical manifestations, their pathophysiology is quite distinct.

Osteoarthritis

Normal joint physiology

Synovial joints consist of articular cartilage (AC), subchondral bone, the synovial membrane, synovial fluid and a joint capsule. The AC lines the underlying (subchondral) bone, forming a smooth surface that provides protection and shock absorption. Articular cartilage is avascular and receives its nutrients from the surrounding synovial fluid, which is produced by the synovial membrane. Synovial fluid also lubricates the joint and acts as a shock absorber. The joint capsule surrounds the joint, providing strength and stability (Antonelli & Starz, 2012; Bullock & Hales, 2012).

Osteoarthritis pathophysiology

Osteoarthritis is a progressive condition that affects the freely moveable synovial (or diarthrodial) joints. It is most commonly seen in the hands, knees and hips (Bijlsma, Berenbaum & Lafeber, 2011). It was traditionally thought to be a non-inflammatory disorder caused by simple wear and tear that primarily affected the articular cartilage. It is now understood that the underlying pathophysiology is much more complex, with a definite inflammatory component and the potential to involve all parts of the joint (Berenbaum, 2013; Bruyere et al., 2015).

Articular cartilage consists of cartilage-forming cells, known as chondrocytes, that are surrounded by a complex extracellular matrix (ECM). This ECM mainly consists of type II collagen, proteoglycans and water. In a healthy joint, homeostatic mechanisms maintain a balance between degradation of the ECM and its synthesis by chondrocytes (Sovani & Grogan, 2013). In OA, chondrocytes respond to biomechanical and biochemical stimuli by increasing the production of proteoglycans and collagen in an initial attempt at repair. Over time, this fails and the chondrocytes start synthesising increased amounts of enzymes (matrix metalloproteinases) that destroy the ECM, therefore shifting the balance from repair to degradation (Bijlsma et al., 2011).

Recent research has found that inflammatory mediators also play a significant role in this process of cartilage degradation (Berenbaum, 2013; Hoff et al., 2013). Pro-inflammatory cytokines, including interleukin-1 (IL-1) and tumour necrosis factor alpha (TNF-α), stimulate both chondrocytes and synovial cells to produce metalloproteinases, while also inhibiting proteoglycan and collagen synthesis, and promoting chondrocyte apoptosis (death) (Goldring & Otero, 2011). Ongoing loss of articular cartilage causes its surface to soften and thin. As a result, it loses its ability to withstand normal mechanical stressors, and cracks or fissures start to develop. Eventually, parts of the subchondral bone are exposed in areas of high pressure. These exposed areas of bone come into contact with each other during movement, resulting in thickening and sclerosis of their surface. Attempts to repair this damage result in cell proliferation and the formation of bony spurs, or osteophytes (see Figure 13.1). Cysts containing synovial fluid can also develop in the subchondral bone (Bullock & Hales, 2012).

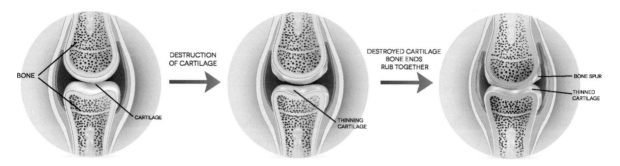

Figure 13.1 A normal joint (left) and loss of cartilage and formation of osteophytes in an abnormal joint (right) in osteoarthritis

Clinical manifestations of osteoarthritis

The loss of cartilage and damage to surrounding joint structures result in pain, stiffness and loss of function. Pain tends to be intermittent and worse after periods of activity. Stiffness is also intermittent and tends to be worse in the mornings and after periods of inactivity. Swelling may also be seen in OA as a result of the inflammatory processes associated with the condition. This inflammation and swelling can be exacerbated when osteophytes break off and accumulate in the synovial fluid, causing irritation to the synovial membrane (Bijlsma et al., 2011). Clinical criteria for the diagnosis of OA include the presence of these clinical manifestations as well as the presence of joint space narrowing and/or osteophytes on X-ray (see Figure 13.2) (Sovani & Grogan, 2013).

Risk factors for osteoarthritis

Modifiable risk factors – factors that can be altered by the patient; for example, cigarette smoking, obesity, and joint injury exposure to joint-loading repetitive tasks.

Non-modifiable risk factors – factors that are beyond the control of the patient; for example, increasing age, female gender and a genetic susceptibility.

While specific risk factors for the development of OA are dependent on the joint involved, it is possible to identify both **modifiable risk factors** and **non-modifiable risk factors** for OA that are common to all joints. Non-modifiable risk factors include increased age, female gender, genetic susceptibility and congenital joint abnormalities. It is important to note that OA does not occur in all older joints. Instead, it is thought that ageing increases a joint's susceptibility to OA, with the condition only developing if other risk factors are present (Anderson & Loeser, 2010). Modifiable risk factors for OA include obesity, injury to the joint, and occupational or recreational exposure to joint-loading repetitive tasks. While obesity is most strongly associated with knee OA, it has also been linked to the development of OA in other joints. Increased mechanical load on the joints is an obvious explanation for this, but it is also thought that a higher body fat percentage can affect the metabolism of cartilage and bone (Garvin, Leung & Kean, 2013). Injuries to joints, such as dislocations, ligament tears and intra-articular fractures, cause ongoing instability in the joint and a progressive loss of articular cartilage, leading to the development of OA,

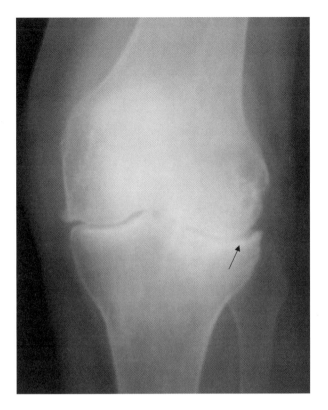

Figure 13.2   Osteoarthritis in the left knee showing osteophytes, narrowing of the joint space and increased subchondral bone density (refer to arrow)

particularly if other risk factors are present (Buckwalter et al., 2013). Examples of physical activities that involve repetitive overuse and impact loading on the joint include squatting, kneeling and heavy lifting, working in cramped spaces, and stair climbing (Richmond et al., 2013).

Rheumatoid arthritis pathophysiology

Rheumatoid arthritis is a progressive autoimmune disease. The autoimmune response seen in RA causes normal antibodies to become autoantibodies (such as rheumatoid factor), which then attack host tissues. Unlike OA, the joint damage seen in RA starts in the synovial membrane. The autoimmune response causes leukocytes and inflammatory mediators (IL-1 and TNF-α) to infiltrate the normally thin synovial membrane in a process that also stimulates the growth of new blood vessels (angiogenesis). The end result of this very complex process is hypertrophy of the synovial membrane and the formation of fibrovascular tissue known as pannus. As it grows, the pannus calcifies, and starts to invade and erode nearby articular cartilage and bone (see Figure 13.3). As in OA, chondrocytes are stimulated to produce metalloproteinases, which further contribute to cartilage degradation. Inflammatory cytokines also trigger an increase in the activity of cells that reabsorb bone (osteoclasts). All of this inflammatory activity also results in increased amounts of synovial fluid within the affected joint (Choy, 2012; Gibofsky, 2012).

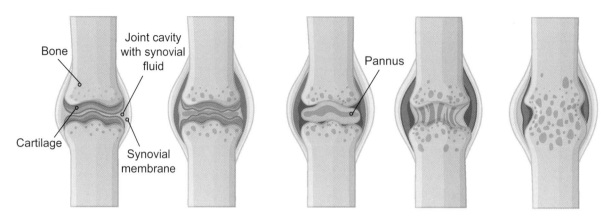

Figure 13.3　Stages of joint deterioration in RA (from left to right): healthy joint, synovitis, pannus, fibrous ankylosis and bony ankylosis

Clinical manifestations and diagnosis of rheumatoid arthritis

Where OA may only affect a few joints, or even a single joint, and is often asymmetrical, RA usually progresses to involve five or more joints and is typically symmetrical in nature. The joints of the hands, wrists and feet are the most likely to be affected in the earlier stages, with the larger synovial joints becoming involved as the disease progresses. Unlike OA, RA is associated with alternating periods of exacerbation and remission, the length of which varies from person to person (Firth, 2011). The cartilage and joint destruction caused by RA results in joint manifestations that include swelling, stiffness, pain, deformity and loss of function. As in OA, this stiffness tends to be worse in the morning or after long periods of inactivity (Walker, 2012). Several characteristic joint deformities are seen in RA (see Figure 13.4), and these occur as a direct result of the ongoing destruction of the joint capsule and surrounding ligaments and tendons. Pain, swelling and stiffness result in decreased use of the affected joint and the subsequent loss of surrounding muscle mass, further reducing function. As the pannus extends through the joint space, complete immobility may occur (Bullock & Hales, 2012).

The systemic effects seen in RA further differentiate it from OA. General systemic manifestations are caused by a systemic inflammatory response and include fatigue, anorexia, weight loss, and generalised aching and stiffness (Walker, 2012). Other, more organ-specific extra-articular manifestations may also occur, particularly in individuals with high levels of circulating rheumatoid factor. Some examples include the development of subcutaneous rheumatoid nodules in areas of the body subject to pressure, anaemia, pericarditis and pleural effusions (Vela, 2014; Walker, 2012). These systemic manifestations can be debilitating, and they contribute to the significant morbidity and mortality associated with RA (Choy, 2012; Firth, 2011). Of particular note is the increasing body of evidence that has identified RA as a very strong risk factor for the development of cardiovascular disease. It is thought that the ongoing systemic inflammatory response associated with RA contributes to the development of atherosclerosis (Palmer & El Miedany, 2013).

Like OA, diagnosis is made primarily on the basis of the presence of these clinical manifestations on physical examination and interview. Other criteria for diagnosis include the presence of changes to joints on X-ray that are not consistent with OA and a positive serum rheumatoid factor test (Gibofsky, 2012).

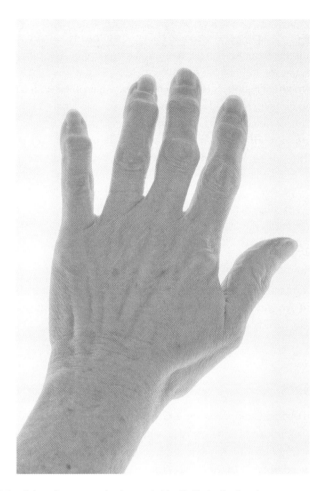

Figure 13.4   Joint deformity as seen in rheumatoid arthritis in the hands

Risk factors for rheumatoid arthritis

Non-modifiable risk factors for RA include increasing age, female gender and a genetic susceptibility (Gibofsky, 2012). Cigarette smoking has been clearly identified as the strongest modifiable risk factor for RA. It is thought that it plays a role in the development of immune system dysfunction early in the course of the disease. Obesity has also been identified as a risk factor, although the link is not as clear as with smoking. A possible explanation for this association is the initiation of pro-inflammatory mediators by adipose tissue (Gerlag, Norris & Tak, 2015).

SKILLS IN PRACTICE

Differentiating between osteoarthritis and rheumatoid arthritis

Bruce is a 53-year-old builder from the Otago Peninsula, New Zealand. In his youth, Bruce was the star fullback for his local rugby team. He has presented to his local medical centre complaining of worsening pain and stiffness in both hands and knees. He states that these symptoms have been troubling him 'on and off' for the last few years. Lately, however, his symptoms have worsened in that the pain is now daily, and this is starting to affect his work. He explains that the pain in his knees is made worse by the repeated bending required in his day-to-day work activities. He also notices the pain more when climbing ladders or stairs, although it does ease with rest. In his hands, the joints most affected by the pain and stiffness are the middle and end finger joints. The stiffness in his knees and hands is always worse for the first half hour after he wakes up. On examination, minimal swelling is noted. Bruce is an otherwise fit, healthy man, with no significant medical history. He has recently started taking ibuprofen and paracetamol for his pain.

QUESTIONS
1. What is the most likely diagnosis for Bruce's joint complaints?
2. How is the diagnosis supported by the clinical picture? In your answer, demonstrate that you clearly understand the underlying pathophysiology, clinical manifestations and possible risk factors.

Osteoporosis

In addition to arthritis, osteoporosis is a chronic, systemic, musculoskeletal condition that presents a significant health burden on the community. The condition causes bones to weaken and become fragile in such a way that even a minor trauma can cause the affected bone to break. Osteoporosis mainly affects people over the age of 50, with 66 per cent of osteoporosis-related hip fractures worldwide occurring in women and 33 per cent in men (AIHW, 2014). In relation to mortality, while not a direct cause of death, the fractures attributed to this disease have been reported to cause premature death, particularly in the elderly. As Australia and New Zealand are ageing populations, an increasing number of Australian and New Zealand people are at risk of developing osteoporosis and sustaining a fracture (AIHW, 2014; Osteoporosis New Zealand, 2015).

Pathophysiology of osteoporosis

Osteoporosis is a metabolic bone disorder in which significant loss of bone mineral density causes the bones to become fragile and brittle, resulting in an increased risk of fractures in the affected bones (Bullock & Hales, 2012). Healthy bone tissue constantly undergoes a remodelling process in which old bone tissue is broken down and reabsorbed by cells called osteoclasts and new bone is formed by cells called osteoblasts. In osteoporosis, there is an imbalance between these two processes in favour of bone destruction due to increased osteoclast activity. Osteoblast activity decreases with age, resulting in decreased formation of new bone, while several factors increase osteoclast activity and bone loss (see Figure 13.5). These include a reduction in the hormone oestrogen, increased levels of corticosteroids and inadequate intake of calcium or vitamin D (International Osteoporosis Foundation, 2015).

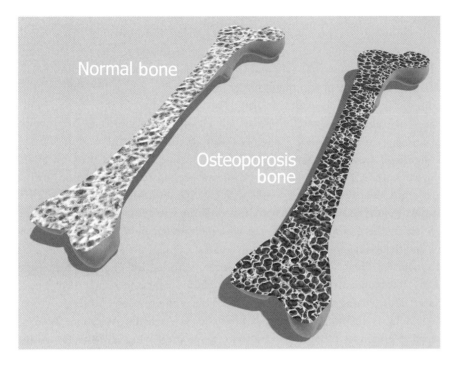

Figure 13.5   Bone tissue degradation seen in osteoporosis

Clinical manifestations and diagnosis of osteoporosis

Osteoporosis is an asymptomatic condition. Insidious pathophysiological changes occur, and in some people a diagnosis will not be made until a fracture is sustained. Common sites for the appearance of osteoporotic fractures are those that are exposed to more stress and include weight-bearing joints such as the hips, pelvis and spine. Bones such as the wrists and forearms are also more prone to fractures as they are frequently used to break falls. As stated earlier, these fractures tend to result from injuries that would not normally cause fractures in people with healthy bones. Diagnosis is based on the assessment of risk factors, clinical examination and the use of medical imaging to measure bone mineral density scanning (Bullock & Hales, 2012).

Risk factors for osteoporosis

There are a number of modifiable and non-modifiable risk factors that can increase the development of osteoporosis. Examples include increasing age, physical inactivity, a familial history of the condition, smoking, reduced calcium intake and long-term steroid use (Osteoporosis Australia Medical and Scientific Advisory Committee, 2015).

Promoting health and reducing risk

The pain and other clinical manifestations of arthritis have the potential to be debilitating. Arthritis is currently one of the leading causes of chronic pain, disability and lost productivity in Australia and New Zealand (Arthritis Australia, 2015b; Bevan, Gunning & Thomas, 2012). The financial burden of arthritis has been discussed earlier in this chapter. This burden is predicted to increase drastically in the future as the population ages and the prevalence of obesity continues to rise. In 2002, the Australian government underlined arthritis and other musculoskeletal conditions as a national health priority. This has resulted in the development of a number of frameworks and initiatives, all of which are aimed at improving and standardising the prevention, detection and treatment of these conditions. This national focus is at the macro level of the Innovative Care for Chronic Conditions Framework (ICCCF), which aims to provide an overall structure to guide health care provision to meet the needs of people with OA, RA and osteoporosis (World Health Organization (WHO), 2002). Despite this ongoing work, there is strong evidence to suggest that there is a significant gap between current best practice recommendations and the management of arthritis in Australia (Australian Commission on Safety and Quality in Health Care, 2017). Problems identified include delays in diagnosis and the commencement of treatment, fragmented care and a lack of psychosocial support. This has led to the development of the Time to Move Strategy, which was launched by Arthritis Australia in March 2014 (Arthritis Australia, 2014). This strategy is aimed at providing a framework for improving all aspects of care for people with arthritis, and contains several key primary prevention and health promotion strategies that address the modifiable risk factors discussed earlier (Arthritis Australia, 2015b). A recent review into the impact of chronic musculoskeletal disorders on New Zealand's workforce has highlighted the need for the implementation of a similar strategy (Bevan et al., 2012).

The key priorities identified by Arthritis Australia are the promotion of a healthy lifestyle and early detection. Maintaining a healthy weight, engaging in regular exercise, injury avoidance and smoking cessation have been universally identified as playing significant roles in the prevention of the onset of all types of arthritis. Specifically, conservative estimates project that up to 70 per cent of OA cases could be prevented through weight loss and injury prevention (Arthritis Australia, 2014). As well as reducing the incidence of arthritis, these measures may also limit disease severity and delay progression, leading to improved patient outcomes and quality of life (Agency for Clinical Innovation, 2012). Early detection is important in all types of arthritis, particularly RA. Research indicates that aggressive treatment in the early stages of the condition can limit severity, progression and subsequent disability (Walker, 2012). Specific strategies that will address these priorities include public awareness campaigns, particularly in relation to modifiable risk factors, and targeted programs aimed at weight reduction and injury prevention.

Additional health promotion and prevention strategies specifically targeted towards osteoporosis include re-fracture prevention and falls prevention. It is very important that those people over the age of 50 who do sustain a fracture receive adequate investigation to prevent further re-fracture. This strategy requires a multidisciplinary approach, including nutritional assessment for calcium intake and general nutrition, and rehabilitation that focuses on physiotherapy and exercise. Of particular importance is falls risk assessment. It is estimated that up to 90 per cent of hip fractures are caused by falls (Osteoporosis Australia, 2014).

The nurse's role in the management of arthritis and musculoskeletal conditions

Two of the main discrepancies between current best practice recommendations and actual clinical practice in relation to arthritis management have been the heavy reliance on non-conservative interventions (pharmacological and surgical), and a tendency towards the delivery of episodic and fragmented care (Agency for Clinical Innovation, 2012). The Time to Move Strategy recommends the implementation of more conservative treatments such as non-pharmacological pain relief and weight reduction, and the increased involvement of the multidisciplinary team (Arthritis Australia, 2015b). Nurses working in all settings have an opportunity to play a key role in the implementation of these changes through the provision of education, support for self-management and participation in the multidisciplinary team.

A recent report commissioned by Australia has identified a clear need for the expansion of the rheumatology nurse workforce. International research has indicated that access to a rheumatology nurse results in improved education and psychosocial care, along with reduced waiting time to see a specialist and improved coordination of care, all of which result in improved outcomes for people rheumatoid and other forms of inflammatory arthritis. This is important in both Australia and New Zealand where it can be difficult to gain timely access to specialist rheumatology care, particularly in rural and remote areas. The report identifies a number of potential areas for growth in the rheumatology nursing workforce, including increased roles for rheumatology nurse practitioners, improved training for nurses who want to specialise in the field, and expansion of the role of the specialist rheumatology nurse in the public and private sectors (Australian Health Care and Hospitals Association, 2017).

As mentioned earlier in relation to osteoporosis, it is vitally important that preventing further secondary fractures is a priority. One recent innovation requiring significant coordination by the nurse is secondary fracture prevention services. These services are directed to patients who have suffered a minimal trauma fracture due to osteoporosis, as these people have a greater risk of sustaining a subsequent fracture. Secondary fracture prevention services are normally delivered by a clinical nurse specialist, who identifies patients with osteoporotic fractures as either orthopaedic in-patients or outpatients managed in a fracture clinic. The nurse initiates treatment for the prevention of subsequent fractures and recommends falls prevention services if appropriate (Osteoporosis Australia, 2015).

REFLECTION

Gaps between current best practice and the actual management of arthritis in the community have necessitated the implementation of the Time to Move Strategy. Can you identify possible reasons for why this gap exists?

Education and support for self-care management

The provision of education regarding arthritis and osteoporosis, and the associated risk factors are essential components of the primary prevention and health promotion strategies discussed earlier in this chapter. Education is also essential in the provision of the support that people with these conditions and their carer networks require to improve the knowledge and skills needed to effectively manage their condition. As discussed throughout this book, self-care management is a model of care that acknowledges the major role of the person in taking responsibility for their own health promotion, disease prevention and management of their chronic condition. When used effectively, self-care management not only reduces the burden on health services, but also improves people's health outcomes and quality of life (De Silva, 2011).

The provision of education and support takes place in a variety of settings. For example, community nurses are more likely to be involved in the implementation of primary prevention and health promotion strategies, and the ongoing monitoring of patients, while nurses working in the hospital setting are more likely to come into contact with people who are experiencing exacerbation of their arthritis symptoms or following joint replacement surgery for osteoarthritis. Effective management of arthritis and other musculoskeletal conditions involves a number of interventions that can be delivered by members of the multidisciplinary team. There is great potential for nurses to improve coordination of care, therefore decreasing the fragmentation identified earlier by them acting as a central point of reference for the patient and making appropriate and timely referrals to allied health professionals, such as physiotherapists, occupational therapists and podiatrists (Bender, Connelly & Brown, 2013).

REFLECTION

Traditionally, there has been a heavy emphasis on the medical model for providing a framework for managing arthritic conditions. Why are contemporary models of care, such as the ICCCF, which encompass a holistic approach, more likely to be beneficial?

Advanced nursing practice for arthritis and musculoskeletal conditions

Within the realm of chronic care, there exist a number of opportunities for nurses wishing to extend their capabilities. As discussed in this chapter, the burden of arthritis-related conditions is only expected to increase, thus placing more demand on already overloaded health services. The management of chronic conditions such as OA, RA and osteoporosis is best achieved using a holistic approach with emphasis placed on the multidisciplinary team (Arthritis Australia, 2015b; Osteoporosis Australia, 2014). This has created opportunities for primary health care nurses in terms of advanced nursing practice that focuses on health promotion, education, self-care management and preventative health within the domain of musculoskeletal conditions. One recent development that extends the nursing role for the primary health care nurse is the implementation of chronic disease nurse clinics. These clinics facilitate a nurse-led model of care for chronic conditions within general practice. As well as advanced skills in assessment and health promotion, this role requires strong leadership and business skills, as well as an environment that is supportive (Arthritis Australia, 2015b).

SKILLS IN PRACTICE

Care of the individual with rheumatoid arthritis

Carol Jones is a 54-year-old accountant who has been admitted to the surgical ward you are working on following an umbilical hernia repair. Carol was diagnosed with rheumatoid arthritis eight years ago. She tells you that she has severe pain and stiffness in both hands, wrists and elbows. You also note obvious swelling in these areas. She states that the pain is constant, that it is slightly worse in the mornings and rates it between 6 and 8 out of 10. Carol takes oral prednisone on and off but has opted not to take Methotrexate due to the unpleasant side effects. She takes ibuprofen regularly in an attempt to manage the pain. A bone density test has also revealed that Carol has osteoporosis.

QUESTIONS

1. Carol has RA. What assessment findings from the case study differentiate this condition from OA?

2. People with RA have a significantly increased risk of developing osteoporosis. What is the underlying pathophysiological link between the two conditions?

3. It is apparent that Carol is experiencing difficulties managing the pain and other symptoms caused by RA. What strategies could be put in place to help her manage her condition better?

4. Identify and explain health promotion strategies to reduce the risk of Carol sustaining a fracture.

SUMMARY

Learning objective 1: Recognise the biopsychosocial impact arthritis has on the individual as well as the community.

The biopsychosocial impact of arthritis and musculoskeletal conditions is considerable. For example, arthritis is a significant contributor to disability because it limits physical activity, subsequently affecting the quality of life of those affected. In addition, the economic burden of this group of diseases on the Australian and New Zealand health systems is enormous.

Learning objective 2: Understand the underlying pathophysiology, and associated modifiable and non-modifiable risk factors relating to OA, RA and osteoporosis.

Osteoarthritis was traditionally thought to be a non-inflammatory disorder caused by simple wear and tear that primarily affected the articular cartilage. It is now understood that the underlying pathophysiology is much more complex, with a definite inflammatory component and the potential to involve all parts of the joint. In contrast, rheumatoid arthritis is a progressive, autoimmune disease in which joint damage starts in the synovial membrane before progressing to other parts of the joint. Systemic effects are also associated with this condition. Osteoporosis is a metabolic disorder in which significant loss of bone mineral density causes the bones to become fragile and brittle, resulting in increased risk of fractures.

Learning objective 3: Identify and discuss health prevention, and promote strategies relevant to these conditions.

Key priorities that have been identified include the promotion of a healthy lifestyle and early detection. Maintaining a healthy weight, engaging in regular exercise, injury avoidance and smoking cessation have been universally identified as playing a significant role in the prevention of the onset of all types of arthritis and musculoskeletal conditions.

Learning objective 4: Highlight the nurse's role in the collaborative management of these conditions.

Nurses working in all settings have the opportunity to play a key role in the collaborative management of chronic musculoskeletal conditions through the provision of education, support for self-care management and participation in the multidisciplinary team.

Learning objective 5: Discuss opportunities for advanced nursing practice in relation to arthritis and osteoporosis.

Workforce projections suggest that general practice will be unable to cope with increasing demand for doctors' visits associated with many chronic conditions such as arthritis and osteoporosis. This has created opportunities for primary health care nurses in terms of advanced nursing practice, with the creation of nurse-led clinics that focus on health promotion, education, self-care management and preventative health.

REVIEW QUESTIONS

1. Write a summary that highlights the reasons why OA, RA and osteoporosis present such significant health and economic burdens both to individuals and the community.
2. Demonstrate you understand the difference in the pathophysiology underlying the conditions discussed in this chapter.

3. Why have the Australian and New Zealand governments emphasised arthritis as being a national health priority?

4. How can nurses play a key role in relation to the management of chronic musculoskeletal conditions?

5. From a primary health care perspective, what opportunities exist for those nurses who wish to extend their scope of practice?

RESEARCH TOPIC

Many people will try a range of complementary and alternative therapies to help manage the pain, stiffness and other symptoms associated with arthritis and musculoskeletal conditions. Complementary therapies are those treatments or therapies that are outside conventional medical or surgical therapy. Some examples include massage, acupuncture and herbal medicines (Arthritis Australia, 2015a). The use of complementary therapies is controversial – some therapies may have good scientific evidence to support their use, but others may not. It is always important to ask patients about their use of other therapies, especially those that may interact with prescribed medications. Below is a list of oral supplements. Conduct your own review of the literature to determine the levels of evidence in relation to the efficacy of:

- green-lipped mussel
- curcumin
- rose hip
- chondroitin
- fish oil
- glucosamine sulphate.

FURTHER READING

Ackerman, I. N., Bohensky, M. A., Pratt, C., Gorelik, A. & Liew, D. (2016). *Counting the Cost Part 1: The Current and Future Burden of Arthritis*. Retrieved from https://arthritisaustralia.com.au/wordpress/wp-content/uploads/2017/09/Final-Counting-the-Costs_Part1_MAY2016.pdf

Arthritis Australia. (2017). Complementary therapies. Retrieved from https://arthritisaustralia.com.au/wordpress/wp-content/uploads/2018/02/ComplementaryTherapies_0118.pdf

Australian Healthcare and Hospitals Association. (2017). *Rheumatology Nurses: Adding Value to Arthritis Care*. Retrieved from https://arthritisaustralia.com.au/wordpress/wp-content/uploads/2017/09/Literature_review_-_Rheumatology_nurses_in_Australia_FINAL_22_Sept_2017-1.pdf

Brand, C., Ackerman, I. & Tropea, J. (2014). Chronic disease management: Improving care for people with osteoarthritis. *Best Practice & Research Clinical Rheumatology*, 28, 119–42.

Palmer, D. & El Miedany, Y. (2013). From guidelines to clinical practice: Cardiovascular risk management in inflammatory arthritis patients. *British Journal of Community Nursing*, 18(9), 424–8.

REFERENCES

Ackerman, I. N., Bohensky, M. A., Pratt, C., Gorelik, A. & Liew, D. (2016). *Counting the Cost Part 1: The Current and Future Burden of Arthritis.* Retrieved from https://arthritisaustralia.com.au/wordpress/wp-content/uploads/2017/09/Final-Counting-the-Costs_Part1_MAY2016.pdf

Agency for Clinical Innovation. (2012). Musculoskeletal network osteoarthritis Chronic care program model of care. Retrieved from www.aci.health.nsw.gov.au/__data/assets/pdf_file/0020/165305/Osteoarthritis-Chronic-Care-Program-Mode-of-Care.pdf

Anderson, A. S. & Loeser, R. F. (2010). Why is osteoarthritis an age related disease? *Best Practice and Research Clinical Rheumatology,* 24(1), 15–26, doi: http://10.1016/j.berh.2009.06.006

Antonelli, M. & Starz, T. (2012). Assessing for risk and progression of osteoarthritis: The nurse's role: Understanding pathophysiology, epidemiology and risk will aid nurses who are seeking to expand their role in management. *Orthopaedic Nursing,* 31(2), 98–102.

Arthritis Australia. (2014). *Time to Move: Arthritis Reports.* Retrieved from www.arthritisaustralia.com.au/index.php/reports/time-to-move-arthritis-reports.html

——(2015a). Complementary therapies. Retrieved from www.arthritisaustralia.com.au/images/stories/documents/info_sheets/2015/Complementary%20therapies/ComplementaryTherapies.pdf

——(2015b). *Osteoarthritis Nurse Clinics: A Resource for Primary Health Care Nurses.* Retrieved from www.apna.asn.au/lib/pdf/Resources/P5%5Bm%5DOsteoarthritis Resource_GML.pdf

Arthritis New Zealand. (2015). Forms of arthritis. Retrieved from www.arthritis.org.r3/information/forms-of-arthritis

Arthritis and Osteoporosis Victoria. (2013). *A Problem Worth Solving: The Rising Cost of Musculoskeletal Conditions in Australia.* Melbourne: Arthritis and Osteoporosis Victoria.

Australian Commission on Safety and Quality in Health Care. (2017). *Osteoarthritis of the Knee Clinical Care Standard.* Retrieved from www.safetyandquality.gov.au/wp-content/uploads/2017/05/Osteoarthritis-of-the-Knee-Clinical-Care-Standard-Booklet.pdf

Australian Institute of Health and Welfare (AIHW). (2014). *Arthritis and Other Musculoskeletal Conditions Across the Life Stages. Arthritis Series No. 18.* PHE 173. Canberra: AIHW.

Bender, M., Connelly, C. D. & Brown, C. (2013). Interdisciplinary collaboration: The role of the clinical nurse leader. *Journal of Nursing Management,* 21, 165–74.

Berenbaum, F. (2013). Osteoarthritis as an inflammatory disease (osteoarthritis is not osteoarthrosis!). *Osteoarthritis and Cartilage,* 21, 16–21.

Bevan, S., Gunning, N. & Thomas, R. (2012). Fit for work? Musculoskeletal disorders and the New Zealand labour market. Retrieved from www.arthritis.org.nz/wp-content/uploads/2012/09/fitforwork.pdf

Bijlsma, J. W., Berenbaum, F. & Lafeber, F. P. (2011). Osteoarthritis: An update with relevance for clinical practice. *The Lancet,* 377, 2115–26.

Bruyere, O., Cooper, C., Arden, N., Branco, J., Brandi, M. L., Herrero-Beaumont, G., ... & Reginster, J.-Y. (2015). Can we identify patients with high risk of osteoarthritis progression which will respond to treatment? A focus on epidemiology and phenotype of osteoarthritis. *Drugs & Aging*, 32, 179–87. doi: http://10.1007/s40266-015-0243-3

Buckwalter, J. A., Anderson, D. D., Brown, T. D., Tochigi, Y. & Martin J. A. (2013). The roles of mechanical stresses in the pathogenesis of osteoarthritis: Implications for treatment of joint injuries. *Cartilage*, 4(4), 286–94. doi: http://10.1177/19476035 13495889

Bullock, S. & Hales, M. (2012). *Principles of Pathophysiology*. Sydney: Pearson.

Choy, E. (2012). Understanding the dynamics: Pathways involved in the pathogenesis of rheumatoid arthritis. *Rheumatology*, 51(Suppl. 5), v3–11. doi: http://10.1093/rheumatology/kes113

De Silva, D. (2011). *Evidence: Helping People Help Themselves*. London: Health Foundation.

Deloitte Access Economics. (2018) *The Economic Cost of Arthritis in New Zealand in 2018*. Retrieved from www2.deloitte.com/content/dam/Deloitte/nz/Documents/Economics/dae-economic-cost-arthritis-nz-2018-v2.pdf

Firth, J. (2011). Rheumatoid arthritis: Diagnosis and multi-disciplinary management. *British Journal of Nursing*, 20(18), 11.

Garvin, J., Leung, K. D. & Kean, W. F. (2013). Osteoarthritis of the hand 1: Aetiology and pathogenesis, risk factors, investigation and diagnosis. *Journal of Pharmacy and Pharmacology*, 66, 339–46. doi: http://10.111/php.12196

Gerlag, D. M., Norris, J. M. & Tak, P. P. (2015). Rheumatology. doi: http://10.1093/rheumatology/ kev347

Gibofsky, A. (2012). Overview of epidemiology, pathophysiology and diagnosis of rheumatoid arthritis. *American Journal of Managed Care*, 18(13), S295–302.

Goldring, M. B. & Otero, M. (2011). Inflammation in osteoarthritis. *Current Opinion in Rheumatology*, 23(5), 471–8. doi: http://10.1097/BOR.0b013e328349c2b1

Hoff, P., Buttgereit, F., Burmester, G.-R., Jakstadt, K., Gaber, T., Andreas, K., … & Rohner, E. (2013). Osteoarthritis synovial fluid activates pro-inflammatory cytokines in primary human chondrocytes. *International Orthopaedics*, 37, 145–51. doi: http://10.1007/s00264-012-1724-1

International Osteoporosis Foundation. (2015). Pathophysiology: Biological causes of osteoporosis. Retrieved from www.iofbonehealth.org/pathophysiology-biological-causes-osteoporosis

New Zealand Ministry of Health (NZMOH). (2018). *Arthritis*. Retrieved from www.health.govt.nz/your-health/conditions-and-treatments/diseases-and-illnesses/arthritis

Osteoporosis Australia. (2014). What you need to know about osteoporosis. . Retrieved from www.osteoporosis.org.au/sites/default/files/files/oa_medical_brochure_2nd_ed.pdf

—— (2015). Refracture prevention. Retrieved from www.osteoporosis.org.au/refracture-prevention

Osteoporosis Australia Medical and Scientific Advisory Committee. (2015). Risk factors. Retrieved from www.osteoporosis.org.au/risk-factors

Osteoporosis New Zealand. (2015). What is osteoporosis? Retrieved from https://osteoporosis.org.nz/osteoporosis-fractures/what-is-osteoporosis

Palmer, D. & El Miedany, Y. (2013). From guidelines to clinical practice: Cardiovascular risk management in inflammatory arthritis patients. *British Journal of Community Nursing*, 18(9), 424–8.

Richmond, S. A., Fukuchi, R. K., Ezzat, A., Schneider, K., Schneider, G. & Emery, C. A. (2013). Are joint injury, sport activity, physical activity, obesity, or occupation activities predictors for osteoarthritis? A systematic review. *Journal of Orthopaedic & Physical Therapy*, 43(8), 515–24. doi: http://10.2529/jospt.2013.4796

Sovani, S. & Grogan, S. P. (2013). Osteoarthritis: Detection, pathophysiology, and current/ future treatment strategies. *Orthopaedic Nursing*, 32(1), 25–36.

Vela, P. (2014). Extra-articular manifestations of rheumatoid arthritis, now. *Emergency Medical Journal Rheumatology*, 1, 103–12.

Walker, J. (2012). Rheumatoid arthritis: Role of the nurse and multidisciplinary team. *British Journal of Nursing*, 21(6), 334–9.

World Health Organization (WHO). (2002) *Innovative Care for Chronic Conditions: Building Blocks for Action*. Retrieved from www.who.int/chp/knowledge/publications/icccglobalreport.pdf?ua=1

Chronic obesity

Amali Hohol, Julia Gilbert and Melissa Johnston

LEARNING OBJECTIVES

After studying this chapter, you should be able to:

1. comprehend the underlying pathophysiology of chronic obesity and the associated risk factors
2. describe strategies that promote health and reduce risk for individuals who are overweight and obese
3. understand the nurse's role in the management of the chronically obese individual
4. appreciate the impact chronic obesity has on the future of health care
5. recognise the importance of advanced nursing practice in the management of obesity.

Introduction

The worldwide prevalence of chronic obesity is rising. In Australia approximately 60 per cent of adults and 25 per cent of children were classified as either overweight or obese (Grima & Dixon, 2013), and in New Zealand one in three adults over the age of 15 years and one in eight children aged between 2−14 years were considered obese (New Zealand Ministry of Health (NZMOH), 2018). The public health burden of obesity is significant as it is closely associated with other chronic conditions, including cardiovascular disease and diabetes mellitus (Schuklenk & Zhang, 2014). Chronic obesity not only has physical implications for the individual – excess weight is closely associated with a reduced quality of life, and an increased risk of morbidity and mortality (Grima & Dixon, 2013).

The nursing workforce spans across a range of clinical settings which place nurses at the forefront of promoting health and reducing the development of obesity. To successfully treat chronic obesity, a person-centred model of care must be followed that aligns with chronic disease management and has the expectation of meeting a variety of health outcomes, not solely weight reduction (Grima & Dixon, 2013). To ensure that care is optimal, nursing interventions should align with the guiding principles of the Innovative Care for Chronic Conditions Framework (ICCCF), including evidence-based decision making, preventative care, and quality and systematic care.

This chapter is aimed at educating nurses and other health professionals about the management of chronic obesity. The underlying pathogenesis of this disease process will be explored, and the associated risk factors identified. Health promotion and prevention strategies that are being utilised in contemporary nursing practice will be discussed, in addition to how nurses can care for obese individuals in different health care environments. The chapter will highlight the potential future impact that this chronic condition may have, as well as provide an overview of the key concepts of advanced nursing practice.

The development of obesity

Obesity is defined as an excessive accumulation of adipose tissue with potentially negative health consequences (Townsend & Scriven, 2014). The development of this chronic obesity involves mechanisms concerning appetite regulation and energy homeostasis. A thorough understanding of the underlying pathological processes involved in chronic obesity enables the development of advanced treatment methods (Shukla, Moreira & Rubino, 2013). The development of obesity occurs progressively and is the result of energy intake exceeding energy expenditure. It is important to understand that a small increase in daily calorie intake can, over time, significantly increase body weight (Baqai & Wilding, 2015).

Hormonal control

The central nervous system regulates both appetite and energy use, and these processes involve complex hormone control. Signals arising from adipose tissue, the pancreas and the gastrointestinal tract will influence feelings of hunger or fullness in an individual. These signals will travel to the hypothalamus and brainstem, and directly or indirectly relay information to the mesolimbic dopamine pathways to influence food intake (Zhang et al., 2014). The ability to gain weight in adulthood may be attributed to alterations to these mechanisms, thus preventing weight loss and subsequently contributing to the development of obesity (Baqai & Wilding, 2015).

Short-term food regulation involves the release of gastrointestinal hormones, including ghrelin and postprandial hormones (such as cholecystokinin, pancreatic polypeptide and glucagon-like peptide-1), which assist in regulating appetite. Ghrelin, the 'hunger hormone', is a peptide hormone which is secreted by the stomach between meals and stimulates food intake. Ghrelin is a significant hormone in the development of obesity as it not only stimulates the release of growth hormone, but also is associated with long-term energy balance since it is released in response to exercise-induced weight loss or reduced calorie intake to protect against lengthy periods of decreased energy production (Cheung, Pucci & Batterham, 2015). Ghrelin production is reduced following a meal when postprandial hormones are released. Postprandial hormones relay signals to the brain to encourage feelings of fullness and cease hunger signals (Baqai & Wilding, 2015) by directly influencing the brain or indirectly acting on the vagus (Rajeev & Wilding, 2015). However, ghrelin can also influence the drive to overeat through the increased consumption of palatable foods, which results in eating in excess of metabolic demand (Howick et al., 2017).

Leptin and insulin regulate long-term appetite and satiety (Zhang et al., 2014). Leptin is an amino acid peptide which is produced by adipocytes (fat cells) and is required to maintain energy balance by reducing appetite-inducing neurons. If there is a reduction of leptin or leptin receptors, hyperphagia will occur, leading to increased calorie intake. Leptin resistance is commonly observed in the obese individual and is the result of dysfunctional leptin receptors, and/or the inability of leptin to enter the interstitial fluid of the brain. Leptin resistance also increases the storage of fat in tissues outside of adipose tissue (Shukla, Moreira & Rubino, 2013). Glucose maintenance requires secretion of the hormone insulin by the pancreas. When there is excess glucose in the body, it is stored in the liver, the muscles or adipose tissue as fat. Insulin and leptin can influence the dopaminergic pathways of the brain and eating patterns. Insulin resistance, similar to leptin-receptor resistance, may also result in an increased intake of palatable foods due to their influence on the dopaminergic reward centre, thereby contributing to the development of the obese person (Zhang et al., 2014).

Leptin – an amino acid that reduces appetite.

Metabolic control

Energy expenditure is related to **basal metabolic rate (BMR)**, **dietary thermogenesis** and physical activity (Rajeev & Wilding, 2015). Basal metabolic rate is the amount of energy required to carry out regular metabolic functions (Baqai & Wilding, 2015) and accounts for 60–70 per cent of total energy expenditure. Dietary thermogenesis refers to the quantity of energy used to digest and store food (Baqai & Wilding, 2015), and represents up to 10 per cent of total energy expenditure (Rajeev & Wilding, 2015). For foods that are high in fat, the degree of dietary thermogenesis is lower than for foods that are rich in carbohydrates, while protein-rich foods have a level of dietary thermogenic action that exceeds high carbohydrate foods (Baqai & Wilding, 2015). In part, this may explain why diets that are high in fats lead to weight gain (Rajeev & Wilding, 2015). People with obesity require significantly greater levels of energy for physical activity and

Basal metabolic rate (BMR) – the level of energy required to keep the body functioning normally.

Dietary thermogenesis – the level of energy required to digest and store food.

sedentary behaviours than non-obese individuals due to their increased body mass (Baqai & Wilding, 2015). Table 14.1 describes the most common causes of chronic obesity and how they contribute to the development of this condition.

Table 14.1 The most common causes of chronic obesity

Risk factors	Description
Diet	• Consumption of energy-dense foods without balance of energy output • Higher satiety response with high fat/sugar foods
Socioecological factors	• Poor environment can disrupt the homeostatic control of food regulation • Social pressures and food marketing increase the consumption of high-energy diets • Increased risk of obesity with low socioeconomic groups due to the availability of more affordable, energy-dense foods
Depression	• Depressed individuals may also partake in 'comfort eating' in response to psychological stress
Physical inactivity	• A reduction in physical activity reduces energy expenditure
Binge eating disorders (BEDs)	• Consumption of large quantities of food without subsequent purging • Food addiction associated with BEDs is a common occurrence in adulthood
Medications	• Specific medications lead to weight gain by disrupting the effects of the central nervous system on appetite • Medications can affect metabolic function resulting in weight gain
Other health conditions	• Prader-Willi syndrome – a genetic disorder characterised by extreme hyperphagia in childhood • Hypothyroidism – reduced thyroid gland activity which slows metabolic function • Physical disability – physical limitations (resulting from previous injury or disease) create a barrier to involvement in physical activity • Cushing's syndrome – growth hormone deficiency can lead to reduced lean body mass and increased body fat • Obesity can be a characteristic of polycystic ovarian syndrome

Sources: Baqai & Wilding (2015); Rajeev & Wilding (2015); Zhang et al. (2014)

There are a number of methods that can be used to measure obesity. Two commonly used methods include abdominal circumference measurement, and the body mass index (BMI) — a weight-for-height calculation which determines weight status (Townsend & Scriven, 2014). However, the limitation of a BMI measurement is that it fails to consider additional factors that can influence weight, including gender, age, bone structure, fat distribution and muscle mass (Schuklenk & Zhang, 2014), and is therefore an inaccurate reflection of adiposity (Townsend & Scriven, 2014). Abdominal circumference measurements, which indicate central obesity, are considered a more accurate reflection of total body fat (Townsend & Scriven, 2014). This specific type of obesity measurement takes into consideration not only the degree of adipose tissue which is present but also where the fat is distributed, and suggests that greater levels of adipose tissue around the mid-section are linked to poorer health outcomes (Rossen & Rossen, 2012).

SKILLS IN PRACTICE

Living with obesity

Sharon is a 54-year-old woman who was admitted to an orthopaedic ward with a fractured ankle following a fall at home. She is 152 cm tall, weighs 110 kg and works behind the ticket counter at the local cinema complex. Sharon suffers from chronic hypertension and frequently experiences shortness of breath on minimal exertion.

Sharon has had a BMI of more than 30 since early childhood and has been unable to lose weight despite many attempts over the years. She has tried fad diets and crash dieting and on one occasion lost 10 kg. Yet the weight rebounded past her baseline weight when she stopped the diet, and she has become progressively heavier over the past five years.

Sharon does not exercise and leads a sedentary life both at home and at work. Her daughter, Jacinta, came to visit Sharon in hospital and approached the nursing staff to request information about strategies to help Sharon better manage her weight. Sharon was at first upset that Jacinta had raised this issue with the nursing staff; however, she was willing to 'give it a go' as she understood the long-term implications her weight could have on her health and wellbeing.

A person-centred management plan was designed for Sharon which focused on following the *Australian Dietary Guidelines* (National Health and Medical Research Council (NMHRC), 2013a) and gently increasing Sharon's level of physical activity. This process was carried out in conjunction with Fiona, a clinical nurse specialist from the community nursing team. Fiona has worked with many obese and overweight clients, and has a thorough understanding of the emotional and physical struggle chronic obesity presents to individuals.

Over a three-month time frame, Sharon has lost 8kg. The journey so far has not been easy, and Sharon has wanted to withdraw from the management plan several times.

However, with encouragement from Jacinta, coupled with psychological support from Fiona and other health professionals, Sharon has continued to adhere to her weight management program. The impact of Sharon's weight loss has resulted in a reduction in her blood pressure and an improvement in her exercise tolerance. These positive outcomes are supporting Sharon in following the treatment strategies implemented for her.

QUESTION

Consider the underlying pathophysiology, in addition to the socioeconomic, physical and psychological factors that may have contributed to Sharon's obesity. How have these factors impacted on Sharon's inability to maintain a healthy body weight?

Promoting health and reducing risk in the management of chronic obesity

No country to date has reversed its obesity epidemic. Roberto and colleagues (2015) highlight an emerging consensus on promotion for healthy diets through core policy actions such as the NOURISHING framework, which was created by the World Cancer Research Fund International and the American Institute for Cancer Research (World Cancer Research Fund International, 2018). This framework focuses on three domains for policy development focused around healthy diets:

1. food environment – includes food labelling, affordability, advertising, retail and food service environment
2. food system – coherence across all sectors of the food supply chain with healthy diets
3. behaviour-change communication – public awareness of food and nutrition, nutrition advice/counselling in health care settings, and nutrition education and skills.

Roberto and colleagues (2015) summarise with the acknowledgement that individuals bear some responsibility for their health; however, policy needs to take into consideration the exploitation by the media of biological, psychological, social economic vulnerabilities that promote overconsumption of unhealthy foods. Multiple strategies for prevention of obesity should be considered in health care; the more an environment consistently promotes healthy behaviours the greater the likelihood that such behaviours will occur (Lobstein et al., 2015). This can also be congruent with prevention and transition from childhood obesity to adult obesity. The World Health Organization (WHO, 2018) discusses the likelihood of overweight and obese children to remain obese into adulthood, with the increased risk of developing chronic diseases such as diabetes and cardiovascular disease at an earlier age. Thus, prevention of childhood obesity is a major consideration in the fight against chronic obesity.

Risk reducing strategies

Environmental causes are prominent in the prevalence of obesity and are potentially open to interventions for prevention (Brauer et al., 2015; NHMRC, 2013Bb). Furthermore, lifestyle interventions such as behavioural therapies, dietary and physical activity programming, and support should be considered the first line of treatment for people who are overweight and/or obese. Prevention strategies for those people who are overweight or obese should therefore include health promotion advice for:

*   maintenance of a healthy weight
*   increased physical activity
*   eating a healthy diet (NHMRC, 2013b).

Prevention strategies and advice around increased physical activity should be consistent with the Australian physical activity and sedentary behaviour guidelines, and/or the eating and activity guidelines for New Zealand adults (Department of Health, 2014; NZMOH, 2015). Advice relating to prevention strategies surrounding healthy eating should be based on the *Australian Dietary Guidelines* (NHMRC, 2013a). In addition to this, BMI calculation and waist circumference is considered an easy and inexpensive tool to measure and monitor weight changes over time to assist with prevention strategies (World Cancer Research Fund International, 2018).

The NHMRC (2013b) and the WHO (2017) discuss other factors that also need to be addressed in the provision of effective prevention strategies, including:

- life stages – childhood, pregnancy and elderly
- sociodemographic factors – cultural background, rural and remote, socioeconomic disadvantage
- individual factors – lifestyle, psychosocial factors, physical and development factors
- environmental factors – food supply, portion size, disrupted sleep and sedentary occupations.

Primary health care professionals across all domains are in an ideal position to provide health promotion and prevention strategies to those who are at risk of becoming overweight or obese. The NHMRC (2013b) suggests primary health care professionals adopt a '5As approach to weight management' (p. 14):

- Ask and Assess – current lifestyle behaviours, BMI, comorbidities
- Advise – healthy lifestyle
- Assist – develop weight management programs; support and provide specific information/referrals
- Arrange – review and follow up, referrals.

In addition to lifestyle modifications, pharmacotherapy may be considered when people with obesity fail to lose excess weight at an acceptable rate. In such cases, weight loss medications may be introduced as an adjunct therapy to lifestyle modification (Hess & Garvey, 2015). Clinicians must also recognise that bariatric surgery is considered an acceptable and appropriate treatment strategy in the management of obesity. Bariatric surgeries; when combined with a healthy diet, exercise and emotional support; are more likely to produce significant weight-loss outcomes than medical therapies alone (McGraw & Wool, 2015).

The nurse's role in the management of obesity

While people with obesity need to be responsible for their own health status, members of the health care team need to ensure that they provide person-centred care, advice and support to achieve optimum health outcomes (Ross et al., 2015). Managing obesity is complex, challenges traditional health strategies and offers unique challenges for health care providers. Collaborative health care involving all members of the health care team and the individual with obesity can foster effective communication, and provide a supportive environment (Patel, 2015).

Managing obesity in the primary care setting

As discussed, person-centred care involves the delivery of treatment and care, which places the person at the centre of their own care and provides the most appropriate interventions for that person given their circumstances and values (Victorian Department of Health, 2014). The provision of person-centred care also aligns with the *Universal Declaration of Human Rights*, the ICCCF and international codes of ethics for nurses (International Council of Nurses, 2016; Phelan et al., 2015; United Nations, 1948). An individual's participation in their medical treatment and nursing care is acknowledged to increase motivation and adherence to treatment regimes in addition to increasing satisfaction with nursing care (Eloranta et al., 2013; Larsson et al., 2011).

Primary health care is the ideal setting in which nurses can engage with obese individuals as it is readily accessible to the general population (Phelan et al., 2015). In primary health care, the person may present with symptoms related to a number of conditions, not necessarily related to their obesity. Presentations such as these provide nurses with the ideal opportunity to discuss not only the condition but also obesity and weight-reduction strategies. A number of factors may impact on the effectiveness of these discussions, including short consultation times, inadequately trained staff members, large client numbers, language or cultural barriers, and poor health literacy (Sturgiss et al., 2017).

The initial step in caring for people with obesity is a baseline assessment, and discussion between the nurse and the individual regarding their perception of obesity, if they want assistance to address it, and their goals and resources. Goal setting involves working with the individual to determine what the person feels they can do, often commencing with simple goals such as walking for 10 minutes, three times a day (Sturgiss et al., 2017). Nurses need to work with the individual's own beliefs, culture and life practices to optimise health outcomes and provide a holistic approach to care. The physical assessment framework assists nurses to produce an individual-ised care plan suitable for the person's needs (Estes, 2014). It also serves as a baseline to determine progress throughout their treatment by providing engagement and motivation.

Nursing the client with obesity in acute care and in the home settings

Clients with obesity, both in acute care and in the home settings, have a wide variety of physical and emotional requirements. There is scant literature relating to how nurses care for people with obesity in the home setting, and they deal with physical and psychological challenges such as lifting equipment, access to resources, client motiva-tion and family support. What is known is that when hospitalised, individuals with obesity require almost twice the staff and material resources required by the non-obese patient, including bariatric commode chairs, wheelchairs and the use of a HoverMatt for transfer from bed to gurney (Walker, Borgstrom & Tsinonis, 2013).

The challenges of nursing people with obesity arise in all health care settings. Physical size can complicate simple procedures regardless of the practice setting, because it requires nurses to consider obesity-related challenges such as skin, pulmon-ary, resuscitation, intravenous access and mobility in their provision of nursing care (Nault, 2015). People with obesity can experience intertrigo (rash in body folds) caused by the presence of large skin folds, increased moisture from perspiration, friction and lack of ventilation (Kalra, Higgins & Kinney, 2014; Sibbald et al., 2013).

Many people with obesity experience respiratory challenges due to reduced total respiratory system function (Barnes et al., 2018). Nursing actions to minimise respira-tory complications include positioning patients in the semi-Fowler position as abdom-inal fat moves away from the thoracic cavity. In the home situation, many people with obesity will require a continuous positive airway pressure (CPAP) machine to facilitate nocturnal respiration (Beijers et al., 2017).

Obesity may interfere with the absorption of medication, resulting in suboptimal treatment outcomes, especially when medications are calculated on the person's weight. Common hazards of immobility for the person with obesity in an acute care setting include skin breakdown, deep vein thrombosis, muscle atrophy, constipation, atelectasis and pneumonia. Regardless of where the nurse encounters the person with obesity, a deep understanding of the complex requirements to manage their care is vital. Many clients with obesity experience stigma, bias and discrimination related to their weight, resulting in feelings of victimisation and bullying. Many individuals develop anxiety, depression, low self-esteem and suicidal tendencies as a result of these experiences (Hayward, Vartanian & Pinkus, 2018).

REFLECTION

What strategies could the nurse caring for the person with obesity utilise to provide holistic, person-centred care? Reflect on how these strategies would facilitate optimum health outcomes in the home care setting.

Implications of chronic obesity on future health care provision

Obesity is a contributing factor in the development of chronic conditions including diabetes and cardiovascular disease, adding increased financial pressure on health care systems (Sharma et al., 2015). As the incidence of individuals with obesity in Australia and New Zealand continues to rise, nurses will care for individuals with obesity more frequently and across a variety of health care settings. To effectively manage people with obesity, health care team members will need to possess a strong understanding of the pathophysiological issues relating to obesity.

Adults with severe obesity may experience physical limitations that impact on their ability to independently perform activities of daily living. These limitations can result in the need for structural changes to their dwellings, including widening of doors, strengthening of toilets and shower bases, and the use of hoists and stair lifts. While chronic obesity raises some considerable environmental challenges, individuals who lose as little as 5–10 per cent of their total body weight can gain significant health benefits, including improved blood pressure, reduced cholesterol and improved blood glucose levels (Phillips, 2017).

Obesity, more than tobacco smoking or alcohol abuse, has emerged as the major factor in the development of chronic conditions and decreased quality of life (WHO, 2015). The projected increase in the incidence of chronic conditions in the ageing population suggests that future health care costs will continue to escalate until they become untenable. The health burden is largely driven by the increased risk of people developing type 2 diabetes, cardiovascular disease and cancer, which have all been linked to the presence of obesity (Beck-Nielsen, 2013).

Advanced nursing practice and the person with chronic obesity

The prevention and reduction of obesity is a global need. Dietz and colleagues (2015) indicate that health professionals are poorly prepared to face this necessity. To facilitate change, there is a need to transform health professionals' education, attitudes and practices towards chronic obesity.

Nurses are at the forefront of providing health promotion to members of the community as they are highly visible in settings such as primary care. The role of general practice nurses has expanded to address the increasing challenges in both the Australian and New Zealand health care systems, including the ageing population and the rapid increase in chronic conditions such as obesity (Stephen, McInnes & Halcomb, 2018).

Education

Studies suggest that nurses need additional education and training in the care of the person with obesity (Stephen et al., 2018). Dietz and colleagues (2015) agree with this statement, signifying the lack of information provided for undergraduate medical education around obesity, with even less available for nursing undergraduates. The information that is available is incorporated into other disease states rather than treated as a unique medical condition and is not integrated well into core coursework. Education and learning opportunities, including those in the role of advanced nursing practice for overweight and obesity prevention and management, can foster critical thinking and problem-solving skills that will improve outcomes among those who are overweight and obese (Stephen et al., 2018).

Nursing bias: professional leadership

Multiple studies have shown that nurses have negative attitudes towards people who are obese, believing that lifestyle factors are the main cause, individuals are non-compliant with treatment, have no willpower, and obesity is preventable and treatable (Dietz et al., 2015; Tanneberger & Ciupitu-Plath, 2018). Weight prejudice in any health care setting is concerning. For the obese individual the outcomes may be poorer care provision, a failure to seek treatment, or a lack of participation in prevention strategies (Smigelski-Theiss, Gampong & Kurasaki, 2017). Advanced practice nurses have an important role in improving health care for the person with obesity through education of their peers and professional leadership. To enable nurses to assist the person with obesity in changing health behaviours, advanced practice nurses are in an ideal position to address and help remove **nursing bias** against these people (Smigelski-Theiss, et al., 2017).

Nursing bias – nursing prejudice against an individual or group of people which could be considered unjust.

REFLECTION

Reflect on your own attitudes and beliefs towards individuals who suffer from chronic obesity. Have you been negatively biased towards these individuals? How might your personal opinions on this chronic condition impact health care delivery?

SKILLS IN PRACTICE

Multidisciplinary support

Edward is a 45-year-old male who attends the pre-admission clinic for an elective left total hip replacement. Edward is 172 cm tall and weighs 150 kg. In his 20s, Edward was a fit and active man with a BMI of 22. However, over the past 15 years his weight has steadily increased as his day-to-day life has become increasingly busy and he has made poorer, more convenient food choices.

Edward has had previous coronary artery bypass graft surgery with three grafts in place and has long-standing hypertension which has been difficult to manage with medication. Edward previously had a right hip replacement and is on the waiting list for elective bilateral knee replacements. He has been recently referred by his general practitioner to have an overnight sleep study, from which he has been diagnosed with obstructive sleep apnoea, requiring nasal CPAP overnight. Edward currently does not have a CPAP machine of his own, stating that he finds the masks uncomfortable and claustrophobic. Edward worked as a machine operator in a factory from the age of 18, but was recently made redundant. Edward currently lives with his wife, Jan, and two teenage daughters, Elise and Sarah.

During Edward's pre-admission clinic visit, the nurse completed a physical examin-ation, including his weight, height, temperature, blood pressure, pulse and respiration rate. Pathology was collected for a blood glucose test, cholesterol, full blood count and electrolyte levels, as Edward is at high risk of developing diabetes and/or cardiovascular disease due to his increased weight and poor lifestyle habits. Risk factors identified by the nurse included Edward's age, environment, inactivity, low socioeconomic status and unhealthy eating behaviours. Jan also attended the visit and was very tearful when the nurse explained the effects of Edward's weight on his health in the future.

The nurse made a number of recommendations to Edward during their conversa-tion, including the importance of weight loss and exercise to improve his general health, operative procedure and post-operative recovery. Edward explained that he had been told this information before, but the hip pain made it difficult for him to exercise which led him to become depressed and increase his emotional eating habits. The nurse discussed the importance of good nutrition and the link to weight loss, and asked Edward if he would like to obtain information on healthy eating. Edward stated that he would like to review the information because he didn't really understand how to eat in a healthy way. Since he had lost his job, money had been short and as fast food is cheap, his family tended to eat this every day rather than fresh fruit and vegetables, which cost more.

QUESTION

How would collaborative multidisciplinary team management support Edward and his family to reduce their obesity risk and promote their understanding of the importance of adopting healthy eating habits?

SUMMARY

Learning objective 1: Comprehend the underlying pathophysiology of chronic obesity and the associated risk factors.

When energy intake outweighs energy expenditure, obesity is likely to develop. This process involves the release of a complex interplay of hormones and is controlled by the central nervous system. Appetite regulation is maintained by both short- and long-term mechanisms, which, when disrupted, can contribute to the development of chronic obesity. Factors including an individual's BMR and rate of thermogenesis must also be considered.

Learning objective 2: Describe strategies that promote health and reduce risk for individuals who are overweight and obese.

Strategies aimed at tackling the growing burden of chronic obesity through programs that promote health and reduce risk are occurring internationally. The NOURISHING framework is an international example of how policymakers are currently working towards reducing the prevalence of chronic obesity. Disease prevention must focus on healthy lifestyle choices in conjunction with addressing individual factors that may be contributing to the development of this chronic condition.

Learning objective 3: Understand the nurse's role in the management of the chronically obese individual.

People with chronic obesity will present differing challenges to nurses. For optimal care provision, nurses must ensure that management plans are individualised and person-centred, and that effective communication is employed throughout all client–nurse interaction. Nurses must have a thorough understanding of the complexity of chronic obesity so that all care needs are met.

Learning objective 4: Appreciate the impact chronic obesity has on the future of health care.

Chronic obesity is associated with, and may contribute to, the development of a number of other chronic health conditions. This has considerable financial implications for health care expenditure at the global level. Nurses must recognise that the growing number of individuals with chronic obesity will result in future strain on health care resources, including nursing staff.

Learning objective 5: Recognise the importance of advanced nursing practice in the management of obesity.

Advanced nursing practice has the potential to improve health outcomes for people who suffer from chronic obesity. Education must occur across the nursing workforce, and also be provided. Nurses must work towards removing negative bias towards sufferers of chronic obesity so that nurse–client relationships can be strengthened.

REVIEW QUESTIONS

1. What are the short-term and long-term metabolic processes that regulate food intake?
2. How would the NOURISHING framework and NHMRC guidelines assist in the reduction of the following risk factors: diet, physical inactivity, depression and environment?

3. How does care of the person with obesity in the acute setting differ from care in the primary health care setting?
4. Compare and contrast how chronic obesity and tobacco smoking can impact on other chronic conditions.
5. What is the importance of advanced nursing practice in the prevention and management of chronic obesity?

RESEARCH TOPIC

The presence of childhood obesity increases the likelihood of developing chronic obesity in adulthood. Given the current statistics on global childhood obesity rates, research what impact will this have on worldwide health service provision and health care expenditure in the future.

FURTHER READING

Australian Institute of Health and Welfare (AIHW). (2017). *Impact of Overweight and Obesity as a Risk Factor for Chronic Conditions: Australian Burden of Disease Study*. Canberra: AIHW. Retrieved from www.aihw.gov.au/getmedia/f8618e51-c1c4-4dfb-85e0-54ea19500c91/20700.pdf.aspx?inline=true

National Health and Medical Research Council (NHMRC). (2013a). *Australian Dietary Guidelines*. Canberra: NHMRC. Retrieved from https://nhmrc.gov.au/about-us/publications/australian-dietary-guidelines

—— (2013b). *Clinical Practice Guidelines for the Management of Overweight and Obesity in Adults, Adolescents and Children in Australia*. Melbourne: NHMRC. Retrieved from https://nhmrc.gov.au/about-us/publications/clinical-practice-guidelines-management-overweight-and-obesity

Opie, C. A., Haines, H. M., Ervin, K. E., Glenister, K. & Pierce, D. (2017). Why Australia needs to define obesity as a chronic condition. *BMC Public Health,* 17(500), 1–4.

Shepherd, A. (2014). Improving treatments for obesity: The concept of self-management. *Nurse Prescribing*, 12(6), 302–6.

REFERENCES

Baqai, N. & Wilding, J. (2015). Pathophysiology and aetiology of obesity. *Medicine*, 43(2), 73–6.

Barnes, R. D., Ivezaj, V., Martino, S., Pittman, B. P., Paris, M. & Grilo, C. M. (2018). Examining motivational interviewing plus nutrition psychoeducation for weight loss in primary care. *Journal of Psychosomatic Research*, 104, 101–7.

Beck-Nielsen, H. (ed.). (2013). *The Metabolic Syndrome: Pharmacology and Clinical Aspects*. London: Springer.

Beijers, R. J., van de Bool, C., van den Borst, B., Franssen, F. M., Wouters, E. F. & Schols, A. M. (2017). Normal weight but low muscle mass and abdominally obese: Implications for the cardiometabolic risk profile in chronic obstructive pulmonary disease. *Journal of the American Medical Directors Association*, 18(6), 533–8.

Brauer, P., Gorber, S. C., Shaw, E., Singh, H., Bell, N., Shane, A., . . . & Canadian Task Force on Preventive Health Care. (2015). Recommendations for prevention of weight gain and use of behavioural and pharmacologic interventions to manage overweight and obesity in adults in primary care. *Canadian Medical Association Journal*, 187(3), 184–95.

Cheung, W., Pucci, A. & Batterham, R. (2015). Gut-derived hormones and energy homeostasis. In S. Agrawal (ed.), *Obesity, Bariatric, and Metabolic Surgery: A Practical Guide* (pp. 21–8). New York: Springer.

Department of Health. (2014). Australia's physical activity and sedentary behaviour guidelines. Canberra: Australian Government. Retrieved from www.health.gov .au/internet/main/publishing.nsf/content/health-pubhlth-strateg-phys-act-guidelines#apaadult

Dietz, W. H., Baur, L. A., Hall, K., Puhl, R. M., Taveras, E. M., Uauy, R. & Kapelman, P. (2015). Management of obesity: Improvement of health-care training and systems for prevention and care. *The Lancet*, 385, 2521–33.

Eloranta, S., Arve, S., Isoaho, H., Aro, I., Kalam-Salminen, L. & Routasalod, P. (2013). Finnish nurses' perceptions of care of older patients. *International Journal of Nursing Practice*, 20(2), 204–11.

Estes, M. E. Z. (2014). *Health Assessment and Physical Examination* (5th edn). Melbourne: Cengage Learning.

Grima, M. & Dixon, J. (2013). Obesity: Recommendations for management in generally practice and beyond. *Australian Family Physician*, 42(8), 532–41.

Hayward, L. E., Vartanian, L. R. & Pinkus, R. T. (2018). Weight stigma predicts poorer psychological well-being through internalized weight bias and maladaptive coping responses. *Obesity*, 26(4), 755–61.

Hess, M. A. & Garvey, W. T. (2015). Assessment and management of patients with obesity. *Women's Healthcare: A Clinical Journal For NPS*, 3(3), 7–13.

Howick, K., Griffin, B. T., Cryan, J. F. & Schellekens, H. (2017). From belly to brain: Targeting the ghrelin receptor in appetite and food intake regulation. *International Journal of Molecular Sciences*, 18(2), doi: http://10.3390/ijms18020273

International Council of Nurses. (2016). *The ICN Code of Ethics for Nurses*. Geneva: International Council for Nurses.

Kalra, M. G., Higgins, K. E. & Kinney, B. S. (2014). Intertrigo and secondary skin infections. *American Family Physician*, 89(7), 569–73.

Larsson, I. E., Sahlsten, M. J. M., Segesten, K. & Plos, A. E. (2011). Patients' perceptions of nurses' behaviour that influence patient participation in nursing care: A critical incident study. *Nursing Research and Practice*, 2, 21–9.

Lobstein, T., Jackson-Leach, R., Moodie, M. L., Hall, K. D., Gortmaker, S. L., Swinburn, B. A., . . . & McPherson, K. (2015). Child and adolescent obesity: Part of a bigger picture. *The Lancet*, 385, 2510–20.

McGraw, C. A. & Wool, D. B. (2015). Bariatric surgery: Three surgical techniques, patient care, risks, and outcomes. *AORN Journal*, 102(2), 141–52. doi: http://10.1016/j.aorn.2014.11.020

National Health and Medical Research Council (NHMRC). (2013a). *Australian Dietary Guidelines*. Canberra: NHMRC.

—— (2013b). *Clinical Practice Guidelines for the Management of Overweight and Obesity in Adults, Adolescents and Children in Australia*. Canberra: NHMRC.

Nault, D. S. (2015). CE nursing consideration when caring for the obese patient. *Michigan Nurse*, 88(2), 10–18.

New Zealand Ministry of Health (NZMOH). (2015). *Eating and Activity Guidelines for New Zealand Adults.* Wellington: Ministry of Health. Retrieved from www.health.govt.nz/system/files/documents/publications/eating-activity-guidelines-for-new-zealand-adults-oct15_0.pdf

—— (2018). Obesity statistics. Wellington: Ministry of Health. Retrieved from www.health.govt.nz/nz-health-statistics/health-statistics-and-data-sets/obesity-statistics

Patel, D. (2015). Pharmacotherapy for the management of obesity. *Metabolism*, 64(11), 1376–85.

Phelan, S. M., Burgess, D. J., Yeazel, M. W., Hellerstedt, W. L., Griffin, J. M. & van Ryn, M. (2015). Impact of weight bias and stigma on quality of care and outcomes for patients with obesity. *Obesity Reviews*, 16(4), 319–26.

Phillips, C. M. (2017). Metabolically healthy obesity across the life course: Epidemiology, determinants, and implications. *Annals of the New York Academy of Sciences*, 1391(1), 85–100.

Rajeev, S. & Wilding, J. (2015). Etiopathogenesis of obesity. In S. Agrawal (ed.), *Obesity, Bariatric, and Metabolic Surgery: A Practical Guide* (pp. 13–20). New York: Springer.

Roberto, C. A., Swinburn, B., Hawkes, C., Huang, T., Costa, S. A., Ashe, M., . . . & Brownell, K. D. (2015). Patchy progress on obesity prevention: Emerging examples, entrenched barriers and new thinking. *The Lancet*, 385, 2400–9.

Ross, R., Blair, S., de Lannoy, L., Després, J. P. & Lavie, C. J. (2015). Changing the endpoints for determining effective obesity management. *Progress in Cardiovascular Diseases*, 57(4), 330–6.

Rossen, L. & Rossen, E. (2012). *Obesity 101.* New York: Springer.

Schuklenk, U. & Zhang, E. (2014). Public health ethics and obesity prevention: The trouble with data and ethics. *Monash Bioethics Review*, 32(1–2), 121–40.

Sharma, A., Lavie, C. J., Borer, J. S., Vallakati, A., Goel, S., Lopez-Jimenez, F., . . . & Lazar, J. M. (2015). Meta-analysis of the relation of body mass index to all-cause and cardiovascular mortality and hospitalization in patients with chronic heart failure. *The American Journal of Cardiology*, 115(10), 1428–34.

Shukla, A., Moreira, M. & Rubino, F. (2013). Pathophysiology of obesity. In C. Thompson (ed.), *Bariatric Endoscopy* (pp. 11–18). New York: Springer Science & Business Media.

Sibbald, R. G., Kelly, J., Kennedy-Evans, K. L., Labrecque, C. & Waters, N. (2013). A practical approach to the prevention and management of intertrigo, or moisture-associated skin damage, due to perspiration: Expert consensus on best practice. *Wound Care Canada*, 11(2), 1–22.

Smigelski-Theiss, T., Gampong, M. & Kurasaki, J. (2017). Weight bias and psychosocial implications for acute care of patients with obesity. *AACN Advanced Critical Care*, 28(3), 254–62.

Stephen, C., McInnes, S. & Halcomb, E. (2018). The feasibility and acceptability of nurse-led chronic disease management interventions in primary care: An integrative review. *Journal of Advanced Nursing*, 74(2), 279–88.

Sturgiss, E. A., van Weel, C., Ball, L., Jansen, S. & Douglas, K. (2017). Obesity management in Australian primary care: Where has the general practitioner gone? *Australian Journal of Primary Health*, 22(6), 473–6.

Tanneberger, A. & Ciupitu-Plath, C. (2018). Nurses' weight bias in caring for obese patients: Do weight controllability beliefs influence the provision of care to obese patients? *Clinical Nursing Research*, 27(4), 414–32.

Townsend, N. & Scriven, A. (2014). *Public Health Mini-Guides: Obesity*. London: Churchill Livingstone Elsevier.

United Nations. (1948). *Universal Declaration of Human Rights*. New York: United Nations.

Victorian Department of Health. (2014). *Maintaining Personal Identity: Respect and Dignity*. Melbourne: State Government of Victoria.

Walker, K., Borgstrom, H. & Tsinonis, H. (2013). Intervening to improve quality and safety of care for the obese in an orthopaedic unit: A collaborative action-orientated quality improvement project in a Magnet recognised facility. *Collegian*, 20(3), 171–7.

World Cancer Research Fund International. (2018). *Diet, Nutrition, Physical Activity and Cancer: A Global Perspective. Continuous Update Project Expert Report*. Retrieved from www.wcrf.org/dietandcancer/resources-and-toolkit

World Health Organization (WHO). (2015). Obesity and overweight. Retrieved from www.who.int/en/news-room/fact-sheets/detail/obesity-and-overweight

—— (2017). *Report of the Commission on Ending Childhood Obesity: Implementation Plan: Executive Summary*. Retrieved from www.who.int/end-childhood-obesity/publications/echo-plan-executive-summary/en/

—— (2018). *Global Strategy on Diet, Physical Activity and Health: Childhood Overweight and Obesity*. Retrieved from www.who.int/dietphysicalactivity/childhood/en/

Zhang, Y., Liu, J., Yao, J., Ji, G., Qian, L., Wang, J., . . . & Liu, Y. (2014). Obesity: Pathophysiology and intervention. *Nutrients*, 6(11), 5153–83. doi: http://10.3390/nu611515

15

Dementia care

Julia Gilbert
and Lyn Croxon

With acknowledgement to Bronwen Ashcroft

LEARNING OBJECTIVES

After studying this chapter, you should be able to:

1. describe the impact of dementia on Australian and New Zealand societies
2. describe various types of dementia and their associated signs and symptoms
3. understand the impact of living with dementia on individuals and families
4. describe strategies to promote health and reduce the risk factors associated with developing dementia
5. understand the role of the nurse in caring for people with dementia.

Introduction

Australia's and New Zealand's ageing populations represent a significant challenge for both nations' health care services, aged care and social policies (Ball et al., 2015; Clancy, 2015). The Commonwealth government of Australia and the New Zealand Ministry of Health have initiated major health reforms by developing action plans for dealing with dementia and increasing dementia services (Clancy, 2015; New Zealand Ministry of Health (NZMOH), 2014). This is consistent with the Innovative Care for Chronic Conditions Framework (ICCCF).

Australia and New Zealand have ageing societies with high life expectancies (Nay et al., 2015). The management of chronic diseases, including the increasing prevalence of dementia, presents a significant challenge for health services, social policy and aged care (Nay, Garratt & Fetherstonhaugh, 2014; Travers, Lie & Martin-Khan, 2015). The number of people living with dementia in rural and regional parts of Australia and New Zealand is increasing rapidly, resulting in an increase on the demands of available services (Clancy, 2015).

Dementia has been recognised as a national health priority area. Strategies are, therefore, crucial to prevent or delay the onset of dementia and to reduce its impact on health care and associated costs (Ball et al., 2015; Travers et al., 2015). The number of people with dementia is predicted to rise by 327 per cent between 2015 and 2050 (Moyle et al., 2011). By 2050, it is expected that there will be 1.1 million people with dementia in Australia and 170 000 people in New Zealand, with an estimated cost of $36 billion AUD and $4.6 billion NZD respectively in health care and lost productivity (Alzheimer's New Zealand, 2018; Dementia Australia, 2016). As the incidence of dementia in Indigenous individuals in both Australia and New Zealand is significantly higher than non-Indigenous individuals, additional services and resources may be required (Taylor & Guerin, 2014).

Dementia should not be regarded as a normal part of ageing; it can happen to anybody, but it is more common after the age of 65. Dementia is the single greatest cause of disability among older Australian and New Zealand people, the third-leading cause of disability burden overall (Alzheimer's New Zealand, 2018; Dementia Australia, 2018), and the second-leading cause of death. There are 1800 people diagnosed with dementia every week in Australia and New Zealand, which equates to approximately one person diagnosed every six minutes. There is no cure for dementia and no effective treatment, even with researchers progressing globally in these areas (Keast, 2015). People with dementia have a heavy dependence on carers, and Australia is expected to face a shortage of more than 150 000 paid and unpaid carers for people with dementia by 2029 (Dementia Australia, 2018).

Dementia is not a single specific condition, but an umbrella term used to describe the loss of memory, intellect, language, social skills, perception, rationality and physical functioning (Dementia Australia, 2018). Common symptoms of dementia include **agnosia, alexia, apraxia**, general confusion, personality changes, withdrawal, apathy and the inability to perform everyday tasks. Although the symptoms vary with the type of dementia, it is generally gradual in onset, progressive and irreversible (Australian Institute of Health and Welfare (AIHW), 2016).

Agnosia – the inability of a person to process sensory information, usually vision or hearing.

Alexia – the inability of a person to understand written or printed information.

Apraxia – an acquired difficulty with motor planning to perform tasks or movements.

Pathophysiology of dementia
Types of dementia

There are many different types of dementia with the most common being Alzheimer's disease, vascular dementia, Lewy body disease and frontotemporal dementia. Other causes of dementia include **Pick's disease**, **Korsakoff syndrome**, **Huntington's disease**, **Creutzfeldt-Jakob disease** and **multi-infarct dementia**. Secondary dementia arises from the human immunodeficiency virus (HIV), intracranial lesions/masses, Parkinson's disease, normal pressure hydrocephalus and pseudodementia. Alzheimer's disease is the most common cause of dementia, accounting for up to 70 per cent of all dementias, followed by vascular dementia (Dementia Australia, 2018; Keast, 2015).

Alzheimer's disease

Alzheimer's disease is characterised by shrinking of the outer layer of the cortex, a decreased brain weight caused by the death of brain cells, and the development of plaque and neurofibrillary tangles. The plaques are external to the brain cells and interfere with the neurotransmission of electrical stimuli. The neurofibrillary tangles destroy brain cells by preventing the transport of nutrients to the brain cells. The increased presence of beta-amyloid, a small protein fragment found in the plaques, is common and thought to initiate the development of Alzheimer's disease (Dementia Australia, 2018).

As Alzheimer's disease progressively inhibits a person's ability to communicate, there is generally several months of decreasing short-term memory and repetitive questioning, declining interest in previously enjoyed activities, such as gardening or listening to music, and difficulty in undertaking activities of daily living (ADL) (Nay et al., 2014).

Vascular dementia

Vascular dementia is a broad term for dementias that are associated with problems of circulation of blood to the brain. Vascular dementia represents the second-largest group of pure dementias and is often associated with defined vascular events; however, it may also be the most under-diagnosed type of dementia (Dementia Australia, 2018; Kalaria, 2016). Two of the most common types of vascular dementia are Binswanger's disease and multi-infarct dementia. Binswanger's disease was previously thought to be rare. However, it has a close association with stroke-related changes and affects the 'white matter' within the brain. It is caused by high blood pressure, atherosclerosis and insufficient circulation. Early symptoms include lethargy and slowness, walking difficulties, emotional highs and lows, and lack of bladder control. Multi-infarct dementia is associated with numerous small strokes or transient ischaemic attacks (TIA), which cause damage to the brain cortex and result in impaired memory, learning and language.

Lewy body disease

Lewy body disease is an overarching term for dementia with Lewy bodies, which are abnormal structures that build up in areas of the brain. It is a chronic progressive

Pick's disease – rare, and typically affects people in their late middle age. It has a genetic link and involves atrophy of the brain. The progressive deterioration involves changes to personality, loss of social skills, and the impairment of intellect, language and memory.

Korsakoff syndrome – usually caused by extensive alcohol use, which leads to a lack of thiamine (vitamin B1) and cognitive decline.

Huntington's disease – inherited and causes the slow degeneration of nerve cells in the brain that affect functional abilities including movement and thinking.

Creutzfeldt-Jakob disease – mental, physical and sensory disturbance caused by prions (a small proteinaceous infectious disease-causing agent) that result in a fatal degenerative disease in the brain, colloquially known as 'mad cow disease'.

Multi-infarct dementia – caused by multiple disruptions of blood flow to the brain; for example, a mild stroke which can cause memory loss.

Presenile – occurring before 65 years of age.

Senile – occurring when a person is 65 years or older.

neuropsychiatric disorder, which is clinically characterised by Parkinsonian symptoms of **presenile** or **senile**, or often younger, onset, and is usually followed by dementia at the later stages. Some of the psychiatric symptoms that may be seen include visual hallucinations and delusions (most common) that are often followed by Parkinsonian symptoms (Kenji, 2014). Parkinsonian symptoms are described in Chapter 17.

Frontotemporal dementia

Frontotemporal lobar degeneration makes up approximately 7 per cent of all dementias (Nay et al., 2014), and is a clinically and pathologically heterogeneous syndrome. It is characterised by progressive decline in behaviour or language associated with degeneration of the frontal and anterior temporal lobes. Patients are often misdiagnosed as having Alzheimer's disease or a psychiatric illness because of the insidious and progressive nature of both Alzheimer's disease and frontotemporal lobar degeneration, and their shared symptoms (Kalaria, 2016).

Risk factors

Both genetic and non-genetic factors have been linked to the development of dementia, including advancing age, gender, biomedical, behavioural, psychological and social factors (Smith, Ali & Quach, 2014).Women are more likely than men to develop Alzheimer's disease because they have a longer life expectancy; therefore, the female gender in itself is not a risk factor once age is taken into consideration. People with fewer years of education are more likely to develop Alzheimer's disease and dementia (Dubois et al., 2016). Biomedical factors include diabetes, hyperlipidaemia, obesity and hypertension (Smith et al., 2014). Hypertension with a systolic blood pressure of greater than 180 mmHg increases the risk of developing Alzheimer's disease by 50 per cent. Similarly, a low diastolic pressure of less than 65 mmHg has an associated 40 per cent increased risk of developing Alzheimer's disease or dementia (Dubois et al., 2016). Decreased physical activity, smoking, excessive dietary and alcohol consumption, depression and reduced cognitive activity are also related to increased dementia risk (Smith et al., 2014).

REFLECTION

Reflect on the common risk factors for dementia that are similar to risk factors for other chronic conditions. Consider the difficulties you may have in assisting people with the comorbidity of dementia in managing other chronic conditions.

Living with dementia

People living with dementia may experience social isolation if their family members feel uncomfortable dealing with the diagnosis, resulting in a reluctance to engage with available resources. As dementia progresses, the individual will experience cognitive changes including difficulty in remembering people, places and where they live; poor concentration, and an inability to think clearly or problem solve. They will experience varying difficulties with completing everyday ADL such as showering, dressing and eating, managing finances, and using appliances safely. Many people will experience loss of social skills, repetitive behaviours and may become physically or verbally aggressive.

The person affected by dementia may find it difficult to engage in conversation due to an inability to comprehend what is being said, and this may result in feelings of loneliness (MacKinlay, 2012). The person's ability to remain connected to familiar people diminishes with an increasing memory loss and inability to engage in social activities, such as cards and bowls with friends, and fewer people continuing to visit. Many people living with dementia are more comfortable with familiar people than with strangers, and prefer to be with family than in day centres with people their own age (Brodaty et al., 2013).

Individuals living with dementia often require assistance with ADL as the condition progresses, with the burden of care falling on family, friends and unpaid carers. Planning care is essential, and must be comprehensive and incorporate physical and psychosocial care, with the involvement of a multidisciplinary team to manage cognitive deficits, behaviours, medical problems, social engagement, legal and financial planning, and support and education for patients, family and carers (Brodaty et al., 2013).

Carers

In 2018 there were 425 416 people in Australia and 62 287 people in New Zealand living with dementia; females had a higher percentage than males (Alzheimers New Zealand, 2017; Dementia Australia, 2018). Approximately 70 per cent of people with dementia live in the community, and it is estimated that Australia has over 200 000 unpaid informal carers, who are predominantly family members and friends (Dementia Australia, 2018); similar experiences are also shown in New Zealand (Alzheimers New Zealand, 2017). Carer strain, due to the need for constant care, is well-documented. Carers are often described as 'the second patient' (Brodaty et al., 2013, p. 40) as their physical and mental health is most often compromised from exhaustion, lack of time for themselves, social isolation, bereavement and depression. Carers of people with dementia are typically women (74 per cent), over the age of 65 (65 per cent), providing more than 40 hours per week of care, often full time, and having a disability themselves (nearly 50 per cent) (AIHW, 2016). The progressive decline associated with dementia is difficult for families as they manage challenging behaviours of the person with dementia and care decisions. Family-based care of an older adult with advanced dementia was found in one study to require 41.5 more hours of care per week as opposed to an older adult with normal cognition, although the same study found that family caregivers may not view their care negatively (Beeber & Zimmerman, 2012).

Family members and carers may experience guilt, grief, loss and anger. It is common for people to feel guilt related to the way the person with dementia has been treated, be embarrassed by the person's changed behaviour or be unable to continue to care for the individual. If the person with dementia is hospitalised or needs to enter 24-hour care, carers may feel guilty because they can no longer manage to care for the person (Bunn et al., 2015). Individuals with dementia and their families may experience grief for the loss of the person that was, and for the loss of the existing relationship or the future that was planned. Family members may experience anger and frustration, including feeling anger towards the person with dementia because of their behaviours and towards support services if they do not assist the person with dementia to remain at home as the condition progresses (Springate & Tremont, 2014).

Support for carers involves health care practitioners educating carers and monitoring how they are coping. Referrals can be made to care or home services, such as aged care packages and respite care. Respite care may be part of the long-term management plan. Institutional care may be needed as the condition progresses. Fifty-three per cent of people diagnosed with dementia will die due to the progression of the disease, and the remaining number will die from comorbidities. Therefore, palliative care or end of life care needs to be considered in the long-term planning (Dempsey et al., 2015).

SKILLS IN PRACTICE

Living with dementia

Doris is 84 years old and widowed; she has lived alone for the past two years in Perth, caring for herself. Her son, Ben, lives in Cairns, and calls Doris every fortnight but has not visited Doris for around eight months. During recent calls, Ben noticed that Doris seemed distracted and unable to follow the conversation, repeatedly asking the same questions and trailing off when answering his questions.

Ben was concerned about Doris and flew to Perth to see her. When he arrived, he was shocked to see the changes in Doris. She was very thin and frail, and had difficulty walking. There was limited food in the house, which was filthy with cobwebs on the walls and food spills on the carpet. Doris was having trouble eating as she didn't feel hungry, and appeared dehydrated and lethargic. Doris had stopped using the oven and the television as she said they didn't work, but Ben found that they were still functioning. Doris was dishevelled, wearing clothes with food stains on them, and her hair was greasy and unwashed. Doris was agitated, getting up from her seat repeatedly and going to the front door and looking out, stating that she had to 'pick up the children'.

Ben took Doris to her general practitioner (GP). During the assessment, Doris was able to say who she was, but did not know her address and thought Ben was her late husband, Frank. She became increasingly agitated, was found to be 10 kg below her ideal weight and was severely dehydrated.

Following the assessment, the GP organised for a community nurse to visit Doris daily to assist her with her ADL. An aged care assessment team was also contacted and visited Doris in her home to complete their assessment. As a result of this assessment, a home services package was approved, providing Doris with meals on wheels and a cleaning service, in addition to ongoing community nurse visits.

QUESTION

Identify the signs of dementia exhibited by Doris. What collaborative interventions are required for her care?

Promoting health and reducing risk
Wellbeing

The person with dementia copes best in a familiar environment. Whether this be their home or a care setting, it is important to create a calm environment with regular routines. In promoting general health and wellbeing, consideration must be given to diet, exercise, social engagement, medication, immunisation and the prevention of falls. Nutrition is a concern as more than half of people with dementia lose some ability to feed themselves. They may also have poor appetite, forget to eat and drink, and experience weight loss due to pacing or wandering (Dementia Australia, 2018; Herke et al., 2015). Strategies to overcome these issues include providing finger foods, regular snacks, foods the individual likes, not arguing over food or eating, using coloured plates and making eating a social occasion.

The person should be encouraged to engage in activities that they enjoy. Over the years, there have been a number of non-pharmacological approaches used to assist those living with dementia. Strategies to encourage engagement in activities include art therapy, behavioural therapy, memory training, distraction techniques, diversional therapy, exercise training, music therapy, reality orientation, relaxation therapy, reminiscence therapy and validation therapy (Hungerford, Jones & Cleary, 2014). There is also evidence that brain exercises or cognitive challenges such as crosswords and computer games can be beneficial for those who have an interest in them (Dawson et al., 2015). Touch, hand and foot massage, and aromatherapy may decrease stress and agitation in dementia, enhance social connectedness and may decrease the sense of feeling alone, which, in turn, improves the quality of life (Moyle et al., 2014). Acupressure combined with aromatherapy has been found to decrease anxiety and agitation in people with dementia (Alm, Danielsson & Porskrog-Kristiansen, 2018). Exercise has been found to increase general wellbeing, balance and cognitive function in all age groups, and evidence is building as to the benefits of physical activity and outdoor activities for the wellbeing and independence of people living with dementia as well as those who care for them (Dawson et al., 2015; Taylor et al., 2017).

There is evidence that **ageing-in-place** has benefits to the quality of life of the person living with dementia and may slow the progression of the disease (Hyde et al., 2015**).** Models of care that reflect a home-like environment, such as the UK's Butterfly Scheme, are receiving positive results and offer an environment that engages the interests of the person (Vogel, 2018). New Zealand has adapted the Dutch model of the 'Dementia Village'. The first opened in 2018 near Rotorua, and incorporates a village of homes, housing six to seven people with similar interests, shops, health facilities, and common outdoor and community facilities. Health care staff visit the residents in their community (O'Connor, 2016). 'Smart homes' may also be useful to maintain independence with the use of memory aids, safety features and remote monitoring (Amiribesheli & Bouchachia, 2017).

Ageing-in-place – where an individual lives in the residence of their choice as they age, for as long as they are able, supported by services to assist this choice.

Challenging behaviours

In Australia, 53 per cent of people living in residential care have shown activity disturbance and 77 per cent have behaved aggressively (Van der Ploeg, Walker & O'Connor, 2014). Other challenging behaviours include mild depression, apathy and repetitive questioning (NSW Health, 2014). In contrast, 20 per cent of people with dementia living in the community have experienced wandering, major depression and verbal aggression, and 10 per cent have shown severe symptoms of aggression, agitation and depression (Hungerford et al., 2014).

Environmental modifications, such as having a secure space to wander and a calm environment, may assist the management of challenging behaviours. While music and recreational therapy have been found to be effective in reducing agitation, it is more useful if the activities are related to the person's former interest and background; for example, music the person enjoyed previously has been found to be more effective than general calming music. The voice of a relative is often more calming than that of a stranger (Looi et al., 2014). Antipsychotic medication can be used to treat behavioural and psychological symptoms, but has been associated with a higher risk of falls, pneumonia, cerebrovascular accident and death (Hungerford et al., 2014).

Challenging behaviours often result when people with dementia feel frustrated that they can no longer do the things they used to do, or they may behave inappropriately if they are unable to express themselves. A dementia-friendly environment in the home will support the person's safety and level of functioning while promoting independence. Compensation for cognitive deficits can take the form of cues, notes, whiteboards, clocks, computers or photos. Velcro can be used instead of buttons and laces on clothes and shoes. Another strategy that can assist individuals with memory impairment to decrease problem behaviours is to incorporate the use of large, coloured signs, prompt questions and cue cards; for example, a coloured sign can indicate the toilet location (Mudge, McRae & Cruickshank, 2015).

Physical exercise of moderate intensity three times a week for a period of 60 minutes each time has been found to decrease challenging behaviours in people with Alzheimer's disease. This would be an appropriate strategy to manage behaviour in those who are able-bodied such as fit, older people or those with younger-onset dementia (Hoffmann et al., 2016).

Legal aspects

The consideration of legal and financial issues includes wills, enduring power of attorney, enduring guardianship and advance care directives (see also Chapter 21). Work arrangements may have to be modified, and a gradual move from work may be a good alternative for the person. Financial advice and assistance in the form of sickness benefits, disability and carer pensions may be appropriate (Brodaty et al., 2013).

As dementia progresses, the ability to drive safely can be compromised. There is not a legal requirement for a medical practitioner to report a diagnosis of dementia; however, the Australian and New Zealand Society of Geriatric Medicine recommends both an on-road and off-road assessment in determining driving ability (Andrew, Traynor & Iverson, 2015).

REFLECTION

What activities would you find soothing if you were to be diagnosed with dementia later in life? Consider what types of music you like and activities that you may be able to participate in when you have a sensory loss such as visual impairment or hearing loss. How do you think nursing homes might change to meet your needs in the future?

SKILLS IN PRACTICE

Early-onset dementia

Keith is a 52-year-old bank executive. Over the past six months he has noticed an accumulation of little things like losing concentration, becoming withdrawn from his family and irritable with his colleagues, losing his car keys and wallet when they were in front of him, and getting lost when driving his usual route home.

Keith thought it was a result of the stress he was under in his job and went to his GP, who treated him for low testosterone levels, but nothing changed. Keith eventually had to resign from his job, and this was stressful for both him and his wife, Wendy.

Progressively Keith's cognition has deteriorated. He got lost going two blocks to the corner store and one day he went to play golf but didn't come home. Wendy drove out to the golf course, but Keith wasn't there and the staff said that he hadn't been there all day. Two hours later, Keith rang Wendy in tears from the corner shop as he didn't know how to get home. This episode served as a trigger for Keith to see a neurologist, who ordered pathology and scans, and eventually diagnosed Keith with dementia. While Keith was relieved at finally getting a diagnosis, Wendy was devastated as she saw their future together disappearing and Keith having to live in a dementia unit.

QUESTIONS

1. What is the impact on family members and carers living with an individual diagnosed with early-onset dementia?
2. Does Keith retain legal competency to make his own decisions, drive or complete legal documentations (for example, a will, advance health directive, or consent for medical procedures)?
3. What strategies could assist both Keith to manage his daily activities and his memory loss, and Wendy to deal with a full-time carer's role at this time?
4. What role does the nurse play in supporting both Keith and Wendy in the community?

The nurse's role in caring for dementia patients

Individuals living with dementia may not access health and community support because they have limited access to information about dementia and the resources available in the community. As dementia is associated with neurogenerative deficits, there is a risk of care becoming depersonalised. Nurses need to individualise care planning by considering the person's life, likes, needs, personality and feelings, and connecting with the person in a meaningful relationship — in fact, to 'know the person' (Chenoweth et al., 2015). Even though there is currently no cure for dementia, support is available for individuals living with dementia and their families to reduce the impact of the physical, emotional and economic pressures. According to the World Health Organization (WHO) (2015), goals for dementia care are:

- early diagnosis
- optimising physical health, cognition, activity and wellbeing
- identifying and treating accompanying physical illness
- detecting and treating behavioural and psychological symptoms
- providing information and long-term support to caregivers.

Nurses work in a variety of roles while caring for individuals living with dementia. Community nurses are members of the primary care team, providing advice and support for individuals with dementia and their family members, and referring the individual to other members of the health care team as required. They assist the individual to engage in daily activities, and provide family caregivers with education and information about dementia (Denning & Hibberd, 2016).

Due to the complexities of the progression of dementia, it is usually helpful if assessment, interventions, and support for family members and caregivers can be effectively managed by a collaborative, interprofessional approach involving members of the health care team. The interprofessional approach in dementia care fosters problem solving, and improves communication between team members, the individual and family members.

Team collaboration incorporates the individual's perspective in the formulation of care to validate their wishes. The nurse can lead the health care team in the provision of individualised holistic care by providing information to the team in collaborative meetings regarding the individual's progress, medication, discharge planning, and therapeutic interventions that may be effective and reduce the incidence of hospital admissions and any issues that could arise. These discussions should include the person with dementia if possible, the caregiver and health care team. (Lewis, Bartlett & Patel, 2016). If the individual with dementia does require 24-hour care within a dementia-specific care unit, the nurse can support family members who may be experiencing emotional stress during the transition (Fortinsky et al., 2014).

Individualised care

Family members are often asked to develop a 'life story' for the patient based on their experiences, preferences and routines to allow staff to enhance their patient inter-actions. This area of practice has been supported for decades in the care of the person with dementia (Kenyan, Clark & de Vries, 2001; Kitwood, 1997). Nurses can discuss with family members how they elicit cooperation from the patient to perform routine care activities such as food and beverage preferences. This information should be incorporated into individualised care plans that reflect the care requirements for the person (Chenoweth et al., 2015; Cooney & O'Shea, 2018). When interacting with individuals with dementia, nurses need to use simple, direct language, gestures, and pictures and cues that have meaning for them. Triggers for agitation and depression, which might include pain, hunger, thirst or lack of social interaction, should also be identified and avoided if possible.

Pain assessment and management

For many individuals with dementia, pain is poorly understood and undertreated, primarily because of the difficulty with communication. Poorly managed pain may result in an increase in adverse behaviours, including aggression, confusion and wandering. Nurses can assist patients by performing frequent patient pain assessments, and administering analgesia in a systematic manner to reduce distress and improve the patients' quality of life. Pain management needs to be tailored to meet the individual patient's needs, circumstances, conditions and risks (Monroe, Parish & Mion, 2015). Pain, as well as other factors such as infection and dehydration, can lead to delirium. Non-pharmacological options should also be considered to support pharmacological pain relief.

Delirium – mental confusion that develops quickly and results from an underlying medical condition, administration or withdrawal from medication or infection.

Advanced nursing practice in dementia care

Advanced nursing practice in the care of people with dementia involves careful monitoring of symptoms (due to the difficulty that people with dementia have in communicating), treatment of comorbidities, monitoring of medication and therapeutic levels, suggestions for non-pharmacological strategies for management, and providing links to community services. Nurses, including nurse practitioners, working at an advanced level are often involved in the assessment of the person with dementia while they are living at home, and play a significant role in maintaining them in this environment. Various comprehensive ADL assessment tools, including the seminal Katz Index of Independence in Activities of Daily Living (Beerens et al., 2015; Katz et al., 1963), can be utilised to measure the individual's overall performance and monitor the impact of the disease progression. These assessment tools capture the erosion of the individual's ability to self-care, such as the inability to self-feed (Amella & Batchelor-Aselage, 2014). In the aged care setting, nurses working at an advanced level frequently work independently, negotiating between the acute care and aged care settings, to provide the best possible care and to avoid their patients having hospital admissions (Fortinsky et al., 2014).

SUMMARY

Learning objective 1: Describe the impact of dementia on Australian and New Zealand societies.

Dementia is an umbrella term for a group of conditions that cause cognitive decline. Its incidence is increasing as the population ages globally. Dementia is progressive and irreversible. Australia and New Zealand are ageing societies with high life expectancies. The number of people living with dementia in rural and regional parts of Australia and New Zealand is increasing rapidly, resulting in an increase on the demands of available services.

Learning objective 2: Describe various types of dementia, and their associated signs and symptoms.

There are many different types of dementia, with the most common being Alzheimer's disease, vascular dementia, Lewy body disease and frontotemporal dementia. Alzheimer's disease is the most common cause of dementia, followed by vascular dementia.

Learning objective 3: Understand the impact of living with dementia on individuals and families.

Individuals with dementia require assistance with ADL as memory loss progresses. The creation of a dementia-friendly environment and the use of cues can increase independence. As the majority of people with dementia live in the community, it is just as important to consider the health and social needs of the carers.

Learning objective 4: Describe strategies to promote health and reduce the risk factors associated with developing dementia.

The general health and wellbeing of the person with dementia includes a consideration of nutrition, exercise, social engagement, medication, immunisation and falling-prevention strategies.

Learning objective 5: Understand the role of the nurse in caring for people with dementia.

Nurses care for individuals living with dementia in a variety of roles. Community nurses and nurses in general practice form part of primary care teams for dementia, and there are nurses in dementia-specific care units, providing advice and support for individuals with dementia and their family members.

REVIEW QUESTIONS

1. What are the factors that can contribute to the development of dementia?
2. What are the symptoms of dementia?
3. Is dementia a normal part of ageing?
4. Are Alzheimer's disease and dementia the same thing?
5. What are the important strategies when communicating with someone with dementia?

RESEARCH TOPIC

While there is no cure or treatment for dementia, there are ways of assisting people to improve life with dementia. Outline what some of these complementary or alternative therapies might be.

FURTHER READING

Chenoweth, L., Stein Parbury, J., Lapkin, S. & Wang, Y. (2015). Organisational interventions for promoting person-centred care for people with dementia (Protocol). *Cochrane Database of Systematic Reviews*, (11). Art. no.: CD011963. doi: http://10.1002/14651858.CD011963

Hungerford, C., Jones, T. & Cleary, M. (2014). Pharmacological versus non-pharmacological approaches to managing challenging behaviours for people with dementia. *British Journal of Community Nursing*, 19(2), 72–7.

Panegyres, P. & Gray, V. (2010). Dementia risk factors for Australian baby boomers. *Neurology International*, 2(2), 57–61.

Springate, B. A. & Tremont, G. (2014). Dimensions of caregiver burden in dementia: Impact of demographic, mood and care recipient variables. *American Journal of Geriatric Psychiatry*, 22(3), 294–300.

Travers, C., Lie, D. & Martin-Khan, M. (2015). Dementia and the population health approach: Promise, pitfalls and progress. An Australian perspective. *Reviews in Clinical Gerontology*, 25, 60–71.

REFERENCES

Alm, A., Danielsson, S. & Porskrog-Kristiansen, L. (2018). Non pharmacological interventions towards behavioural and psychological symptoms of dementia – An integrated literature review. *Open Journal of Nursing*, 8, 434–7. doi: http://10.4236/ojn.2018.87034

Alzheimers New Zealand. (2017). *Dementia Economic Impact Report 2016*. Wellington: Alzheimers New Zealand. Retrieved from www.alzheimers.org.nz/getmedia/79f7fd09-93fe-43b0-a837-771027bb23c0/Economic-Impacts-of-Dementia-2017.pdf/

Amella, E. J. & Batchelor-Aselage, M. B. (2014). Facilitating ADLs by caregivers of persons with dementia: The C3P model. *Occupational Therapy in Health Care*, 28(1), 51–61.

Amiribesheli, M. & Bouchachia, H. J. (2017). A tailored smart home for dementia care. *Journal of Ambient Intelligence and Humanized Computing*, 9, 1755–82. doi: http://.org/10.1007/s12652-017-0645-7

Andrew, C., Traynor, V. & Iverson, D. (2015). An integrative review: Understanding driving retirement decisions for individuals living with a dementia. *Journal of Advanced Nursing*, 71(12), 2699–3018. doi: http://10.1111/jan.12727

Australian Institute of Health and Welfare (AIHW). (2016). *Dementia*. Canberra: AIHW.

Ball, L., Jansen, S., Desbrow, B., Morgan, K., Moyle, W. & Hughes, R. (2015). Experiences and nutrition support strategies in dementia care: Lessons from family carers. *Nutrition & Dietetics*, 72(1), 22–9.

Beeber, A. S. & Zimmerman, S. (2012). Adapting the family management style framework for families caring for older adults with dementia. *Journal of Family Nursing*, 18(1), 123–45. doi: http://10.1177/1074840711427144

Beerens, H. C., Zwakhalen, S. M. G., Verbeek, H., Ruwaard, D., Ambergen, A. W., Leino-Kilpi, H., ... & Hamers, J. P. H. (2015). Change in quality of life of people with dementia recently admitted to long-term facilities. *Journal of Advanced Nursing*, 71(6), 1435–47.

Brodaty, H., Connors, M., Pond, D., Cumming, A. & Creasey, H. (2013). Dementia: 14 essentials of management. *Medicine Today*, 14(5), 29–41.

Bunn, F., Sworn, K., Brayne, C., Iliffe, S., Robinson, L. & Goodman, C. (2015). Contextualizing the findings of a systematic review on patient and carer experiences of dementia diagnosis and treatment: A qualitative study. *Health Expectations*, 18(5), 740–53.

Chenoweth, L., Stein Parbury, J., Lapkin, S. & Wang, Y. (2015). Organisational interventions for promoting person-centred care for people with dementia (Protocol). *Cochrane Database of Systematic Reviews*, (11). Art. no.: CD011963. doi: http://10.1002/14651858.CD011963

Clancy, A. (2015). Practice model for a dementia outreach service in rural Australia. *Australian Journal of Rural Health*, 23(2), 87–94.

Cooney, A. & O'Shea, E. (2018). The impact of life story work on person-centred care for people with dementia living in long-stay care settings in Ireland. *Dementia*. doi: http://.org/10.1177/1471301218756123

Dawson, A., Bowes, A., Kelly, F., Velzke, K. & Ward, R. (2015). Evidence of what works to support and sustain care at home for people with dementia: A literature review with a systematic approach. *BMC Geriatrics*, 15(59). doi: http://.org/10.1186/s12877-015-0053-9

Dementia Australia. (2016). Economic cost of dementia. Retrieved from www.dementia .org.au/dementia-news/issue-07/economic-cost-of-dementia

——(2018). Dementia – key facts and statistics. Retrieved from www.dementia.org.au/ files/documents/Key-facts-and-statistics.pdf

Dempsey, L., Dowling, M., Larkin, P. & Murphy, K. (2015). The unmet palliative care needs of those dying with dementia. *International Journal of Palliative Nursing*, 21(3), 126–33. doi: http://10.12968/ijpn.2015.21.3.126

Denning, K. & Hibberd, P. (2016). Exploring the community nurse role in family–centred care for patients with dementia. *British Journal of Community Nursing*, 21(4), 198–202. doi: http://org/10.12968/bicn.2016.21.4.198

Dubois, B., Hampel, H., Feldman, H. H., Scheltens, P., Aisen, P., Andrieu, S., ... & Broich, K. (2016). Preclinical Alzheimer's disease: Definition, natural history, and diagnostic criteria. *Alzheimer's & Dementia*, 12(3), 292–323.

Fortinsky, R. H., Delaney, C., Harel, O., Pasquale, K., Schjavland, E., Lynch, J., ... & Crumb, S. (2014). Results and lessons learned from a nurse practitioner-guided dementia care intervention for primary care patients and their family care givers. *Research Gerontological Nursing*, 7(3), 126–37.

Herke, M., Burckhardt, M., Wustmann, T., Watzke, S., Fink, A. & Langer, G. (2015). Environmental and behavioural modifications for improving food and fluid intake in people with dementia. *Cochrane Database of Systematic Reviews 2018. Issue 7*. Art. no. CD011542. doi: http://10.1002/14651858.CD011542.pub2

Hoffmann, K., Sobol, N. A., Frederiksen, K. S., Beyer, N., Vogel, A., Vestergaard, K., ... & Hasselbalch, S. G. (2016). Moderate-to-high intensity physical exercise in patients with Alzheimer's disease: A randomised controlled trial. *Journal of Alzheimer's Disease*, 50, 443–53. doi: http://org/10.3233/JAD-150817

Hungerford, C., Jones, T. & Cleary, M. (2014). Pharmacological versus non-pharmacological approaches to managing challenging behaviours for people with dementia. *British Journal of Community Nursing*, 19(2), 72–7.

Hyde, J., Perez, R., Doyle, P., Forester, B. P. & Whitfield, T. (2015). The impact of enhanced programming on aging in place for people with dementia in assisted living. *American Journal of Alzheimer's Disease and Other Dementias,* 30(8), 733–7.

Kalaria, R. N. (2016). Neuropathological diagnosis of vascular cognitive impairment and vascular dementia with implications for Alzheimer's disease. *Acta Neuropathologica*, 131(5), 659–85.

Katz, S., Ford, A. B., Moskowitz, M. D., Jackson, B. A. & Jaffe, M. W. (1963). The Index of ADL: A standardised measure of biological and psychosocial function. *Journal of the American Medical Association*, 185(12), 914–19.

Keast, K. (2015). Australia's dementia diagnosis. *Australian Nursing and Midwifery Journal*, 22(11), 18–23.

Kenji, K. (2014). Latest concept of Lewy body disease. *Psychiatry and Clinical Neurosciences*, 68(6), 391–4.

Kenyan, G. M., Clark, P. & de Vries, B. (eds). (2001). *Narrative Gerontology: Theory, Research and Practice*. New York: Springer.

Kitwood, T. (1997). *Dementia Reconsidered: The Person Comes First*. Oxford: Oxford University Press.

Lewis, L., Bartlett, R. & Patel, H. (2016). Improving verbal communication between older adults with dementia, care givers and the inter-professional team within the hospital setting: A literature review and qualitative analysis. *Age and Ageing*. 45(Suppl 1), i7–8. doi: http://10.1093/ageing/afw024.31

Looi, J. C., Byrne, G. J., Macfarlane, S., McKay, R. & O'Connor, D. W. (2014). Systemic approach to behavioural and psychological symptoms of dementia in residential aged care facilities. *Australian and New Zealand Journal of Psychiatry*, 48(2), 112–15. doi: http://10.1177/0004867413499078

MacKinlay, E. (2012). Resistance, resilience, and change: The person and dementia. *Journal of Religion, Spirituality & Aging*, 24(1/2), 80–92. doi: http://0.1080/15528030.2012.633048

Monroe, T. B., Parish, A. & Mion, L. C. (2015). Decision factors nurses use to assess pain in nursing home residents with dementia. *Archives of Psychiatric Nursing*, 6, 21–5.

Moyle, W., Cooke, M., Beattie, E., Shum, D., O'Dwyer, S. & Barrett, S. (2014). Foot massage versus quiet presence on agitation and mood in people with dementia: A randomised controlled trial. *International Journal of Nursing Studies*, 52(6), 856–64.

Moyle, W., Kellett, U., Ballantyne, A. & Gracia, N. (2011). Dementia and loneliness: An Australian perspective. *Journal of Clinical Nursing,* 20(9/10), 1445–53.

Nay, R., Bauer, M., Fetherstonhaugh, D., Moyle, W., Tarzia, L. & McAuliffe, L. (2015). Social participation and family carers of people living with dementia in Australia. *Health & Social Care in the Community*, 23(5), 550–8. doi: http://10.1111/hsc.12163

Nay, R., Garratt, S. & Fetherstonhaugh, D. (2014). *Older People: Issues and Innovations in Care* (4th edn). London: Elsevier.

New Zealand Ministry of Health (NZMOH). (2014). *Improving the Lives of People with Dementia*. Wellington: Ministry of Health.

NSW Health. (2014). *Aged Care – Working with People with Challenging Behaviours in Residential Aged Care Facilities: GL2006_014*. Sydney: Department of Health, NSW. Retrieved from www.health.nsw.gov.au/policies/gl/2006/pdf/GL2006_014.pdf

O'Connor, T. (2016). Revolutionising aged care. *Kai Taiki: Nursing New Zealand*, 22(10), 22–3.

Smith, B., Ali, S. & Quach, H. (2014). Public knowledge and beliefs about dementia risk reduction: A national survey of Australians. *BMC Public Health*, 14(661).

Springate, B. A. & Tremont, G. (2014). Dimensions of caregiver burden in dementia: Impact of demographic, mood and care recipient variables. *American Journal of Geriatric Psychiatry*, 22(3), 294–300.

Taylor, K. & Guerin, P. (2014). *Health Care and Indigenous Australians: Cultural Safety in Practice* (2nd edn). Melbourne: Palgrave Macmillan.

Taylor, M., Lord, S. R., Brodaty, H., Kurrie, S. E., Hamilton, S., Ramsay, E., ... & Close, J. C. (2017). A home-based, carer-enhanced exercise program improves balance and falls efficacy in community-dwelling older people with dementia. *International Psychogeriatrics*, 29(1), 81–91. doi: http://10.1017/S1041610216001629

Travers, C., Lie, D. & Martin-Khan, M. (2015). Dementia and the population health approach: Promise, pitfalls and progress. An Australian perspective. *Reviews in Clinical Gerontology*, 25, 60–71.

Van der Ploeg, E. S., Walker, H. & O'Connor, D. W. (2014). The feasibility of volunteers facilitating personalized activities for nursing home residents with dementia and agitation. *Geriatric Nursing*, 35(2), 142–6.

Vogel, L. (2018). Pilot project delivers dementia care that feels like home. *Canadian Medical Association Journal*, 190(23), E729. doi: http://10.1503/cmaj.109-5610

World Health Organization (WHO). (2015). *Dementia Fact Sheet No. 362*. Geneva: WHO.

16

Chronic kidney disease

Melissa Arnold-Chamney, Maryanne Podham
and Judith Anderson

LEARNING OBJECTIVES

After studying this chapter, you should be able to:

1. describe the underlying pathophysiology and risk factors of chronic kidney disease (CKD)
2. describe the different treatment options for people with CKD
3. understand the health prevention and health promotion requirements for people with CKD
4. identify issues affecting quality of life related to the treatment of CKD
5. understand the nurse's role in working with people with CKD.

Introduction

Tackling chronic conditions and their causes is a huge challenge facing Australia's health system (Australian Health Ministers' Advisory Council, 2017). Chronic kidney disease also continues to be an under-recognised condition globally, and occurs in both adults and children. Kidney Health Australia (2015a) suggests that around 1.7 million Australians over the age of 18 have clinical evidence of CKD, and less than 10 per cent of people with the condition are aware that they have it, as CKD typically has no symptoms. Unfortunately, up to 90 per cent of kidney function can be lost before symptoms become evident The Australian Institute of Health and Welfare (AIHW, 2017) stated 1.7 million hospitalisations during 2015–16 were associated with CKD, which accounted for 16 per cent of all hospitalisations in Australia. These results are similar in New Zealand with an estimated 7–10 per cent (approximately 210 000 people in 2015) of the total population living with some degree of CKD. The New Zealand Ministry of Health (NZMOH, 2015) states that there was an increase of 84 per cent in 12 years of reported cases of end stage CKD within the New Zealand population.

Chronic kidney disease is diagnosed when a person has evidence of kidney damage and/or a reduced kidney function which lasts longer than three months (Sandilands et al., 2013). Chronic kidney disease can be categorised into five stages (increasing from stage 1 to 5 stage), in accordance with the **glomerular filtration rate (GFR)** and the presence of albuminuria. **End-stage kidney disease (ESKD)** is the most severe form of CKD, with those affected often requiring **renal replacement therapy (RRT)**, either in the form of dialysis or kidney transplantation, without which they would not survive (Hite & DeBellis, 2009).

The health care and economic burden of CKD on individuals, communities and globally is high, and is predicted to further increase as the population ages and the prevalence of diabetes increases. In Australia, the health care cost for people with CKD was 85 per cent more than for people without CKD, costs increasing incrementally with each stage of the disease. For example, the annual health care cost for people with stage 4 or 5 CKD was $14 545 AUD compared with $1829 AUD for people without the disease (Wyld et al., 2015). In New Zealand, the cost of treatment for a person with ESKD on RRT, such as **haemodialysis,** ranged from $30 000 to $60 000 per person per year (NZMOH, 2015). This cost is not only measured in monetary terms – CKD also impacts on education, employment, family responsibilities, reduced quality of life and life expectancy (AIHW, 2014). In Australia, Aboriginal and Torres Strait Islander peoples are more than twice as likely as non-Indigenous people to have indicators of CKD. They are three times as likely to have indicators of stage 1 CKD, and more than four times as likely to have indicators of stages 4–5 CKD (Australian Bureau of Statistics, 2014). In New Zealand, the disparity in incidence of ESKD for Māori people also persists. The rate of haemodialysis commencement for non-Māori, non-Pacific individuals was 4.5-fold lower than for Māori, similar to Indigenous Australians who were five times more likely than non-Indigenous Australians to begin haemodialysis (ANZDATA Registry, 2017; NZMOH, 2016).

To effectively promote the health and wellbeing of a person with CKD, nurses and multidisciplinary teams need to have an understanding of how the function of the kidney is altered in CKD, the complexities of care when a person has CKD, other

Glomerular filtration rate (GFR) – the amount of fluid filtered from the blood through the kidney per minute.

End-stage kidney disease (ESKD) – the most severe form of CKD, with those affected often requiring RRT, either in the form of RRT or kidney transplantation.

Renal replacement therapy (RRT) – a therapy that replaces the normal blood filtering of the kidney. It can involve dialysis (haemodialysis or peritoneal dialysis) or renal transplantation.

Haemodialysis – involves the filtration of blood across a semi-permeable membrane (the dialyser) to remove toxins from the body, via the dialysate. Excess toxins are removed via diffusion and excess fluid by ultrafiltration.

chronic conditions including diabetes and cardiovascular disease, and the physical, physiological and social aspects of the person and their family who are affected by a diagnosis of CKD.

Underlying pathophysiology and risk factors for chronic kidney disease

The kidneys are resilient organs (see Figure 16.1) and are responsible for several functions, many of which are interlinked. The kidneys' functions include the regulation of water and electrolytes, waste product excretion, hormone secretion and acid–base homeostasis (Copstead & Banasik, 2013; Sandilands et al., 2013).

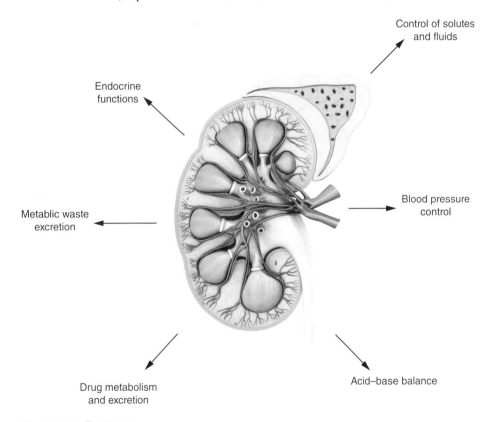

Figure 16.1 The kidney

The progression of CKD involves glomerulosclerosis, interstitial leukocyte infiltration, tubular atrophy and tubulointerstitial fibrosis (Schlondorff, 2008). There are a number of theories surrounding the actual cause of CKD, including immunological-mediated reaction or injury, renal cell tissue hypoxia and ischaemia, the effects of exogenic agents such as pharmaceutical drugs, the effects of endogenous substances such as glucose, and congenital defects (Matovinovic, 2009). The kidneys' response to these factors always leads to localised tissue damage and the formation of scar tissue or fibrosis. Fibrosis, in turn, leads to disruption in the structure and function of the nephrons, which then affects the ability of the kidneys to maintain homeostasis (Schlondorff, 2008).

Chronic kidney disease, cardiovascular disease and diabetic kidney disease

In countries worldwide, including Australia and New Zealand, diabetes is the leading cause of ESKD. In 2012, 4727 Australians, who had type 2 diabetes and ESKD, were receiving either dialysis or living with a functional transplant (donor kidney). It was also estimated that during the same period 250 000 Australians had early stages of both diabetes and kidney disease, which in turn put them at a high risk of cardiovascular events and dying prematurely (White & Chadban, 2014). Hyperglycaemia, hypertension and dyslipidaemia cause microvascular complications, which cause changes in the function of the renal system. Hyperglycaemia leads to kidney hypotrophy, causing increased pressure within the glomerulus; this pressure causes hyperfiltration of the glomerular capillaries, allowing the excretion of albumin into the urine. Prostaglandin release in response to hyperglycaemia leads to vasodilation, and increased renal perfusion and glomerular pressure, resulting in hyperfiltration and proteinuria. Hypertension causes an increase in afferent arteriole pressure, which over time leads to increases in glomerular pressures. This pressure increase impacts on the facilitation of proteinuria. Dyslipidaemia leads to oxidative stress, which causes structural damage to the kidney. Collectively, these three pathways cause damage to the glomerular and scar tissue develops. Renal function is lost, proteinuria results and irreversible kidney damage occurs (Hite & DeBellis, 2009).

Chronic kidney disease classification system

Each of the five stages of CKD (see Table 16.1) is predominantly linked to the person's estimated glomerular filtration rate (eGFR), as well as identifiers of kidney damage including proteinuria (Sandilands et al., 2013). Stage 1 and stage 2 are considered a silent form of CKD as the person is usually asymptomatic. At stages 3 and 4 symptoms include a lower eGFR. They also include a mild feeling of being unwell, and electrolyte disturbances of phosphate and potassium. Stage 5 is ESKD. This is diagnosed when the person's eGFR is recorded at 15 mL/min or less. At this level the person requires RRT of either dialysis or a kidney transplant (Hite & DeBellis, 2009).

Table 16.1　Stages of CKD

Stage	eGFR mL/min	Description	Symptoms	Treatment suggestions
1	> 90	• Normal GFR • Comorbidities can affect kidney function	• Nil – mild renal • Possibly those related to comorbidities	• Identify and address risk factors • Education and treatment of comorbid conditions
2	60–89	• Evidence of kidney damage with mild reduction of GFR	• Increase in serum creatinine • Abnormal urinalysis • Mild proteinuria	• Continue comorbid education and treatment to slow progression of damage

Stage	eGFR mL/min	Description	Symptoms	Treatment suggestions
3	30–59	• Half of kidney function lost and moderate reduction of GFR	• As above and nocturia • Hypertension • Anaemia	• Increase in treatment of comorbid conditions • Encourage diet and lifestyle changes • Addition of medications and possible surgical interventions
4	15–29	• Severe reduction of GFR	• As above and fatigue • Cold intolerance • Shortness of breath	• Continue management of comorbid conditions • Discussion of RRTs
5	< 15	• End stage kidney failure	• As above and malaise • Pruritus • Leg cramps • Nausea and vomiting	• Initiation of dialysis • Consideration of kidney transplantation • Conservative treatment

Sources: Adapted from Hite & DeBellis (2009); Sandilands et al. (2013)

Risk factors for chronic kidney disease

As with all risk factors it is unknown at what time the risk causes the chronic condition or when the condition can lead to the risk factor; for example, high blood pressure can lead to CKD, as well as being the result of it (AIHW, 2015). Modifiable behavioural risk factors associated with CKD include tobacco smoking, limited physical activity, excessive alcohol consumption and a nutritionally poor diet. Non-modifiable biomedical risk factors include: being overweight or obese, hypertension or cardiovascular disease, type 2 diabetes or impaired fasting glucose (also known as prediabetes), being over the age of 50, being of Aboriginal or Torres Strait Islander heritage, recurrent urinary tract infections, exposure to non-steroidal anti-inflammatory drugs (NSAIDs), aminoglycoside antibiotics such as gentamicin, and radiological contrast agents such as iodine (AIHW, 2015; Campbell, Woods & Sankey, 2008).

A group of risk factors known as the metabolic syndrome have been strongly linked to the development of CKD. The metabolic syndrome is characterised as the presence of abdominal obesity, low levels of high-density lipoprotein cholesterol, high triglyceride levels, hypertension and fasting hyperglycaemia. Those individuals with metabolic syndrome also have a higher risk of microalbuminuria, which greatly increases the likelihood of rapid progression to ESKD (Campbell et al., 2008).

Children and chronic kidney disease

Risk factors for CKD in children differ from that of adults. Harambat and colleagues (2012) suggest that in children under 12 years of age, congenital abnormalities of the kidney and urinary tract, and hereditary neuropathies are the most common cause. In children 12 years and older, glomerulonephritis is the leading cause of the development of CKD. Interestingly, children who are found to have any major structural anomalies are considered to have CKD without having to meet the usual three-month-with-symptoms criteria, as used in the adult population (Harambat et al., 2012).

Treatment options

Treatment options for someone with CKD are known as renal replacement therapies (RRTs). Ideally, people should be referred to a nephrologist for assessment a minimum of one year prior to needing RRT (Thomas, 2014). Renal replacement therapy is the term used to encompass the life-sustaining but non-curative treatments which are required for people with CKD. It includes three modalities: haemodialysis, **peritoneal dialysis (PD)** and transplantation. A fourth option of supportive or palliative treatment is also available. No matter what option is chosen, the nurse will be at the forefront of health care, and will be there to undertake nursing assessment and carry out the treatment, and to be an advocate and educator. This includes further disease prevention if applicable, and assessing the health needs of individuals, their carers and their families.

Haemodialysis

Haemodialysis (HD) involves the filtration of blood across a semi-permeable membrane (the dialyser) to remove toxins from the body, via the dialysate. Excess toxins are removed by **diffusion** and excess fluid by **ultrafiltration** (Thomas, 2014). People can undertake their HD treatment in hospital, stand-alone HD centres or at home. Stand-alone HD centres are in the community and largely managed by nurses. This is also the same within rural and remote areas of Australia, where HD centres have been established so that people can remain living close to their homes and not be required to move to a larger town for treatment. Haemodailysis treatment is usually undertaken for four hours three times a week, but individuals can also have alternate day HD, daily HD or nocturnal HD.

There are three main forms of vascular access available for those requiring HD for long-term RRT. In order of preference, these are: arteriovenous fistulae (AVF), arteriovenous grafts (AVG) using prosthetic or biological material, and either tunnelled or non-tunnelled catheters placed in a central vein. Arteriovenous fistulae have been shown to have better patency rates, access survival and the lowest number of interventions during the lifespan of the access. Arteriovenous fistulae also have lower rates of access-related sepsis, and overall morbidity and mortality is lower compared to AVG and central venous haemodialysis catheters (Padberg, Calligaro & Sidawy, 2008). Hospitalisation frequency is also diminished and costs are the lowest with AVF access (Ravani et al., 2013).

There are numerous types of HD that can be undertaken and each has its own benefits, but there are also negative aspects which can include additional costs to the

Peritoneal dialysis (PD) – involves the removal of excess toxins and fluids via diffusion, convection and ultrafiltration from the blood (Levy, Brown & Lawrence, 2016). There are two types of PD available: continuing ambulatory peritoneal dialysis and continuous cycler peritoneal dialysis.

Diffusion – the movement of a substance from an area of higher to lower concentration.

Ultrafiltration – achieved by the application of positive and negative hydrostatic pressure.

renal unit. HD is often performed via two needles if using an AVF or AVG, or double lumen catheter (see Figure 16.2). Occasionally, single lumen dialysis is required however, this is not recommended practice due to increased recirculation reducing the efficiency of the treatment.

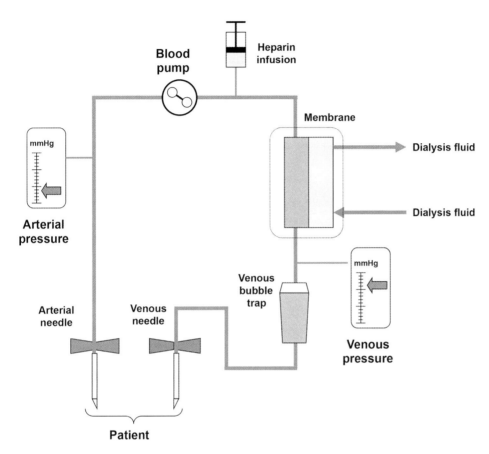

Figure 16.2 Haemodialysis circuit

Peritoneal dialysis

Peritoneal dialysis involves the removal of excess toxins and fluids via diffusion, **convection** and ultrafiltration from the blood (Levy et al., 2016). There are two types of PD available (see Figure 16.3); these are continuing ambulatory peritoneal dialysis – where the person needs to undertake an exchange four to five times per day – and continuous cycler peritoneal dialysis, which is an automated form of peritoneal dialysis, where a machine performs exchanges while the person sleeps. At times people may also require another daytime exchange, but many can have the daytime free from PD requirements. Continuous cycler peritoneal dialysis is becoming more common than continuing ambulatory peritoneal dialysis and both forms of PD can be undertaken at home.

Convection – the movement of molecules (for example, waste products) through a semi-permeable membrane which is associated with fluid during ultrafiltration. This is also known as solvent drag.

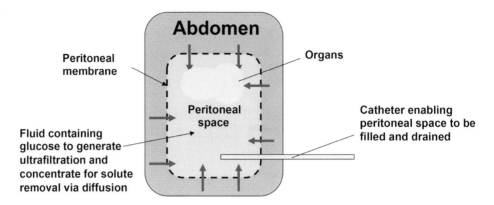

Figure 16.3   Peritoneal dialysis

Transplantation

Transplantation is where a healthy kidney from one person (the donor) is transferred into the body of a person who has little or no kidney function (the recipient). A healthy kidney can come from either a living donor or deceased donor. One form of living donation that is increasing is the use of altruistic donation. The donor will have no connection with the recipient but wishes to donate a kidney to a stranger in need (Morrissey et al., 2005).

Supportive or palliative treatment

Supportive or palliative treatment is required when the person with advanced CKD (stage 5) decides to forgo RRT, recognising that the burden of RRT may outweigh their likely survival and quality of life benefits (Noble, 2008). It is an important role of those involved in the care of individuals and their families after a diagnosis of CKD that a discussion surrounding the end of life care wishes of the person are discussed early and documented in an advanced care plan. Chronic kidney disease is known to be a progressive and life-limiting condition that can lead to cognitive impairment in the advanced stages. An advanced care plan allows clarification and communication of a person's wishes, which can promote increased compliance with treatment options and improved satisfaction for families in relation to treatment trajectories and psychological outcomes during the bereavement process (Luckett et al., 2017). This option should ensure that individuals, and their families, are supported and fully informed of their options and of the type of care they wish to receive up until the end of their life. More on the care of the person at the end of their life is provided in Chapter 21.

SKILLS IN PRACTICE

Treatment modalities for stage 5 chronic kidney disease

Hamza is a 32-year-old male with stage 4 CKD. He has been admitted to the ward this morning following a routine outpatient appointment with his nephrologist. As you are admitting Hamza to the ward, he asks you about his future and the possible treatment modalities he may require if his CKD progresses to stage 5.

QUESTION

What would you would tell Hamza about the positives and negatives of different treatments which may be an option for him? Consider the differing education formats you will be able to use to provide this information to him.

Promoting health and reducing risk for people with chronic kidney disease

Health promotion is 'the process of enabling people to take control over those factors that determine their health' (Keleher & MacDougall, 2011). Unfortunately, often signs and symptoms of kidney disease do not appear until late in progressive CKD. These symptoms can include raised blood pressure, fluid retention, tiredness, nausea and vomiting, weight loss, and itchy skin. Due to the delay in recognition of CKD, some health promotion strategies can be difficult to achieve, as the signs and symptoms are already affecting how a person is able to function in their daily life.

Delaying chronic kidney disease progression

There are a number of ways to assist in delaying the progression of CKD. This is suitable for people who present to their general practitioner (GP) and are referred to a nephrologist at least 12 months prior to reaching ESKD. Unfortunately, at least one-fifth of people present less than one month before requiring RRT, and therefore it is not possible to delay their progression from one stage to another stage of CKD. Late referral of patients to specialist renal services is associated with poor clinical outcomes (Thomas, 2014).

Aspects that can help in delaying CKD progression are for a person to aim for a blood pressure below 140/90, or 130/80 mmHg if the person has diabetes (Thomas, 2014). First-line therapy for hypertension is either **ACE inhibitor** or **angiotensin receptor blocker**, as both are associated with a reduction in proteinuria and slowing the progression of CKD (Cardiovascular Expert Group, 2012). Regular measurement, assessment and management of the person's cardiovascular risk (smoking cessation, weight loss and exercise) is crucial. It is also important for patients to avoid nephrotoxic medication (for example, NSAIDs) as these can cause further damage to the kidneys. Another important aspect is to avoid adding salt to food.

The health promotion strategies that are available will also depend upon the stage of CKD. If the person is still in stage 3 then medication review, diabetes management, blood pressure control and cardiovascular disease management can be effective in delaying progression to stage 4. If the person is at stage 4 they already have moderate to severe kidney damage and will require additional input. Here, the focus should start on the preparation for RRT once the person's eGFR drops below 20 mL/min/1.72 m^2 (Thomas, 2014).

Early referral and attendance at a low clearance clinic can assist in improving issues of anaemia, poor nutrition, bone disease management, **access creation** such as AVF or Tenckhoff catheter (if needed), and the opportunity for the person to make informed choices about the type of RRT, transplantation, or palliative or supportive treatment they

ACE inhibitor – a medication that blocks the body from producing angiotensin II. When angiotensin II enters the bloodstream, blood vessels become narrower and blood pressure is consequently raised.

Angiotensin receptor blocker – a medication that blocks the body from producing angiotensin II.

Access creation – describes the creation of access for haemodialysis or peritoneal dialysis.

need. It is essential that the individual and family work collaboratively with the renal staff so that a personalised education program is implemented that improves their understanding of the individual's CKD and its possible outcomes.

REFLECTION

Consider what other health professionals you might include in a discussion with the person and their family dealing with the progression of CKD to ESKD and requiring RRT.

SKILLS IN PRACTICE

Requiring renal replacement therapy

Archie is an 11-year-old Caucasian boy who has been admitted to the renal ward of the local children's hospital. Archie has been diagnosed as stage 5 CKD secondary to haemolytic uraemic syndrome, after a recent *E. coli* infection that he contracted from eating contaminated beef. On admission to the ward the following was determined about Archie:

- weight – 27 kg – his parents state this was 25 kg two weeks ago; he also had vomiting and bloody diarrhoea for three days after eating the beef
- height – 145 cm
- blood pressure – 160/94
- diet – home-cooked meals and sandwiches, chips and apple juice for school lunches. Archie states that he likes drinking lemonade instead of water on the weekends, and that his favourite foods include strawberries, bananas, tomatoes and popcorn
- eGFR – 16 ml/min
- visual – pale, irritable and needing to rest frequently. Not able to stay awake at school this past week.

During this admission, Archie and his parents meet Jasper the nephrologist. Jasper recommends that Archie has a subclavian vein catheter inserted and commence three-times-a-week haemodialysis. He also wishes to commence testing of Archie's parents for a possible kidney donation.

QUESTIONS

1. What education would you provide to Archie and his parents about the management of his subclavian catheter and the haemodialysis treatment?
2. What education is needed for Archie about his dietary requirements?
3. Archie is concerned that he will miss school and his friends will think he is weird for having a catheter. How can you ease his concerns?
4. What education would you provide about live donation versus cadaveric donation so that everyone is clear about the options available?

Issues affecting quality of life related to treatment of chronic kidney disease
Physical and mental health

In the context of health, quality of life relates to the holistic wellbeing of a person and should address physical, functional, psychological and social aspects of their life (Randall & Ford, 2011). One issue that affects people of all ages is quality of life, and there is a need for nurses to focus on both physical and mental health care needs. Elderly people, in addition to the illness burden of their CKD, encounter multiple sociological and psychological issues, which can impact on their wellbeing and quality of life (Brown et al., 2015). Thomas (2014) states that good nutrition has emerged as playing a vital role in reducing RRT morbidity and mortality, yet there is an increasing awareness that any comprehensive evaluation of health outcomes should assess patient-based outcomes, and not just morbidity and mortality (Levy et al., 2016).

The way CKD is experienced by the individual and their family is influenced not only by the stage of the disease process, but also by family structure, the role of the individual in the family, their professional status, and their personal and family status (Lubkin, 2015). Renal failure needs to be recognised as a family concern, as it not only affects the person's mental health and wellbeing but can also affect their family and friends; so, it is important that individuals, families and carers are supported (Hope, 2012). This is consistent with the triad at the core of the Innovative Care for Chronic Conditions Framework (ICCCF) adopted by the World Health Organization, which focuses on the relationship between the health professional, client/family and community and, as noted throughout this book, is the preferred model for chronic care management internationally (Nuño et al., 2012).

Multidisciplinary and individualised education that ensures knowledge of the condition and treatment options available are imperative to assist quality of life, which is known to improve if a person is given the freedom of choice in relation to their RRT modality. Health-related quality of life is the impact of a chronic disease and its related treatment on individuals' perceptions of their own physical and mental function. There are numerous measures that are used within the renal specialisation, such as the Medical Outcomes Study Short Form-36 (SF-36) and Sickness Impact Profile (SIP). The impact of ESKD on quality of life has been recognised as an important outcome measure. The Kidney Disease Quality of Life Short Form (KDQOL-SF™) is an example of a validated and widely used tool that is a renal specific measure of quality of life.

Depression is experienced in less than 10 per cent of the general population, but is prevalent in 20–30 per cent of people on RRT (Levy et al. 2016). People who are depressed have decreased quality of life, increased hospitalisation, **concordance** issues with treatments and greater mortality (Dobbels et al., 2010). Sexual difficulties can be an issue, with approximately 75 per cent of men on RRT experiencing erectile dysfunction and 30–80 per cent of women on RRT experiencing symptoms associated with sexual dysfunction (Thomas, 2014). Body image is interwoven with sexuality as those on RRT will have had at least one form of vascular access surgery that will have

Concordance – where the person with the health issue and the health practitioner work in partnership to make decisions together.

caused them to have scars, or in the case of a peritoneal or vascular catheter, a foreign body that is visible to them and can have a negative effect on their quality of life.

Renal transplantation

Renal transplantation is the treatment of choice for many people and, in general, will provide better quality of life than a life with RRT. However, organs available for transplantation are in short supply and there are transplant waiting lists in both Australia and New Zealand. Overall, quality of life is better for transplant recipients than those on RRT, with 80 per cent of transplant recipients performing at normal physiological levels, compared to 50 per cent on RRT (Thomas, 2014). Transplant recipients no longer need to undertake RRT so they have increased freedom, and their life satisfaction, and physical and emotional wellbeing, are significantly better than people on HD or PD (Danovitch, 2017).

The nurse's role in working with people with chronic kidney disease

In Australia, nurses play a key role in providing care for all people with CKD. Nurses work across a range of health care and community services in urban, rural and remote settings, interacting with individuals and family members, who have diverse personal and cultural needs (Kelly et al., 2016). Aggressive and ongoing assessment, treatment and management options are often considered first without taking into consideration the individual's and their family's understanding of the diagnosis, and, in turn, what the prognosis actually means. Aside from an understanding of what CKD is, it is imperative that nurses also have skills in educating individuals and their families to become active collaborators in dealing with any chronic condition, including kidney disease (Alikari et al., 2015). Nurses need to enquire into both the physical and psychological wellbeing as psychological issues, such as depression and anxiety-related fears, can create a barrier where the person does not feel these issues are important enough to broach with health care professionals (Randall & Ford, 2011). Nurses need to be aware that renal disease can have an impact upon the person and their education/career prospects, their social life and their lifestyle, including religious and cultural needs (Thomas, 2014). The ideal approach when dealing with a diagnosis of any stage of CKD is to include a multidisciplinary and collaborative approach which identifies behavioural and problem-solving skills that involve the person and support networks in an empowering manner (Rice, Kocurek & Snead, 2010).

Nurses need to ensure that cultural aspects of care are taken into account and consider cultural safety of all individuals. A New Zealand Māori and nursing council developed a model (Papps & Ramsden, 1996) endorsed by the Congress of Aboriginal and Torres Strait Islander Nurses and Midwives (2014). Care can only be safe if it is identified as such by the people themselves. Nurses also need to consider social determinants of health, power imbalances and the impact of racism, assumptions and colonisation impacts (Kelly et al., 2016).

Medical treatments alone do not address personal issues, such as the psychological and behavioural choices a person makes. Part of the nurse's role is to ensure that people are aware that CKD is lifelong and will impact on all aspects of their life, and that of their family and support networks. When developing a management plan, it is important to consider many self-care behaviours, including those explained in Table 16.2.

Table 16.2   Management plan for the person with chronic kidney disease

Self-care behaviour	Considerations	Who to collaborate with
Diet	• Consider understanding of portion size, when to eat and how often to eat • What are healthy choices (especially in limited availability areas)? • Include family in these discussions	• Dietitian/nutritionist • Consider community groups to have cooking classes
Activity	• Discuss importance of activity to weight management • Discuss that activity can be free and does not need to be arduous	• Exercise physiologist • Physiotherapist/occupational therapist • Community groups to have group sessions
Self-monitoring	• Discuss importance of measuring blood pressure weekly • Monitoring weight changes • Monitoring urine for protein and/or infection	• Pharmacist/local chemist • GP
Medication compliance	• Discuss the importance of taking medications as directed • Discuss possible interactions between medications and food • Explain that medications and changes to diet and activity can affect progression of disease	• Pharmacist • GP
Risk reduction/consideration	• Discuss use of alcohol, tobacco, illicit substances • Discuss over-the-counter preparations • Discuss importance of having regular screening for other conditions including diabetes, heart disease and cancer • Discuss how risk reduction can maximise quality of life	• GP • Nurse practitioner/renal nurse specialist • Pharmacist
Problem solving	• Develop a 'sick day' plan and ensure family are aware of the plan, too • Develop a network that can assist with change-in-life situations • Develop a plan for dealing with the ageing process	• Social worker • GP
Coping strategies	• Develop skills to reinforce motivation and adherence to treatment plan • Discuss and develop a 'what if' plan and share this with support network	• Social worker • GP • Nurse practitioner/renal nurse specialist

Source: Adapted from Mobley (2009); Rice et al. (2010)

REFLECTION

Create a table that discusses the advantages and disadvantages of the various RRTs you could use in the education of a person with ESKD.

Advanced nursing practice

Clinical nurse specialists can play a significant role in caring for the client who has CKD. A thorough assessment can indicate the presence of comorbidities, such as anaemia, which can have serious consequences if not treated effectively. During treatment, clinical nurse specialists also assess client responses such as haemoglobin or iron levels. Nurses play a large part in supporting the work of the multidisciplinary team and ensuring consistency of health service provision and implementation of evidence-based practice. They assist with the education of other staff, and the development of local policies and procedures to contextualise the care provision to the local community and assist with education (Bejjani, 2015). Nurse-led CKD management programs have been found to be effective in improving client outcomes and satisfaction (Bejjani, 2015).

The risk factor of high blood pressure is significant, not only in developing CKD, but also in increasing morbidity and death as it progresses. For this reason, managing blood pressure is one of the targets frequently set with clients who have this chronic condition. Blood pressure control has been independently associated with a person's knowledge of the goal blood pressure (less than 130/80 is recommended), clearly demonstrating the benefits of an informed, collaborative relationship with these clients, and the need for clear goal setting and frequent discussion of each goal (Wright-Nunes et al., 2012). Multidisciplinary care has been demonstrated to reduce overall care costs for both adults and children with CKD by slowing its progression, and thereby making it a worthwhile investment at the micro level of the ICCCF. These multidisciplinary services are frequently led by nurses (especially those functioning at an advanced level); they can have a significant impact in managing nutrition, anaemia and hypertension, and often involve pharmacists, dieticians, social workers and physicians (Filler & Lipshultz, 2012); and have also been demonstrated to be effective in Indigenous Australian populations (Barrett & Salem, 2015). The addition of a nurse practitioner to the multidisciplinary team caring for people with CKD has been shown to improve management of blood pressure, low-density lipoprotein and parathyroid hormone (McCrory et al., 2018). Clinical practice guidelines exist for improving quality of care and health outcomes for clients with kidney disease in Australia and New Zealand; for example, see the *KHA-CARI Guidelines* (Kidney Health Australia, 2015b).

SKILLS IN PRACTICE

Living with chronic kidney disease

James is a 42-year-old Caucasian male who has been a frequent patient in the renal ward of the local hospital. James was first admitted at the age of 32 with stage 3 CKD secondary to idiopathic glomerulosclerosis. James was managed with diet, exercise and monitoring of blood pressure which maintained his renal health until the age of 38. After James' spouse died, there was a decline in his diet and exercise regime, and overall physical and mental health.

During a medical check-up at the age of 42, the following was found (see Table 16.3).

Table 16.3   Comparison of patient results at 38 years and 42 years

	Last visit at 38 years	Findings at current visit/notes
Weight	62 kg	85 kg – increase of 23 kg in 4 years
Height	182 cm	182 cm
Blood pressure	126/78	158/92
Diet	• Good intake of fresh fruit and vegetables, fish, chicken, lean red meat, • No high fat foods (takeaways, etc.) • Low sugar intake • Brown rice • Minimal alcohol • No energy drinks or soft drinks consumed • Prefers water and tea	• Mostly takeaway food since wife died; no time to cook or doesn't want to cook • Increase in alcohol consumption (now daily, was weekly previously) • Increase in high sugar, white starch breads • Drinking soft drinks instead of water
Smoking status	Nil	Nil
eGFR	48 mL/min	15 mL/min

Following this visit, James was referred to a nephrologist, who recommended James have a Tenckhoff catheter inserted and commence continuous ambulatory peritoneal dialysis.

QUESTION

What education would you provide to James about the management and treatment of his CKD? Don't forget to take a holistic perspective, and address promoting health and reducing risk aspects of his care.

SUMMARY

Learning objective 1: Describe the underlying pathophysiology and risk factors of CKD.

Damaged kidneys form scar tissue or fibrosis, leading to disruption in the structure and function of the nephrons, which then affects the ability of the kidneys to maintain homeostasis (Schlondorff, 2008). There are five stages of CKD ranging from normal to end stage kidney disease (ESKD). Modifiable behavioural risk factors associated with CKD include tobacco smoking, limited physical activity, excessive alcohol consumption and a nutritionally poor diet. Non-modifiable biomedical risk factors include being overweight or obese, hypertension or cardiovascular disease, type 2 diabetes or impaired fasting glucose (also known as prediabetes), being over the age of 50, being of Aboriginal or Torres Strait Islander heritage, recurrent urinary tract infections, and exposure to non-steroidal anti-inflammatory drugs (NSAIDs), aminoglycoside antibiotics such as gentamicin and radiological contrast agents such as iodine.

Learning objective 2: Describe the different treatment options for people with CKD.

Treatment options for people with CKD are known as RRT. Renal replacement therapy includes three modalities: haemodialysis, peritoneal dialysis and transplantation. A fourth option of supportive or palliative treatment is also available.

Learning objective 3: Understand the health prevention and health promotion requirements for people with CKD.

Early referral and attendance at a low clearance clinic, as required, can help improve issues of anaemia, poor nutrition, bone disease management and access creation (if needed). It also enables individuals to have the opportunity to make informed choices about the type of RRT they want, which can either result in transplantation, or palliative or supportive treatment.

Learning objective 4: Identify issues affecting quality of life related to the treatment of CKD.

Quality of life will affect people with CKD of all ages, and there is a need for nurses to focus on both the physical and mental health care needs of those in their care. Elderly people, in addition to the illness burden of their CKD, encounter multiple sociological and psychological issues which can impact on their wellbeing and quality of life.

Learning objective 5: Understand the nurse's role in working with people with CKD.

Nurses play a pivotal role in encouraging and supporting the person and their family following a diagnosis of CKD. Renal disease can impact on all aspects of daily life including the physical, mental, social and cultural aspects. Management plans need to address the biomedical symptoms, as well as support adaption and coping strategies for this condition (Thomas, 2014). Clinical nurse specialists can play a significant role in caring for people with CKD. This should include a thorough assessment to indicate the presence of comorbidities which can have serious consequences if not treated effectively. Nurse-led CKD programs assist with education of other staff and the development of local policies, and can improve client outcomes and satisfaction (Bejjani, 2015).

REVIEW QUESTIONS

1. What are the differences between each of the five stages of CKD?
2. What are the three forms of RRT? Describe them.
3. How would you educate a person with mild kidney disease in order to prevent their condition from worsening?
4. Identify five social or psychological issues that could impact on someone with CKD.
5. Describe three significant aspects of the role of the nurse in caring for a person with CKD.

RESEARCH TOPIC

Find clinical guidelines for the management of CKD and identify three new strategies that you could implement into your practice.

FURTHER READING

Australian Institute of Health and Welfare (AIHW). (2015). *Cardiovascular Disease, Diabetes and Chronic Kidney Disease – Australian Facts*. Canberra: AIHW.

Dobbels, F., Duerinckx, N., Breunig, C. & De Geest, S. (2010). What every renal nurse should know about depression. *Journal of Renal Nursing*, 2(1), 6–11.

Levy, J., Brown, E. & Lawrence, A. (2016). *Oxford Handbook of Dialysis* (4th edn). Oxford: Oxford University Press.

Thomas, N. (2014). *Renal Nursing* (4th edn). Oxford: Wiley Blackwell.

Wright-Nunes, J. A., Luther, J. M., Ikizler, T. A. & Cavanaugh, K. L. (2012). Patient knowledge of blood pressure target is associated with improved blood pressure control in chronic kidney disease. *Patient Education and Counseling*, 88(2), 184–8. doi: http://10.1016/j.pec.2012.02.015

REFERENCES

Alikari, V., Matziou, V., Tsironi, M., Theofilou, P. & Zyga, S. (2015). The effects of nursing counselling on improving knowledge, adherence to treatment and quality of life of patients undergoing hemodialysis. *International Journal of Caring Sciences*, 8(2), 514–18.

ANZDATA Registry. (2017). *The 40th Annual ANZDATA Report*. Adelaide: Australia and New Zealand Dialysis and Transplant Registry. Retrieved from www.anzdata.org.au

Australian Bureau of Statistics. (2014). *Australian Aboriginal and Torres Strait Islander Health Survey: Biomedical Results, 2012–13*. Report No.: 4727.0.55.003. Canberra: Australian Bureau of Statistics.

Australian Health Ministers' Advisory Council. (2017). *National Strategic Framework for Chronic Conditions*. Canberra: Australian Government.

Australian Institute of Health and Welfare (AIHW). (2014). *Projections of the Prevalence of Treated End-Stage Kidney Disease in Australia: 2012–2020*. Cat. no. PHE 176. Canberra: AIHW.

—— (2015). *Cardiovascular Disease, Diabetes and Chronic Kidney Disease – Australian Facts*. Canberra: AIHW.

—— (2017). Chronic kidney disease compendium. Canberra: AIHW. Retrieved from www .aihw.gov.au/reports/chronic-kidney-disease/chronic-kidney-disease-compendium/ contents/how-many-australians-have-chronic-kidney-disease

Barrett, E., Salem, L. & Wilson, S. (2015). Chronic kidney disease in an Aboriginal population: A nurse practitioner-led approach to management. *Australian Journal of Rural Health,* 23(6). doi: http://org/10.1111/ajr.12230

Bejjani, R. (2015). Anemic control in patients with chronic kidney disease: A controversial issue. *MEDSURG Nursing*, 24(1), 23–6.

Brown, M. A., Collett, G. K., Josland, E. A., Foote, C., Li, Q. & Brennan, F. P. (2015). CKD in elderly patients managed without dialysis: Survival, symptoms, and quality of life. *Clinical Journal of the American Society of Nephrology*, 10(2), 260–8.

Campbell, S., Woods, M. & Sankey, J. (2008). Chronic kidney disease and the primary health care network. *Renal Society of Australia*, 4(3), 81–9.

Cardiovascular Expert Group. (2012). *Therapeutic Guidelines: Cardiovascular. Version 6.* Melbourne: Therapeutic Guidelines Ltd.

Congress of Aboriginal and Torres Strait Islander Nurses and Midwives. (2014). Cultural safety position statement. Retrieved from http://catsinam.org.au/static/uploads/ files/cultural-safety-endorsed-march-2014-fginzphsxbz.pdf

Copstead, L. & Banasik, J. (2013). *Pathophysiology* (5th edn). St Louis, MO: Elsevier.

Danovitch, G. (2017). *Handbook of Kidney Transplantation* (6th edn). Philadelphia, PA: Lippincott Williams & Wilkins.

Dobbels, F., Duerinckx, N., Breunig, C. & De Geest, S. (2010). What every renal nurse should know about depression. *Journal of Renal Nursing*, 2(1), 6–11.

Filler, G. & Lipshultz, S. (2012). Why multidisciplinary clinics should be the standard for treating chronic kidney disease. *Pediatric Nephrology*, 27(10), 1831–4. doi: http:// 10.1007/ s00467-012-2236-3

Harambat, J., van Stralen, K., Kim, J. & Tizard, J. (2012). Epidemiology of chronic kidney disease in children. *Pediatric Nephrology*, 27, 363–73.

Hite, P. F. & DeBellis, H. F. (2009). Diabetic kidney disease: A renin-angiotensin-aldosterone system focused review. *Journal of Pharmacy Practice*, 22(6), 560–70.

Hope, J. (2012). Call for action on mental and emotional health. *Journal of Renal Nursing*, 4(1), 5.

Keleher, H. & MacDougall, C. (2011). Concepts of health and primary health care. In H. Keleher & C. McDougall (eds), *Understanding Health*. Melbourne: Oxford University Press.

Kelly, J., Wilden, C., Chamney, M., Martin, G., Herman, K. & Russell, C. (2016). Improving cultural and clinical competency and safety of renal nurse education. *Renal Society of Australasia Journal,* 12(3),106–12.

Kidney Health Australia. (2015a). *State of the Nation: 2015 Kidney Health Week: Chronic Kidney Disease in Australia*. Retrieved from www.kidney.org.au/LinkClick.aspx? fileticket=wCrYByDnxxg%3d&tabid=635&mid=1590

—— (2015b). *KHA-CARI Guidelines*. Retrieved from www.kidney.org.au/Health Professionals/KHACARIGuidelines/tabid/637/Default.aspx

Levy, J., Brown, E. & Lawrence, A. (2016). *Oxford Handbook of Dialysis* (4th edn). Oxford: Oxford University Press.

Lubkin, I. (2015). *Chronic Illness: Impact and Interventions* (9th edn). London: Jones and Bartlett.

Luckett, T., Spencer, L., Morton, R. L., Pollock, C. A., Lam, L, Silvester, W., . . . & Clayton, J. M. (2017). Advance care planning in chronic kidney disease: A survey of current practice in Australia. *Nephrology*, 22, 139–49.

Matovinovic, M. S. (2009). Pathophysiology and classification of kidney disease. *The Journal of the International Federation of Clinical Chemistry and Laboratory Medicine*, 20(1), 2–11.

McCrory, G., Patton, D., Moore, Z., O'Connor, T. & Nugent, L., (2018). The impact of advanced nurse practitioners on patient outcomes in chronic kidney disease: A systematic review. *Journal of Renal Care*, 44(4), 197–209. doi: http://org/10.1111/jorc.12245

Mobley, A. M. (2009). Slowing the progression of chronic kidney disease. *Journal for Nurse Practitioners*, 5(13), 188–94.

Morrissey, P., Dube, C., Gogh, R., Yango, A., Gautam, A. & Monaco, A. (2005). Good Samaritan kidney donation. *Transplantation*, 80(10), 1369–73.

New Zealand Ministry of Health (NZMOH). (2015). *Managing Chronic Kidney Disease in Primary Care: National Consensus Statement*. Wellington: Ministry of Health. Retrieved from www.health.govt.nz

—— (2016). *New Zealand Health Strategy: Future Direction*. Wellington: Ministry of Health.

Noble, H. (2008). Supportive and palliative care for the patient with end-stage renal disease. *British Journal of Nursing*, 17(8), 498–504.

Nuño, R., Coleman, K., Bengoa, R. & Sauto, R. (2012). Integrated care for chronic conditions: The contribution of the ICCC Framework. *Health Policy*, 105(1), 55–64. doi: http://dx.doi.org/10.1016/j.healthpol.2011.10.006

Padberg, F. T., Jr., Calligaro, K. D. & Sidawy, A. N. (2008). Complications of arteriovenous hemodialysis access: Recognition and management. *Journal of Vascular Surgery*, 48(5), S55–80. doi: http://10.1016/j.jvs.2008.08.067

Papps, E. & Ramsden, I. (1996). Cultural safety in nursing: The New Zealand experience. *International Journal of Quality Health Care*, 8(5), 491–7.

Randall, S. & Ford, H. (2011). *Long-Term Conditions: A Guide for Nurses and Healthcare Professionals*. Oxford: Wiley-Blackwell.

Ravani, P., Palmer, S., Oliver, M., Quinn, R., MacRae, J., Tai, D., . . . & James, M. (2013). Associations between haemodialysis access type and clinical outcomes: A systematic review. *Journal of the American Society of Nephrology*, 24(3), 465–73.

Rice, D., Kocurek, B. & Snead, C. A. (2010). Chronic disease management for diabetes: Baylor health care system's coordinated efforts and the opening of the Diabetes Health and Wellness Institute. *Baylor University Medical Center Proceedings*, 23(3), 230–4.

Sandilands, E. A., Dhaun, N., Dear, J. W. & Webb, D. J. (2013). Measurement of renal function in patients with chronic kidney disease. *British Journal of Clinical Pharmacology*, 76(4), 504–15.

Schlondorff, D. (2008). Overview of factors contributing to the pathophysiology of progressive renal disease. *Kidney International*, 74(7), 860–6.

Thomas, N. (2014). *Renal Nursing* (4th edn). Oxford: Wiley-Blackwell.

White, S. & Chadban, S. (2014). *Kidneys in Diabetes Report.* Kidney Health Australia. Retrieved from www.kidney.org.au/LinkClick.aspx?fileticket=wCrYByDnxxg%3d& tabid=635&mid=1590

Wright-Nunes, J. A., Luther, J. M., Ikizler, T. A. & Cavanaugh, K. L. (2012). Patient knowledge of blood pressure target is associated with improved blood pressure control in chronic kidney disease. *Patient Education and Counseling*, 88(2), 184–8. doi: http://10.1016/j.pec.2012.02.015

Wyld, M. L., Lee, C. M., Zhuo, X., White, S., Shaw, J. E., Morton, R. L., ... & Chadban, S. J. (2015). Cost to government and society of chronic kidney disease stage 1-5: A national cohort study. *Internal Medicine Journal*, 45(7), 741–7. doi: http://10.1111/imj.12797

17

Parkinson's disease and multiple sclerosis

Sally-Anne Wherry
and Marguerite Bramble

LEARNING OBJECTIVES

After studying this chapter, you should be able to:

1. understand the impact of Parkinson's disease and multiple sclerosis (MS) on people living with these chronic conditions
2. describe the signs, symptoms and pathophysiology of Parkinson's disease and MS
3. describe health promotion and prevention strategies which are appropriate for people living with Parkinson's disease or MS
4. describe nursing assessment and management strategies of the person living with Parkinson's disease or MS
5. understand advanced nursing practice in relation to Parkinson's disease and MS.

Introduction

Multiple sclerosis and Parkinson's disease are complex disorders. Patients with these diseases require strong links and communication between community organisations, such as patient support groups and acute health care systems. There is a need for collaborative, multidisciplinary care, and it is a large part of the nursing role that nurses act as advocates and educators for patients, as well as their caregivers and families (Chaplin, Hazan & Wilson, 2012). This collaborative link allows patients to be informed and motivated to self-manage their conditions, seeking support appropriately from the health care team and community partners. The incidence of these disorders is provided in Table 17.1.

Table 17.1   Incidence and prevalence of Parkinson's disease and multiple sclerosis in Australia and New Zealand

Disorder	Incidence	Prevalence per 100k population
Parkinson's disease	Between 0.01% (aged 45–54) and 0.81% (aged 85+)	294 – Australia 210 – New Zealand
MS	0.1%	1 – Australia and New Zealand

Sources: Deloitte Access Economics (2015); MS Queensland (2018); Multiple Sclerosis New Zealand (2017); Palmer et al. (2013); Taylor et al. (2010)

Parkinson's disease: risk factors, pathophysiology and diagnosis

Neurodegenerative – conditions that primarily affect neurons in the brain.

Dopamine neurons – main source of dopamine in the central nervous system (CNS).

Parkinson's disease is an incurable, **neurodegenerative** disease, in which the progressive loss of **dopamine neurons** causes the disease's classic motor symptoms, alongside a background of cognitive, mood, autonomic and sensory symptoms. It is the most common neurodegenerative disease after Alzheimer's disease. In Australia, it is reported that more than 80 000 people live with Parkinson's disease (Deloitte Access Economics, 2011). The burden of Parkinson's disease in Australia is estimated at $775.4 million per year (Deloitte Access Economics, 2015), a figure that includes health system costs at $478.5 million, loss of productivity at $107.3 million and informal care at $11.2 million. Over the course of the disease (most commonly 12 years in length) the average cost, therefore, would be $144 000 per person living with Parkinson's disease.

The risk factors for Parkinson's disease are not fully understood, with both genetic and environmental factors increasing the chances of experiencing the disorder. Ageing is the highest risk factor, but little is understood of the processes behind this, since it is not part of normal ageing. The current theories suggest an increased vulnerability of the dopaminergic neurons to toxic insults (Schapira & Jenner, 2011). Additionally, a number of genes have been identified as factors modulating the likelihood of developing Parkinson's disease (Bonifati, 2014). Other factors such as exposure to pesticides, consumption of daily products, a history of melanoma or traumatic brain injury are known to increase risk. However, conversely, a reduced risk is associated with smoking, caffeine consumption, physical activity, use of ibuprofen and higher serum urate concentrations (Ascherio & Schwarzschild, 2016)

The progression of Parkinson's disease is thought to start at the brain stem in the substantia nigra (where dopamine disease is produced), spreading from there throughout the brain. This widely accepted theoretical model is known as the Braak hypothesis (Visanji et al., 2013) (see Figure 17.1).

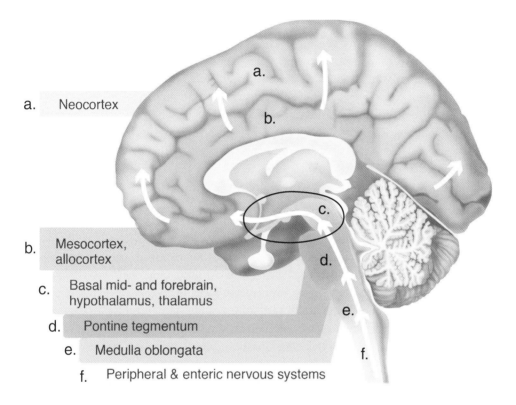

a.   Neocortex

b.   Mesocortex, allocortex

c.   Basal mid- and forebrain, hypothalamus, thalamus

d.   Pontine tegmentum

e.   Medulla oblongata

f.   Peripheral & enteric nervous systems

Figure 17.1   The Braak hypothesis
Source: Visanji et al. (2013)

Diagnosis and symptoms

Diagnosis of Parkinson's disease is through clinical criteria (Wirdefeldt et al., 2011) but is supported by new neuroimaging technology, such as radionuclide imaging and magnetic resonance imaging. There are also imaging methods that work by binding to the dopamine transporter, known as DaTscans; these allow exclusion of other disorders with similar symptoms to Parkinson's (Fang et al., 2015). According to the Movement Disorder Society criteria, **differential diagnosis** requires the presence of two or more of the cardinal motor symptoms to diagnose idiopathic (cause unknown) Parkinson's disease (Postuma et al., 2015). These include **bradykinesia** plus 4–6 Hz per second **resting tremor**, postural instability or **muscular or cogwheel rigidity** (Postuma et al., 2015). However, it is important to ensure that other potential disorders are considered and the diagnosing specialist must look for exclusion criteria, which includes symptoms such as cerebellar abnormalities (cerebellar gait, limb ataxia or

Differential diagnosis – distinguishing one particular condition from another which has similar signs and symptoms.

Bradykinesia – slowness in initiating and executing movement.

Resting tremor – typically Parkinsonian tremor occurring when the body part is at rest. Frequency of 4–7 Hz per second.

Muscular or cogwheel rigidity – rigidity felt on passive movements around a joint, specific to Parkinson's disease.

cerebellar oculomotor abnormalities), downward vertical supranuclear gaze palsy, or absence of response to levodopa (Postuma et al., 2015). There are also a number of symptoms that pre-date the diagnosis by up to 20 years, which often include anxiety, constipation or loss of sense of smell (Knudsen et al., 2015).

The symptoms of Parkinson's disease are varied and unique to the individual. They can be physical, neuropsychiatric, autonomic or sensory. The physical symptoms include bradykinesia, tremor, rigidity and gait changes. The neuropsychiatric symptoms may include apathy, depression, anxiety, insomnia and dementia. Autonomic changes may include postural hypotension, urinary and bowel issues, and erectile dysfunction. Sensory symptoms may include pain, tingling or aches (Chaudhuri et al., 2014).

People living with Parkinson's disease are vulnerable to a number of health-related complications, including falls (Allen, Schwarzel & Canning, 2013), chest or urinary infections, cognitive changes, adverse responses to changes in medication, or prescription of contraindicated medications. A rapid increase in confusion, hallucinations or paranoia, or a decrease in mobility could indicate an issue that needs urgent attention (Munhoz, Scorr & Factor, 2015).

Promoting health and reducing risk

Health promotion for people with Parkinson's disease is focused on the maintenance and improvement of health, and this requires collaborative work between the person and their health care team. All people living with chronic conditions have varying levels of information resources and support available to them. Everyone self-manages, but not necessarily in the manner the health care team would prefer. A refusal to engage with services could be considered self-management, and the nursing role is often central to the provision of information that allows health promotion and self-care, alongside the focus that nurses can bring to the individual's strengths (Connor et al., 2015).

Patient education, support and collaborative health care increase quality of life, improve concordance with medication, and allow the person, their families and caregivers to maintain control over their lives to a certain extent (Malek & Grosset, 2015; Tickle-Degnen et al., 2010). Learning to manage symptoms reduces the risk of hospital admissions; the main causes of hospital admissions include falls, fractures, neuropsychiatric symptoms, issues related to medication and infections (Muzerengi et al., 2016). Patients with a better understanding of their condition often have improved medication adherence and self-management skills (Eneanya et al., 2016). Additionally, the support patients gain by having open access to their health care team, and more frequent contact, is correlated with reduced unplanned admissions to hospital (Muzerengi et al., 2016).

In the acute care or home setting, medication errors can be problematic. Contra-indicated medications, such as many anti-emetics or antipsychotics that are frequently prescribed in error, block dopamine uptake and worsen Parkinsonian symptoms (Hou et al., 2012). Anti-Parkinsonian medications can be given late, causing an increase or return of the symptoms. The timing of these medications is vital, with patients in the later stages often having multiple doses during the day and night. Where possible, people living with Parkinson's disease should be encouraged to self-administer their medication, as this ensures timely doses and improved understanding of their medication regime (Richardson et al., 2014).

REFLECTION

When designing a health promotion program for an older person with Parkinson's disease who comes from a cultural and linguistically diverse background, what are some of the important considerations you would include?

The nursing role

In any location, the nursing role in caring for the person with Parkinson's disease has some fundamental similarities. A holistic nursing assessment frequently uncovers vital issues, improving quality of life for the person living with this chronic condition through information provision, health promotion and early interventions. The assessment should cover all realms of life, including physiological, psychological and emotional aspects. It should also include environment and social situations. It is vital to ensure that the assessment, and the plan of care, is based on a good-quality evidence base and underpinning knowledge. The nurse should also be aware of and work within the scope of their practice and role.

The care coordination component of the nursing role entails referral to appropriate multidisciplinary services; often these will be physiotherapy, occupational therapy, speech pathology or social work. There may be times when these referrals must be prioritised to prevent the patient from becoming overwhelmed or when the patient rejects the suggestions, despite information on the reasoning behind them (Cowen, Harrison & Burns, 2012). The complexity of health, social care and non-government organisation systems can be problematic for people living with chronic conditions. It is part of the care coordination role for nurses to advocate and guide patients in order to meet their needs. Appropriate multidisciplinary working will assist the nurse in this area of practice; for example, social workers have a wealth of knowledge on how and when to access local and national services. The needs of the person and their family may vary; people who are from culturally and linguistically diverse populations are known to require additional support in accessing services (Zhou, 2016), rural communities have issues accessing local services (Dew et al., 2013), and people with dementia and their carers require increased community support (Vecchio et al., 2016). All patients are assumed to have the capacity to make decisions, unless proven otherwise, and have the absolute right to decline services (NSW Government, 2008).

The nursing role for people living with Parkinson's disease often focuses on medication administration; patient, caregiver and family education on management and health promotion; and basic assessment appropriate to the environment. Awareness of the risks of constipation and infection in this condition is important for both acute and community settings, with preventing deterioration a vital goal. Screening for these issues, alongside medication concordance, should be considered a priority if there are signs of deterioration, prior to assuming additional diagnoses (Magennis & Corry, 2013).

Support of independence in activities of daily living (ADL) is another vital nursing role, and the nurse can provide encouragement for the person to do as much as they are capable of doing. Episodes of immobility and freezing may be improved by medication, and so interventions such as showering and mealtimes should be arranged with the person's abilities in mind. A basic understanding of the medications will allow assessment of potential problems, such as side effects, and a reduction of the potential impacts of them. Side effects can include impulsive behaviour, gastric issues and hallucinations (Factor & Weiner, 2007).

SKILLS IN PRACTICE

Supporting a person living with Parkinson's disease

Harold, a 65-year-old male with Parkinson's disease, lives with his wife, Gloria, in a two-storey house. They have three children, two sons and a daughter, none of whom live locally, but one of the sons, George, is regularly in contact and visits monthly.

Harold and Gloria have been independent until recently, but now Harold is having trouble walking and has had several 'near miss' falls. He does not currently use a walking aid. He is having episodes where he finds it hard to start walking when he has sat for a long period of time or when he is in a confined space.

He regularly forgets his Parkinsonian medication and is having periods of immobility when he does so. He has been unwilling to leave the house and has stopped going to his exercise group. Gloria complains that he sits in his armchair all day and is miserable. He says he is often sad and sometimes cries.

Gloria is obviously tired, concerned and tearful. She has given up her weekly coffee with her friends and her knitting circle. She is also suffering from arthritis.

Harold currently has urgency and frequency of urine, and Gloria mentions that it is very smelly. He sees a geriatrician for his Parkinson's disease and other conditions, which includes diabetes. He also has a number of other hospital appointments regularly which he struggles to get to.

A comprehensive nursing assessment is made of Harold, and the following results are received.

- Harold has a urinary tract infection.
- His depression screening is positive.
- His standing blood pressure reveals postural hypotension.
- His memory test shows obvious deficits.

QUESTIONS

Consider the background and assessment information and answer the following questions.

1. What signs may be caused by the infection as opposed to disease progression?
2. Who would you consider to be Harold's caregiver?
3. What support might Harold, his family and caregivers need to support independent living?
4. What are the potential barriers to good-quality health care for Harold and his family?
5. What multidisciplinary team members would be useful to involve in his care?

Multiple sclerosis: risk factors, pathophysiology and diagnosis

Multiple sclerosis (a Greek term meaning 'scars') is an incurable **autoimmune** disease of the central nervous system (CNS), where the myelin becomes damaged and scarred with **glial scars** (these lesions are known as plaques), impacting on the conduction of nerve impulses. This causes problems with motor, sensory and cognitive functions. Multiple sclerosis is the most common cause of neurological disability in young adults, affecting those in their most productive years (Serono Symposia International, 2008). It not only impacts the person diagnosed but family, caregivers and society as well. Living with a chronic, unpredictable and progressive disease such as MS, results in a lifetime of social, financial and personal loss (Maloni, 2013).

Autoimmune – system of immune responses of an organism against its own cells and tissues.

Glial scars – (sclerosis) occur as the body attempts to repair the neuronal cellular damage.

In 2018, it was estimated that approximately 2.3 million people globally have been diagnosed with MS (Mulitple Sclerosis International Foundation, 2018). There is no known cure and on average most people with MS live about seven years less than the general population (Palmer et al., 2016; Weatherspoon, 2018). Epidemiological studies show incidence and prevalence of the disease continue to rise, as does the burden of disease, because individuals with MS experience high levels of disability and impaired quality of life for many years (Melcon, Correale & Melcon, 2014). The burden of this disease in Australia is estimated at $1.75 billion per year, which includes direct costs of $30 346 per person, and indirect costs of $21 858 per person from lost wages. Total costs have increased by 41 per cent from 2010 to 2017 due to an increase in the number of people living with MS in Australia and increased costs per person (Menzies Health Economics Research Group, 2018). This represents an enormous economic impact on the individual and a similar economic burden of disease as Parkinson's. The economic burden of disease is three times higher than that of a person living with type 2 diabetes (Maloni, 2013).

The average age of onset of MS is between 20 and 40 years, with 75 per cent of those affected being women (Palmer et al., 2013). As with those people living with Parkinson's disease, people living with MS will require education and support to assist with the debilitating effects of the disease over time (Tan et al., 2011). This includes adherence to therapies, particularly medications; specialised understanding of the motor, cognitive and sensory changes associated with the condition; and prevention of caregiver stress (Tan et al., 2011). The creation of the National Disability Insurance Scheme in Australia has allowed younger people living with such chronic conditions to access appropriate and person-centred resources in the community. For example, a person with MS may choose to spend their money on transport to and from work, or equipment to enable them to fulfil ADL (Council of Australian Governments, 2015). It is important that nurses support both person-centred approaches and appropriate self-management, such as treatment adherence, to improve both clinical and economic outcomes (Tan et al., 2011).

Multiple sclerosis is currently believed to be an autoimmune disorder, triggered by a viral infection (Nicol et al., 2015). However, the risk factors include genetic susceptibility and environmental factors, such as latitude location, with a higher prevalence in

Demyelination – damage to the myelin sheath of neurons, impairing the conduction of signals in the affected nerves.

Remyelination – process of propagating new cells to create new myelin sheaths.

Northern Europe and North America, and a lower prevalence in Asia and South America (Tullman, 2013). The loss of myelin (**demyelination**) and axons is shown in the neurological deficits, resulting in inefficient conduction or conduction block. Although the loss of axons – occurring during the acute inflammatory phase of the disease – explains the permanent disability, the clinical recovery is more difficult to explain. Limited **remyelination** occurs but does not fully explain the remission periods. Neurological deficits from the acute MS plaque are related to both the loss of myelin and axons, and inflammation and oedema around the lesion (Agamanolis, 2014).

Diagnosis and symptoms

The primary assessment of history and clinical presentation is vital in diagnosing MS. Diagnosis requires evidence of lesions in more than one site in the CNS and that they emerged at different times. As with Parkinson's disease, differential diagnosis must be considered. The characteristic signs and symptoms of MS include visual disturbances, muscle weakness and paralysis of one or more limbs, unsteadiness of gait or poor coordination, involuntary eye movements, difficulties with speech, spastic paraparesis, pain or altered sensory perceptions, bowel and bladder function changes, and mood and intellectual capacity changes (Serono Symposia International, 2008).

There are considered to be four manifestations of MS:

Relapsing remitting – most common form of MS defined by attacks of worsening neurological function.

Primary progressive – less common but symptoms more progressive and unremitting.

Clinically isolated syndrome – a single incidence of neurological symptoms that does not fit the criteria for the diagnosis of MS (Porten & Carrucan-Wood, 2017).

1. **relapsing remitting**
2. secondary progressive
3. **primary progressive**
4. **clinically isolated syndrome** (Porten & Carrucan-Wood, 2017).

Relapsing remitting is the most common form of the disease and accounts for 85 to 90 per cent of new diagnoses (Porten & Carrucan-Wood, 2017). It is thought that 60 per cent of people who have relapsing remitting MS will eventually develop what is known as the secondary progressive form of the disease; with this secondary form, people do not experience remission from the symptoms, resulting in increasing disability or impairment. Half of those diagnosed with MS will require either a walking aid or help with mobility within 15 years of diagnosis (Coleman, Rath & Carey, 2001). A smaller cohort (10 to 15 per cent) will experience primary progressive MS. This is a progressive, unremitting neurological deterioration from the point of the first symptoms (Coleman et al., 2001).

Promoting health and reducing risk

Similar to Parkinson's, the nursing role in health promotion for people with MS is to provide person-centred management strategies aimed at maintaining and improving health, and supporting collaborative work between the person and their multidisciplinary health care team. The holistic nursing assessment is focused on improving the quality of life for the person living with MS. The nurse should also be aware of, and work within the scope of, their practice and role.

Management of the daily aspects of living with MS requires self-care management. Activity and exercise are vital components of this, balanced against the fluctuating nature of the disorder. Exercise helps control pain, stiffness, balance, weakness, depression, anxiety, insomnia and fatigue (Maloni, 2013). The choice of exercise should suit the person, and it is important that they remain cool, since their ability to moderate their own temperature is impaired, and this can lead to overheating and dehydration (Serono Symposia International, 2008).

Dietary management should involve avoidance of antioxidants, including herbs; these stimulate the immune system, which is not advised in MS, since the immune system is attacking the person's body. A varied diet should provide all the vitamins required to avoid nutritional deficits. Alcohol should be limited or avoided, as it leads to dehydration, which exacerbates the symptoms of MS (Serono Symposia International, 2008).

Development of coping strategies to manage and reduce stress is an important part of self-care management in this disorder. Mindfulness, stress diaries, relaxation, prioritising, and other stress reduction techniques can be learned and supported by the health care team (Senders et al., 2014).

The nursing role

Nurses have a central role for people living with MS, with a focus on supporting activities that may improve health or recovery and encouraging independence as far as possible. Nurses also support behavioural changes, education and self-care management, alongside the multidisciplinary team (American Association of Neuroscience Nurses, Association of Rehabilitation Nurses & International Organisation of Multiple Sclerosis Nurses (AANN, ARN & IOMSN), 2011). The goals of this education should include understanding of the type of manifestation and how this may impact upon the person's life (Porten & Carrucan-Wood, 2017). This will empower the person and their family to make informed decisions about the future, including employment, family and lifestyle. As with all education, the content and depth of information must depend on the wishes of the person and their family; some may not wish for in-depth discussions or may wish for detailed data (AANN, ARN & IOMSN, 2011).

Supporting and encouraging adherence to the therapies that patients may be on is a vital day-to-day role of the nurse. Establishment of a relationship, supporting realistic expectations and plans, and performing regular follow up and monitoring are key parts of that role (Serono Symposia International, 2008).

REFLECTION

How might you, as a nurse, encourage a patient with MS to self-manage their condition? Identify three aspects of self-care that you would consider important for most people with MS.

Advanced nursing practice for Parkinson's disease and multiple sclerosis

Both Parkinson's disease and MS, as areas of practice, require similar skills and postgraduate qualifications for the specialist neurologist nurse (Nursing and

Midwifery Board of Australia, 2016). Such training and expertise are congruent with the scope of practice identified for a clinical nurse specialist and clinical nurse consultant. The specialist neurological nurse then has the capacity to clinically manage patients; recognise acute changes and deterioration; provide education; undertake nursing assessments, nursing decisions and referrals; analyse and interpret clinical data; and contribute to policies affecting the patients they care for (NSW Health, 2017).

Support of the carers and family, through active listening and meeting those needs in a tailored manner, is as integral to this area of advanced practice as symptom management (see Figure 17.2). The provision of case management services in the form of referral management, coordination of care, organising, and emotional and psychological support, is also a central part of these advanced roles (Maloni, 2013; Parkinson's NSW, 2016). This may involve initiating referrals to other services, such as community nursing, to allow others to meet these needs (Hellqvist & Berterö, 2015).

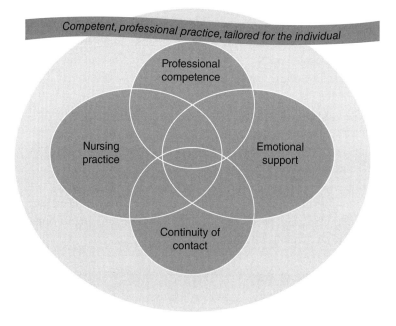

Figure 17.2 The role of the specialist nurse
Source: Hellqvist & Berterö (2015)

The advanced nursing practice role also requires that the nurse functions at a broader level, creating two-way links between the community, specialist doctors and acute care teams. This may be achieved by conducting nurse-led clinics and working within a multidisciplinary team, receiving referrals from and referring to other clinicians (Maloni, 2013; Royal College of Nursing, 2017). These complex therapies require supported decision making, education, assessment prior to and during the procedures, and follow up.

Parkinson's disease

The role of the Parkinson's disease nurse specialist in the care of people living with Parkinson's disease extends to the complex therapies, including apomorphine, levodopa–carbidopa intestinal gel and deep brain stimulation. These therapies are appropriate for patients whose oral therapy is no longer covering their Parkinsonian symptoms, and who have a confirmed response to levodopa and are cognitively able to manage their therapy (Worth, 2013).

Apomorphine is an agonist that works on the dopamine receptors in the CNS and is absorbed through a subcutaneous injection or pump. Initiation often requires an overnight admission to assess the response to the medication and titrate the appropriate dosage (Worth, 2013). Levodopa–carbidopa intestinal gel is levodopa infused directly into the small intestine. Initiation requires a hospital admission to allow a percutaneous gastrostomy tube with an inner jejunostomy tube to be inserted. A pump is then attached to allow a steady rate of infusion (Worth, 2013). Deep brain stimulation involves electrical stimulation of targets within the basal ganglia. A pulse generator, similar to a pacemaker, is implanted subcutaneously below the clavicle, with permanently implanted electrodes connected subcutaneously to the pulse generator (Worth, 2013).

The specialist nurse is often involved in these treatments, providing education, support and practical arrangements, such as titration of medication (alongside the medical team), arrangements for admissions and troubleshooting after the procedures. These treatments are often long term and the nurse remains a large part of the review and support processes throughout.

Multiple sclerosis

As with Parkinson's disease nurses, the MS nurses have a specialist role in **immunotherapy**, to slow down or stop the demyelinating process. Barring a cure, safe and effective therapies with tolerable adverse reactions are the ideal treatment regime (Maloni, 2013). These therapies cannot reverse damage but can be used to shorten attacks or slow progression. Immunotherapies use interferons, a group of proteins produced by cells in response to viral infections, which are divided into three types: interferons beta and alpha, produced by white blood cells and fibroblasts, and interferon gamma which is produced by activated T cells. These are usually given by intramuscular injection, subcutaneous injection or intravenous infusion (Serono Symposia International, 2008). During the titration and treatment, the management of the side effects becomes the primary reason for contact with their specialist nurse (Coleman et al., 2001; Maloni, 2013). The primary side effects can include injection-site reactions, systemic reactions and flu-like symptoms (Serono Symposia International, 2008).

Immunotherapy – treatment designed to boost the body's natural defences to fight disease.

Outside the realm of conventional medications, 75 per cent of people with MS use **complementary and alternative medicine**, such as yoga, acupuncture, vitamin D, psyllium/calcium for constipation, and valerian and cranberry for urinary tract infection (Maloni, 2013). Nurses should be aware that substances that activate the immune system should be avoided in MS, such as echinacea, zinc, Asian ginseng, garlic, alfalfa and melatonin. Other alternative treatments such as changing diet, bee-sting therapy, hyperbaric oxygen therapy, Prokarin, magnets, and having amalgam fillings removed have been shown to have no effect on disease outcomes (Maloni, 2013).

Complementary and alternative medicine – forms of treatment that are used in addition (complementary) or instead of (alternative to) standard treatments.

SKILLS IN PRACTICE

Supporting a person living with MS

Julia, a 55-year-old woman diagnosed relapsing-remitting MS five years ago, continues to work as a secretary. She is married and has two children aged 25 and 28. Although she has been independent until recently, a recent relapse has reduced her mobility and she has been struggling to sleep. Her husband, George, works full-time. Her eldest daughter, Gloria, is often available to take her mother to appointments and sometimes takes her shopping.

Julia has noticed that she is experiencing significant fatigue, and that her vision has changed. She has also had an increase in her unpredictable and frequent falls.

Her husband has found that he has also had to take more time off work to support her, and that their social life and hobbies are being impacted on by the change. He does not identify as a carer and is often frustrated by the change in their lives.

A comprehensive nursing assessment is made and the following results are received.

- Julia's fatigue is a primary symptom of her MS.
- Due to the change in her vision, Julia can no longer drive and is unable to complete her usual tasks at work.
- Julia often feels isolated and unsupported by her husband.

QUESTIONS

Consider the background and assessment information, and answer the following questions.

1. Who would you consider to be Julia's caregiver?
2. What support might Julia, her family and caregivers need to support independent living?
3. What are the potential barriers to good-quality health care for Julia and her family?
4. What multidisciplinary team members would be useful to involve in Julia's care?

SUMMARY

Learning objective 1: Understand the impact of Parkinson's disease and MS on people living with these chronic conditions.

The impact of these neurodegenerative diseases has been described in this chapter, highlighting the emotional, social, physical and financial costs.

Learning objective 2: Describe the signs, symptoms and pathophysiology of Parkinson's disease and MS.

The signs and symptoms of Parkinson's disease include rigidity, tremor, postural instability, cognitive changes and autonomic issues. The signs and symptoms of MS include visual disturbances, muscle weakness and paralysis, unsteadiness of gait or poor coordination, difficulties with speech, spastic paraparesis, pain or altered sensory perceptions, autonomic issues, and cognitive changes.

Learning objective 3: Describe health promotion and prevention strategies which are appropriate for people living with Parkinson's disease or MS.

The health promotion and prevention strategies include patient education, diet, exercise, and the recognition of deterioration and its causes.

Learning objective 4: Describe nursing assessment and management strategies of the person living with Parkinson's disease or MS.

The nurse's role includes assessment and management of a person living with Parkinson's disease or MS, and the advanced nurse is also involved in these areas of practice. Nurses encourage self-management, coordinate care, support behavioural changes and work with the patient to identify early signs of deterioration.

Learning objective 5: Understand advanced nursing practice in relation to Parkinson's disease and MS.

Advanced nursing practice in this area supports complex therapies, coordinates complex cases, and provides education and support to the patient.

REVIEW QUESTIONS

1. What are the impacts of Parkinson's disease and MS on family members?
2. What are the primary diagnostic symptoms of Parkinson's disease?
3. What self-management activities can be undertaken by someone living with Parkinson's disease or MS?
4. Which part of the brain produces dopamine?
5. What are the components of a holistic assessment?

RESEARCH TOPICS

1. In his book on unforgettable cases and lessons, *Movement Disorders*, Hubert Fernandez reflects upon cases of Parkinson's disease impulse control issues (Fernandez & Merello, 2012). This side effect of medication is often a hidden face of treatment.

Consider how this may manifest. How may the patient and those close to them experience this? What impact does this have on their lives? What role does the nurse have in this issue? Consider also the legalities of behaviour performed under the influence of medication.

2. In their practice paper on caring for a patient with MS, Porten and Carrucan-Wood (2017) describe the impacts of overheating on acute exacerbation of neurological symptoms, known as Uhthoff's syndrome. Discuss the pathophysiology of this phenomenon in MS and how it might best be resolved. What do we mean by acute exacerbations (relapses)? What role does the nurse have in the treatment and management of relapses?

FURTHER READING

American Association of Neuroscience Nurses, Association of Rehabilitation Nurses & International Organisation of Multiple Sclerosis Nurses (AANN, ARN & IOMSN). (2011). Nursing Management of the Patient with Multiple Sclerosis. Retrieved from https://rehabnurse.org/uploads/about/cpgms.pdf

Halper, J. & Harris, C. (2016). *Nursing Practice in Multiple Sclerosis: A Core Curriculum* (4th edn). New York: Springer Publishing Company.

Hou, J. G., Wu, L. J., Moore, S., Ward, C., York, M., Atassi, F., . . . & Lai, E. C. (2012). Assessment of appropriate medication administration for hospitalized patients with Parkinson's disease. *Parkinsonism & Related Disorders*, 18(4), 377–81. doi: http://10.1016/j.parkreldis.2011.12.007

Kessler, D. & Liddy, C. (2017). Self-management support programs for persons with Parkinson's disease: An integrative review. *Patient Education Counseling*, 100(10), 1787–95.

Parkinson's Australia. (2015). Welcome to Parkinson's Australia. Retrieved from www.parkinsons.org.au

REFERENCES

Agamanolis, D. (2014). Demyelinative diseases. Retrieved from http://neuropathologyweb.org/chapter6/chapter6aMs.html

Allen, N. E., Schwarzel, A. K. & Canning, C. G. (2013). Recurrent falls in Parkinson's disease: A systematic review. *Parkinson's Disease*. doi: http://10.1155/2013/906274

American Association of Neuroscience Nurses, Association of Rehabilitation Nurses & International Organisation of Multiple Sclerosis Nurses (AANN, ARN a& IOMSN). (2011). *Nursing Management of the Patient with Multiple Sclerosis.AANN, ARN and IOMSN Clinical Practice Guideline Series.* Retrieved from https://rehabnurse.org/uploads/about/cpgms.pdf

Ascherio, A. & Schwarzschild, M. A. (2016). The epidemiology of Parkinson's disease: Risk factors and prevention. *The Lancet Neurology*, 15(12), 1257–72. doi: http://10.1016/S1474-4422(16)30230-7

Bonifati, V. (2014). Genetics of Parkinson's disease – State of the art, 2013. *Parkinsonism & Related Disorders*, 20, S23–8.

Chaplin, H., Hazan, J. & Wilson, P. (2012). Self-management for people with long-term neurological conditions. *British Journal of Community Nursing*, 17(6), 250–7.

Chaudhuri, K. R., Tolosa, E., Schapira, A. H. V. & Poewe, W. (2014). *Non-Motor Symptoms of Parkinson's Disease* (2nd edn). Oxford: Oxford University Press.

Coleman, J., Rath, L. & Carey, J. (2001). Multiple sclerosis and the role of the MS nurse consultant. *Australian Nursing Journal*, 9(3), CU1.

Connor, K., Cheng, E., Siebens, H. C., Lee, M. L., Mittman, B. S., Ganz, D. A. & Vickrey, B. (2015). Study protocol of "CHAPS": A randomized controlled trial protocol of Care Coordination for Health Promotion and Activities in Parkinson's Disease to improve the quality of care for individuals with Parkinson's disease. *BMC Neurology*, 15(1), 258.

Council of Australian Governments. (2015). *National Disability Insurance Scheme (NDIS) – Bilateral Agreement between Commonwealth and NSW*. Canberra: CAOG.

Cowen, P., Harrison, P. & Burns, T. (2012). *Shorter Oxford Textbook of Psychiatry*. Oxford.: Oxford University Press.

Deloitte Access Economics. (2015). *Living with Parkinson's Disease – An Updated Economic Analysis 2014*. Retrieved from www.parkinsonsvic.org.au/images/site/publications/Research/Living_with_Parkinsons_Disease.pdf

Dew, A., Bulkeley, K., Veitch, C., Bundy, A., Gallego, G., Lincoln, M., . . . & Griffiths, S. (2013). Addressing the barriers to accessing therapy services in rural and remote areas. *Disability and Rehabilitation*, 35(18), 1564–70.

Eneanya, N. D., Winter, M., Cabral, H., Waite, K., Henault, L., Bickmore, T., . . . & Paasche-Orlow, M. K. (2016). Health literacy and education as mediators of racial disparities in patient activation within an elderly patient cohort. *Journal of Health Care for the Poor and Underserved*, 27(3), 1427–40.

Factor, S. A. & Weiner, W. (2007). *Parkinson's Disease: Diagnosis & Clinical Management* (2nd edn). New York: Demos Medical Publishing.

Fang, Y.-H. D., Chiu, S.-C., Lu, C.-S., Yen, T.-C. & Weng, Y.-H. (2015). Fully automated quantification of the striatal uptake ratio of [^{99m}Tc] – TRODAT with SPECT Imaging: Evaluation of the diagnostic performance in Parkinson's Disease and the temporal regression of striatal tracer uptake. *BioMed Research International*. doi: http://10.1155%2F2015%2F461625

Fernandez, H. H. & Merello, M. (2012). *Movement Disorders: Unforgettable Cases and Lessons from the Bedside*. New York: Demos Medical Publishing.

Hellqvist, C. & Berterö, C. (2015). Support supplied by Parkinson's disease specialist nurses to Parkinson's disease patients and their spouses. *Applied Nursing Research*, 28(2), 86–91.

Hou, J. G., Wu, L. J., Moore, S., Ward, C., York, M., Atassi, F., . . . & Lai, E. C. (2012). Assessment of appropriate medication administration for hospitalized patients with Parkinson's disease. *Parkinsonism & Related Disorders*, 18(4), 377–81. doi: http://10.1016/j.parkreldis.2011.12.007

Knudsen, K., Flensborg Damholdt, M., Mouridsen, K. & Borghammer, P. (2015). Olfactory function in Parkinson's disease – Effects of training. *Acta Neurologica Scandinavica*, 132(6), 395–400. doi: http://10.1111/ane.12406

Magennis, B. & Corry, M. (2013). Parkinson's disease: Top 10 causes of sudden deterioration. *British Journal of Neuroscience Nursing*, 9(5), 234–9.

Malek, N. & Grosset, D. G. (2015). Medication adherence in patients with Parkinson's disease. *CNS Drugs*, 29(1), 47–53. doi: http://10.1007/s40263-014-0220-0

Maloni, H. W. (2013). Multiple sclerosis: Managing patients in primary care. *The Nurse Practitioner*, 38(4), 24–35.

Melcon, M. O., Correale, J. & Melcon, C. M. (2014). Is it time for a new global classification of multiple sclerosis? *Journal of the Neurological Sciences*, 344(1), 171–81.

Menzies Health Economics Research Group. (2018). *Health Economic Impact of Multiple Sclerosis in Australia in 2017*. Retrieved from https://msra.org.au/wp-content/uploads/2018/08/health-economic-impact-of-ms-in-australia-in-2017_ms-research-australia_web.pdf

MS Queensland. (2018). What is MS? Symptoms, diagnosis and treatments. Retrieved from www.msqld.org.au/site/about-ms/what-is-ms

Multiple Sclerosis New Zealand. (2017). What is MS? Retrieved from www.msnz.org.nz/about

Munhoz, R. P., Scorr, L. M. & Factor, S. A. (2015). Movement disorders emergencies. *Current Opinion in Neurology*, 28(4), 406–12.

Muzerengi, S., Herd, C., Rick, C. & Clarke, C. E. (2016). A systematic review of interventions to reduce hospitalisation in Parkinson's disease. *Parkinsonism & Related Disorders*, 24, 3–7.

Nicol, B., Salou, M., Laplaud, D.-A. & Wekerle, H. (2015). The autoimmune concept of multiple sclerosis. *La Presse Médicale*, 44(4), e103–12.

NSW Government. (2008). *Capacity Toolkit*. Sydney: NSW Government.

NSW Health. (2017). Information bulletin: Clinical nurse /midwife consultants - List of domains and functions. Retrieved from www1.health.nsw.gov.au/pds/ActivePDSDocuments/IB2017_002.pdf

Nursing and Midwifery Board of Australia. (2016). *Advanced nursing practice and speciality areas within nursing*. Melbourne: Nursing and Midwifery Board of Australia.

Palmer, A. J., Colman, S., O'Leary, B., Taylor, B. V. & Simmons, R. D. (2013). The economic impact of multiple sclerosis in Australia in 2010. *Multiple Sclerosis Journal*, 19, 1640–6.

Palmer, A. J., Taylor, B., Van der Mei, I., Si, L. & Ahmad, H. (2016). Life expectancy, quality-adjusted life years, and total lifetime costs for Australian people with multiple sclerosis. *Value in Health*, 19(7), A808. doi: http://10.1016/j.jval.2016.08.722

Parkinson's NSW. (2016). A rationale for the increased utilisation of Parkinson's Disease Nurse Specialists across regional areas of NSW. Sydney: Parkinson's NSW.

Porten, L. & Carrucan-Wood, L. (2017). Caring for a patient with multiple sclerosis. *Kai Tiaki: Nursing New Zealand*, 23(6), 16–18.

Postuma, R. B., Berg, D., Stern, M., Poewe, W., Olanow, C. W., Oertel, W., . . . & Lang, A. E. (2015). MDS clinical diagnostic criteria for Parkinson's disease. *Movement Disorders*, 30(12), 1591–601.

Richardson, S. J., Brooks, H. L., Bramley, G. & Coleman, J. J. (2014). Evaluating the effectiveness of self-administration of medication (SAM) schemes in the hospital setting: A systematic review of the literature. *PLOS ONE*, 9(12), e113912.

Royal College of Nursing. (2017). *Competencies: A Competency Framework for Nurses Working in Parkinson's Disease Management*. London: Royal College of Nursing.

Schapira, A. H. & Jenner, P. (2011). Etiology and pathogenesis of Parkinson's disease. *Movement Disorders*, 26(6), 1049–55.

Senders, A., Bourdette, D., Hanes, D., Yadav, V. & Shinto, L. (2014). Perceived stress in multiple sclerosis: The potential role of mindfulness in health and well-being. *Journal of Evidence-Based Complementary & Alternative Medicine*, 19(2), 104–11.

Serono Symposia International. (2008). *The Australian Multiple Sclerosis Nursing Manual* (2nd ed.). Sydney: PharmaGuide.

Tan, H., Cai, Q., Agarwal, S., Stephenson, J. J. & Kamat, S. (2011). Impact of adherence to disease-modifying therapies on clinical and economic outcomes among patients with multiple sclerosis. *Advances in Therapy*, 28(1), 51–61.

Taylor, B. V., Pearson, J. F., Clarke, G., Mason, D. F., Abernethy, D. A., Willoughby, E. & Sabel, C. (2010). MS prevalence in New Zealand, an ethnically and latitudinally diverse country. *Multiple Sclerosis Journal*, 16, 1422–31.

Tickle-Degnen, L., Ellis, T., Saint-Hilaire, M. H., Thomas, C. A. & Wagenaar, R. C. (2010). Self-management rehabilitation and health-related quality of life in Parkinson's disease: A randomized controlled trial. *Movement Disorders*, 25(2), 194–204. doi: http://10.1002/mds.22940

Tullman, M. J. (2013). Overview of the epidemiology, diagnosis, and disease progression associated with multiple sclerosis. *The American Journal of Managed Care*, 19, S15–20.

Vecchio, N., Fitzgerald, J. A., Radford, K. & Fisher, R. (2016). The association between cognitive impairment and community service use patterns in older people living in Australia. *Health & Social Care in the Community*, 24(3), 321–33.

Visanji, N. P., Brooks, P. L., Hazrati, L.-N. & Lang, A. E. (2013). The prion hypothesis in Parkinson's disease: Braak to the future. *Acta Neuropathologica Communications*, 1(2). doi: http://10.1186/2051-5960-1-2

Weatherspoon, D. (2018). Multiple sclerosis prognosis and your life expectancy. Retrieved from www.healthline.com/health/multiple-sclerosis/prognosis-and-life-expectancy

Wirdefeldt, K., Adami, H.-O., Cole, P., Trichopoulos, D. & Mandel, J. (2011). Epidemiology and etiology of Parkinson's disease: A review of the evidence. *European Journal of Epidemiology*, 26(1), 1. doi: http://10.1007/s10654-011-9581-6

Worth, P. F. (2013). When the going gets tough: How to select patients with Parkinson's disease for advanced therapies. *Practical Neurology*, 13(3). doi: http://10.1136/practneurol-2012–000463.

Zhou, Q. (2016). Accessing disability services by people from culturally and linguistically diverse backgrounds in Australia. *Disability and Rehabilitation*, 38(9), 844–52.

18

Chronic bowel conditions

Maryanne Podham, Judith Anderson
and Patience Moyo

LEARNING OBJECTIVES

After reading this chapter, you should be able to:

1. identify and describe the most common chronic bowel conditions in Australia and New Zealand
2. describe the underlying pathophysiology and risk factors associated with chronic bowel conditions
3. discuss the different treatment options for people with a chronic bowel condition
4. identify ways to promote health and address the quality of life related to living with a chronic bowel condition
5. discuss the nurse's role in working with individuals who have a chronic bowel condition.

Introduction

Chronic bowel conditions can be due to one of two disease processes inflammatory bowel disease (IBD) or irritable bowel syndrome (IBS). Irritable bowel disease involves idiopathic, relapsing and remitting inflammations of the gastrointestinal tract, with the most common being Crohn's disease and ulcerative colitis (Gastroenterological Society of Australia (GESA), 2017). Irritable bowel syndrome is described as a functional gastrointestinal disorder, characterised by symptoms such as abdominal pain and altered bowel function that do not have any link to structural abnormalities (Crocker, Chur-Hansen & Andrews, 2013).

The Gastroenterological Society of Australia (2017) estimates that approximately 75 000 Australians are living with IBD, and over 1000 new cases are diagnosed each year. In New Zealand there are approximately 15 000 people living with IBD (New Zealand Ministry of Health (NZMOH), 2018). The global prevalence of IBD conditions is difficult to determine due to the variance in diagnostic criteria; however, Canavan, West and Card (2014) suggest that around 11 per cent of the global population are affected by one of these conditions, with a predominance of female sufferers, between the ages of 5 and 40 (Canavan et al., 2014).

Irritable bowel syndrome is linked to almost 50 per cent of the visits people make to a specialist gastroenterologist worldwide (GESA, 2006). The Gastroenterological Society of Australia (2006) suggests that the Australian incidence of this syndrome is approximately 15 per cent, and in New Zealand it affects approximately 10–20 per cent of the population (Health Navigator, 2018). Irritable bowel syndrome prevalence varies in different countries, but risk factors are not clearly defined, although it is more prevalent in women (Lovell & Ford, 2012), and more likely in people who have depression and insomnia (Lee et. al., 2017). Like IBD, the tools used to diagnose this condition differ between medical practitioners. However, the standardised Rome IV Criteria have assisted in the consistency of diagnosis.

There is no cure for these chronic bowel conditions and management should address direct issues such as symptom management, psychosocial wellbeing and nutritional information. Indirect issues such as economic loss to the person due to time off work and repeated visits to medical specialists, and the associated costs involved in the use of pharmacological and alternative treatments to sustain an optimal quality of life, also need to be considered (Canavan et al., 2014).

The role of the nurse in the care of a person who is living with a chronic bowel disorder is dependent on where they are along their disease trajectory. Multidisciplinary team members including, for example, a general practitioner, gastroenterologist, dietitian, stomal therapist nurse and pharmacist may also need to be involved (Thompson & Read, 2015). Regardless of where the person is along their disease trajectory, a clear understanding of the pathophysiology of these conditions is required.

Underlying pathophysiology of chronic bowel conditions

Irritable bowel disease

Irritable bowel disease has traditionally been linked to the industrial Westernised populations of the world, with epidemiological studies of the condition linking the cause to the environment one lives in (Kaplan, 2015). Risk factors are difficult to pinpoint, but it is thought that exposure to food additives, tobacco smoke, pesticides; the use of non-steroidal anti-inflammatory drugs (NSAIDS); and a pre-existence of immune or allergy disorders puts people at greatest risk. Genetic or familial history of IBD further increases the risk (French, 2017). Both ulcerative colitis and Crohn's disease have similar clinical and pathological features, with the main difference being the location and extent of the inflammation in the gastrointestinal tract (GESA, 2017). Table 18.1 identifies the distinct features of both conditions.

Table 18.1   Distinct features of ulcerative colitis and Crohn's disease

Feature	Ulcerative colitis	Crohn's disease
Symptoms	Severe rectal bleeding, inflamed rectum, lower left quadrant pain, diarrhoea, fever, weight loss, **anorexia**, vomiting, dehydration, frequency of urgent need to defecate (up to 20 times a day), faeces usually contains blood and mucous.	Infrequent rectal bleeding, fever, anorexia, fatigue, **anaemia**, lower right quadrant pain not relieved with defecation, weight loss
Location of inflammation	Colon to anus	Anywhere from mouth to anus, predominantly in small intestine (ileum)
Course of disease	Exacerbations, remissions	Long and variable
Mucosal involvement	Mucosal layer only	Transmural (full thickness)
Cure	Total colectomy only	Incurable

Source: French (2017)

Anaemia – a condition that results from less than the normal number of red blood cells, which affects the oxygen-carrying capacity of the blood.

Anorexia – an eating disorder leading to persistent restriction of energy intake and obsession about food being consumed.

The onset of Crohn's disease is usually insidious, and begins with oedema and thickening of the mucosa, leading to the development of ulcerations on the inflamed mucosa in multiple areas, separated by normal bowel tissue (Hendrickson, Gokhale & Cho, 2002). This can lead to the development of **fistulas**, fissures and abscess formation through to the peritoneum as inflammation increases. As the disease advances, the intestinal lumen narrows due to thickening of the bowel wall (French, 2017). Symptoms are more common **postprandial** due to **peristalsis** attempting to move food through a narrowed lumen, leading to crampy lower abdominal pain that is somewhat relieved through defecation (French, 2017; Hendrickson et al., 2002). To address these events occurring, the person often reduces what they eat and when they eat, leading to nutritional deficits and associated issues (GESA, 2017).

Ulcerative colitis characteristically appears in exacerbations and remissions. Inflammation begins in the anus due to the development of multiple and continuous ulcerations that travel throughout the colon. The ulcerations bleed, with the mucosa becoming oedematous and inflamed, causing diarrhoea that contains blood and

Fistulas – abnormal connections between two hollow spaces such as blood vessels, intestines or hollow organs.

Postprandial something which occurs or is attended to after a meal.

Peristalsis – wavelike muscular contractions which move food through the digestive tract.

mucous. As the condition progresses, the bowel characteristically narrows, shortens and thickens, due to muscular **hypotrophy** (French, 2017).

Hypotrophy – degeneration of an organ due to a progressive loss of cells.

Irritable bowel syndrome

Research indicates strong links between an alteration in gastrointestinal tract micro-biota following an episode of gastroenteritis (leading to **dysbiosis**), and the develop-ment of IBS symptoms (Canavan et al., 2014; Ghoshal et al., 2012). In IBS, peristalsis is predominantly affected, leading to changes in the movement of faecal matter in the intestine. There is usually no inflammation or tissue change within the gastrointestinal tract. Symptoms fluctuate between constipation and diarrhoea or both, with associated pain, bloating and abdominal distention, and the passage of mucus with stools. Abdominal pain is often precipitated by eating and relieved by defecation (Barboza, Talley & Moshiree, 2014; French, 2017).

Dysbiosis – the adhesion of pathogenic bacteria to the gastrointestinal tract wall.

SKILLS IN PRACTICE

Recurrent abdominal pain: Sharon

Sharon is a 36-year-old woman who presents with symptoms of recurrent abdominal pain, bloating and frequency of loose stools. Sharon states that she has had these symptoms on and off since she was 18. Over the past year, her symptoms have been occurring more frequently and with greater severity. On assessment of her pain, Sharon states she rates the pain at 7 out of 10 and it appears to be related to defecation. Sharon says that her bowel movements are loose more than half the time and she will often have two to three bowel movements per day, depending on her dietary intake. Sharon is married and works as a dental nurse part time; she has two young children aged four and six.

QUESTION
What are the symptoms of Sharon's IBS?

REFLECTION

Consider how Sharon's condition could affect her lifestyle, including work commit-ments and family outings.

Treatment options for chronic bowel conditions

The goals of treatment for any chronic bowel disorder require individual assessment and planning, and are dependent on the phase and location of the disease process, and the impact the disorder is having on a person's quality of life (Wilhelm & Love, 2017). Treatment may involve: addressing acute inflammations; improving and/or reducing symptoms, inducing a chemical (pharmaceutical) remission; improving extra-intestinal complications; reviewing and evaluating the person's response to previous treatments; and surgical palliation or cure in the case of ulcerative colitis (Schwartz, 2016).

Non-pharmacological treatments

While nutritional support is paramount for a person with a chronic bowel condition, so too is the need to monitor the person's psychological and psychosocial wellbeing. Chronic bowel conditions can cause psychological and psychosocial issues, such as social isolation, difficulties in maintaining employment and diminished self-esteem (Trindade, Ferreria & Pinto-Gouveria, 2017).

The formation of therapeutic relationships between health care providers is important to allow the person to openly (and safely) discuss their concerns relating to their condition. These discussions should encourage the person to: review their interpersonal relationships; surround themselves with friends and family who are supportive and encouraging (this can assist the person in developing resiliency); and develop coping mechanisms to deal with stressful situations such as symptom flair ups or treatment changes (Purc-Stephenson, Bowlby & Qaqish, 2014). The therapeutic relationship can also allow discussion of the availability of support groups, including online communities, which can further develop acceptance and understanding of the person's condition through the sharing of experiences and situations (Purc-Stephenson et al., 2014). Complementary and alternative medicine and psychological therapies – including **cognitive behavioural therapy**, psychotherapy, acupuncture and Chinese medicine – have yielded mixed results in addressing symptom distress (Chey, Kurlander & Eswaran, 2015).

Monitoring and maintaining a nutritional balance should be a major focus in the treatment of chronic bowel conditions. Reduced dietary intake, anorexia, malabsorption and food avoidance are some of the factors which can lead to nutritional issues. Malnutrition is a serious side effect that can lead to other issues, including increased fatigue and malaise, which impacts on the person's ability to maintain their activities of daily living. For this reason, an accurate and thorough nutritional assessment should be conducted at least annually and during any hospital admission for acute exacerbation of symptoms and their management (Mowat et al., 2011).

Nutritional deficits are common in chronic bowel conditions, due to malabsorption, which occurs because of the involvement of all layers of the gastrointestinal wall and the resultant damage to intestinal mucosa. A common consequence for people with chronic bowel disorders is to develop lactose intolerance, where a dairy-free diet is prescribed to help reduce gas and bloating (Mowat et al., 2011).

Common nutritional deficits include:

- protein and fats
- calcium
- fat-soluble vitamins: A, D, E & K
- iron
- folic acid
- vitamin B12
- electrolytes including potassium and magnesium.

Cognitive behavioural therapy – a practical collaborative approach which involves active steps taken to assist an individual to challenge negative thoughts, feelings and behaviours by providing positive, fulfilling solutions aimed at improving one's quality of life (Duff et al., 2018).

While there is no specific diet that has been proven to reduce the manifestations of chronic bowel conditions, new research is indicating that restricting short-chain carbohydrates (FODMAP foods) can be effective in reducing symptoms such bloating, flatus and abdominal pain (Barrett, 2013). A low FODMAP (fermentable oligosaccharides, disaccharides, monosaccharides and polyols) diet has been shown to be effective in reducing the amount of water and fermentable substances in the colon of people with and without functional bowel disorders such as Crohn's disease (Barrett, 2013). Further research has linked the osmotic load of high FODMAP carbohydrates as the likely cause of diarrhoea in both IBS and IBD (Zhan, Zhan & Dai, 2018).

Table 18.2 identifies foods which have a high FODMAP content and suitable low FODMAP alternatives.

Table 18.2 Food groups of high FODMAP with low FODMAP alternatives

Food group	High FODMAP	Low FODMAP alternative
Fruit	• Apples • Apricots • Cherries • Mangos • Pears • Watermelons	• Bananas • Grapes • Lemons • Limes • Oranges • Strawberries
Vegetables	• Asparagus • Cauliflower • Garlic • Mushrooms • Onion • Snow peas	• Carrots • Chilli • Cucumber • Green beans • Olives • Tomato • Zucchini
Protein	• Legumes • Pistachio nuts • Cashews	• All fresh beef, pork, chicken and lamb • Macadamias, peanuts, walnuts and pine nuts • Eggs • Tofu
Breads and cereals	• Wheat • Rye • Barley	• Corn • Oats • Polenta • Quinoa • Rice • Spelt
Dairy	• Condensed or evaporative milk • Cottage or ricotta cheese • Custard	• Butter • Lactose-free products • Rice milk • Other cheese
Other	• Honey • Fructose syrup • Sorbitol/mannitol	• Golden syrup • Maple syrup • Regular sugar • Glucose

Source: Adapted from Barrett (2013)

Increasing ingestion of liquid, particularly fibre such as psyllium or bran, is an initial treatment of IBS with constipation. It assists in reducing abdominal pain and discomfort, but can lead to bloating and abdominal pain, so should be incorporated into the diet gradually (Barboza et al., 2014).

Pharmacological treatments

The goal of any treatment of a chronic bowel condition is aimed at healing the mucosa, relieving symptoms and reducing potential complications from occurring.

Pharmacological treatment options belong to five categories:

1. aminosalicylates (5-ASA)
2. corticosteroids
3. antibiotics (metronidazole, ciprofloxacin)
4. immunomodulators (azathioprine, methotrexate)
5. biological agents (infliximab, adalimumab).

As remission and symptom-free intervals are the predominant goal, anti-inflammatory and immunosuppressive agents are first-line options.

Anti-inflammatory medications used to maintaining remission in ulcerative colitis are 5-ASA drugs, such as sulfasalazine and mesalazine. These medications work by suppressing the production of pro-inflammatory mediators in the colonic mucosa and controlling inflammation (GESA, 2017). Their use in Crohn's disease remains controversial, but these drugs are supportive in some instances in reducing the reoccurrence of symptoms after a surgical bowel resection (Mowat et al., 2011).

Acute flare ups of symptoms respond well to the use of corticosteroids. This group of medications provide rapid and significant reduction in inflammation. Due to significant side effects, predominantly immunosuppression, the duration of these medications should be limited, and the person monitored during treatment. When a person ceases use of these medications, it should be done slowly over weeks rather than days. These medications should not be used for long-term management (GESA, 2017; Mowat et al., 2011).

Antibiotics like metronidazole and ciprofloxacin are used during exacerbations of conditions such as fistulas, infective colitis and post-operative wound infections. In some instances, antibiotic therapy is also used in long-term symptom management, such as the prevention of abscess formation. The role antibiotics play relates to their ability in reducing the bacterial load in the gut lumen and altering the composition of the microbiota of the bowel (Nitzan et al., 2016).

Long-term use of medication therapy is required for the maintenance of remission and symptom control. Immunomodulators, such as azathioprine, mercaptoprurine and methotrexate, are used to control inflammation and to prevent or reduce corticosteroid dependence. These medications can take up to two to three months for an optimal response to be achieved. As with corticosteroids, this group of medications affects the immune system by reducing the inflammatory response, so close monitoring of the person is required as they have a higher risk of contracting opportunistic infections (GESA, 2017; Mowat et al., 2011).

Anti-tumour necrosis factor-α (anti-TNFα) medications, such as infliximab (Remicade) can promote mucosal healing, which leads to a long remission from symptoms and improves the quality of life for the individual who is unresponsive or intolerant of corticosteroids, thiopurines and aminosalicylates (Amiot & Peyrin-Biroulet, 2015; GESA, 2017).

Pain is a common complaint in people with a chronic bowel condition due to active inflammation or infection, secondary complications, or functional pain caused by diarrhoea and/or constipation, which is usually visceral in nature (Docherty, Jones & Wallace, 2011). Medication that may be used to treat visceral pain include antispasmodics, antidepressants and anticonvulsants such as gabapentin or pregabalin. Simple analgesics such as paracetamol and short-term use of NSAIDs may also be effective in the treatment of acute pain. Opiate preparations like morphine may be considered, but their common side effects of nausea and constipation should be monitored and treated (Docherty, Jones, & Wallace, 2011). Antispasmodics such as hyoscine can be effective in the treatment of abdominal pain and cramping, as can peppermint oil, which has also been found to have smooth muscle relaxation properties (Barboza et al., 2014). Antidepressants can be useful in treating both pain and bowel dysfunction, as they can improve the dysregulation of neurogenetic pathways; for example, tricyclic antidepressants, including imipramine, assist in slowing the colonic transit of food as a result of the anticholinergic actions (Barboza et al., 2014).

Surgical options

Mowat and colleagues (2011) suggest that up to 30 per cent of people with ulcerative colitis will require bowel surgery. Surgery is indicated: for those who do not respond to intensive pharmaceutical therapies; if there is a presence of carcinoma or dysplasia; if the disease is poorly controlled; if there are recurrent acute exacerbations of fistulas, strictures, obstructions, perforations, or abscesses; or to control bleeding (GESA, 2017). In Crohn's disease, surgery does not cure the condition and the disease can, and frequently does, recur after surgery. Ulcerative colitis is considered cured after surgery removes the entire colon, but this requires the formation of an ileostomy or ileal pouch (GESA, 2017) (see Figure 18.1).

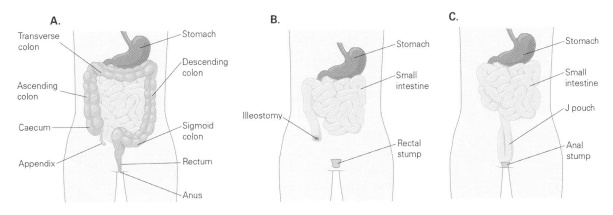

Figure 18.1   A. normal anatomy; B. subtotal colectomy formation of illeostomy; C. subtotal colectomy and formation of J pouch

Promoting health and reducing risk

Health maintenance programs are essential for people with chronic bowel conditions as many pharmacological treatments involve long-term immunosuppressive medications, which increase the risk of developing infections and other conditions. For this reason, individuals with chronic bowel conditions should be encouraged to practise health maintenance, which includes immunisations, screening interventions such as cervical cancer, identification of depression and anxiety, and smoking cessation programs (Farraye et al., 2017).

Smoking is a risk factor for Crohn's disease, worsening its course and increasing the need for pharmacological interventions. However, smoking protects against ulcerative colitis, improves its course and decreases the need for colectomies. So, smoking cessation is important in people with Crohn's disease, but in ulcerative colitis its benefits must be balanced against other risks which can be more significant. Interestingly, nicotine replacement therapy does not modify the progression of ulcerative colitis, indicating that the benefits of smoking in this condition are not related to nicotine pathways (Abegunde, Muhammad & Ali, 2016).

Moderate exercise has been demonstrated to reduce some symptoms of IBD and obesity, and low levels of fitness are linked to higher IBD activity (Abegunde et al., 2016). Regular physical exercise also helps generally with chronic bowel conditions to improve intestinal gas clearance, which decreases abdominal bloating and constipation (Anastasi & Capili, 2013).

As a result of malabsorption, there is tendency for a large fluid loss with resultant electrolyte imbalance. Consequentially, malnutrition leads to fatigue and decreased ability to perform self-care activities. It is, therefore, essential to maintain fluid balance and optimise the person's nutritional status (Pullen & Julian, 2012). Diets high in polyunsaturated fats and low in fibre can increase the risk of IBD. Diets high in fibre, especially fruit and cruciferous vegetables, decrease the risk of Crohn's disease but not ulcerative colitis. People with IBD are at risk of malnutrition, particularly in relation to several micronutrients, such as folate and iron. Those with Crohn's disease and extensive bowel resections are particularly at risk for vitamin B12 deficiencies (Abegunde et al., 2016).

Issues relating to quality of life

People with chronic bowel conditions resulting in constipation have a better disease-specific quality of life than those with chronic bowel disorders resulting in diarrhoea. Issues include gastrointestinal symptoms such as heartburn/regurgitation, feelings of fullness, nausea, vomiting, bloating and abdominal pain. These can lead to: interference with activities and body image; food avoidance; and negative effects on social interactions, relationships and sexual health (Singh et al., 2015; Trindade et al., 2016).

Anaemia is common in people with IBD with 30 per cent having haemoglobin levels below 12g/dL and many having iron deficiency. Screening every three months is recommended, and extensive testing may be required to identify the cause and suitable treatment to avoid hospitalisation, improve quality of life and ability to work, and to reduce the associated costs of treatment (Abegunde et al., 2016).

Osteoporosis and osteopenia are more common in people with IBD due to corticosteroid use and malnutrition, and the impact of fractures can be significant on quality of life (Abegunde et al., 2016). Physical exercise not only reduces symptoms of IBD, but also has the potential to improve psychological health, nutritional status, immunological responses and bone mineral density, as well as increasing muscle mass and strength – all of which improve quality of life (Abegunde et al., 2016).

The psychological impact of having a chronic relapsing condition and medication side effects can be significant, with rates of depression being particularly high in this group. Frequent screening, and the provision of counselling and medication as required can assist. Antidepressant medications such as selective serotonin reuptake inhibitors, although used for the treatment of anxiety and depression, have also been found to decrease pain, gut irritability and the urgency of defecation (Abegunde et al., 2016).

The nurse's role in caring for the patient with a chronic bowel condition

The nurse needs to be conversant with assessment and management requirements for a person with chronic bowel condition. The nurse's responsibility includes providing comprehensive systematic assessments, planning, and providing holistic care to manage the disease processes and reduce the frequency of symptoms; this is done in collaboration with the person, who will benefit from being empowered to self-manage their conditions more effectively. **Shared decision making** allows both the person and those providing treatment options to openly discuss and evaluate disease knowledge and treatment intentions, suggest behaviour modifications and psychological well-being, and optimise health outcomes (GESA, 2017; Pullen & Julian, 2012; Veilleux et al., 2018). Support and education are essential to help the person understand the rationale for the treatment that they are receiving in order to promote self-management.

Shared decision making – integrating the individual's values, goals and concerns with treatment options to achieve appropriate health care decisions.

The nurse should provide information to the person so that they are informed about the disease process and the need for lifestyle modifications. Certain food and drink can exacerbate the symptoms of chronic bowel conditions; cereals, dairy products, spicy foods, high-fat foods, alcohol and caffeine can be problematic so education will be needed to enable people with chronic bowel conditions to make necessary dietary modifications (Duff et al., 2018). Nurses can also refer people with these conditions to dieticians who conduct nutritional assessments and plan diets, in collaboration with the person, to ensure that nutritional requirements are met. Nutritional assessment should include a consideration of dietary intake, body mass index and the patient's weight, and any weight loss or gain.

Nutritional strategies could include reducing or preventing gastrointestinal symptoms through avoidance of trigger foods, adequate oral fluid intake (sipping rather than gulping), eating small frequent meals, supplementary multivitamins and iron supplements (Pullen & Julian, 2012). A high-protein, high-fibre, low animal fat, low FODMAP diet could be recommended to reduce inflammation, and help relieve bloating, pain and diarrhoea (Duff et al., 2018). Total parenteral nutrition may be indicated in severe cases of chronic bowel disorders where there is intestinal failure and nurses will need to ensure safe administration if it is required (Pullen & Jullian, 2012). One strategy is to encourage the person to keep a daily food, fluid and stool (frequency, consistency, urgency, straining and pain) diary to keep track of symptoms, recording the severity with each food or fluid consumed in order to exclude the trigger foods from the diet (Anastasi & Capili, 2013). Noting non-dietary triggers, such as mood or stress, can also be useful to allow them to be managed. Relaxation techniques and exercise can contribute to stress reduction (Anastasi & Capili, 2013).

Person-centred care focuses on the nurse building a relationship with the person who has a chronic bowel condition, and identifying goals and management strategies with them, such as the plan outlined in Table 18.3.

Table 18.3   Management plan for a person with a chronic bowel condition

Self-care strategy	Considerations	Collaborations

Diet	• Consider:
	  – foods which do not trigger symptoms
	  – a low FODMAP diet
	  – avoiding trigger foods
	  – eating small, frequent meals
	  – adequate fluid intake to maintain hydration (sipping rather than gulping)
	  – vitamin and iron supplements
	• Regularly monitor weight
	• Family involvement in discussions related to dietary requirements
		• Dietician/ nutritionist Community groups for cooking classes

Physical activity	• Discuss the importance of regular exercise to improve intestinal gas clearance and therefore decrease chances of bloating and constipation
	• Exercise:
	  – to help control the occurrence and severity of symptoms
	  – to help relieve stress
		• Exercise physiologist physiotherapist/ occupational therapist/ community exercise groups

Risk reduction	• Discuss:
	  – avoidance of trigger foods, alcohol, caffeine, etc.
	  – avoidance of trigger over-the-counter drugs
		• Dietician/GP/ pharmacist

Self-monitoring	• Discuss:
	  – regular weight checks
	  – daily food and fluid diaries to keep track of the symptoms noting the severity with each food or fluid consumed so that they can be excluded from the diet
	  – daily stool diaries to track frequency, consistency, urgency, straining and pain
		• GP/community nurse

Medication use	• Discuss:
	  – the importance of following instructions when taking medications
	  – possible medication and food interactions
		• Pharmacist/GP

Self-care strategy	Considerations	Collaborations
Coping strategies	• Discuss self-relaxation techniques to manage stress/anxiety • Develop a network of support systems to assist in life crisis • Establish a 'what if' plan and share with support networks	• Social worker/GP/community nurse

Source: Adapted from Duff et al. (2018); Pullen & Julian (2012)

SKILLS IN PRACTICE

Holistic assessment: Holly

Holly is a 38-year-old female who has presented to the nurse-led clinic at the doctor's practice you work at today. Holly states that she has a six-year history of a 'bowel' disease which, up until the last 12 months, was being managed well with diet, exercise and medications. Unfortunately, over the last year, Holly's symptoms have become worse and her last exacerbation (which began two weeks ago) has not responded to the prescribed medications. She has lost 20 kilograms in weight over the last 12 months (weight 62 kg, height 170 cm) and is constantly tired.

Holly states that she is constant pain (crampy in nature) in her umbilical area, has frequent lower abdominal cramping, and a tender perianal area due to having her bowels open up to 20 times a day. Holly describes her bowel motions as loose, with frequent mucous and blood, and defecation as painful, with it presenting as sharp in nature immediately prior to needing to defecate and then returning to a dull cramp afterwards.

Holly mentions that it has had a huge impact on her family and work life. She has no sick leave left and is unable to be too far away from a toilet as she can never predict when she needs to go. She asks you if there are any surgical options to treat the disease, so she can get her life back.

QUESTIONS

1. From the information provided does Holly have Crohn's disease or ulcerative colitis?

2. What is the significance of Holly's weight loss?

3. What other information would you consider relevant to collect from your initial assessment of Holly?

4. Which multidisciplinary team members would you involve in Holly's management planning?

5. Using the above multidisciplinary team members, what care plan would you develop that would holistically address Holly's needs?

SUMMARY

Learning objective 1: Identify and describe the most common chronic bowel conditions in Australia and New Zealand.

Irritable bowel disease can be due to either Crohn's disease or ulcerative colitis; it is estimated that around 75 000 Australians and 15 000 New Zealanders are living with either of these conditions. The incidence of IBS is linked to approximately 15 per cent of the Australian population. Irritable bowel disease is more common in females and can affect women across the lifespan, predominantly those between 5 and 40 years of age.

Learning objective 2: Describe the underlying pathophysiology and risk factors associated with chronic bowel conditions.

Both IBD and IBS are described as idiopathic relapsing and remitting inflammations of the gastrointestinal tract. These conditions are often considered to be an immune reaction to the environment. Symptoms of both conditions include abdominal pain, bloating, and fluctuations between diarrhoea and constipation.

Learning objective 3: Discuss the different treatment options for people with a chronic bowel condition.

As with diagnosis, treatment options are developed on an individual basis, and rely on both pharmaceutical and non-pharmaceutical options. Irritable bowel syndrome and Crohn's disease cannot be cured, but ulcerative colitis can be cured with a surgical intervention such as a subtotal colectomy, which may result in either a stoma (ileostomy) or J pouch. It is important that a multidisciplinary team approach is taken when treating a person with either IBD or IBS as these conditions also pose many psychosocial issues.

Learning objective 4: Identify ways to promote health and address the quality of life related to living with a chronic bowel condition.

Holistic and multidisciplinary-focused care and education is the key in ensuring the individual and their family receive the best treatment options available to them. Pharmaceutical-based treatments require education on the importance of medication compliance, while non-pharmaceutical options include reviewing diet and nutritional needs, maintaining physical activity, self-monitoring (including a symptom diary), and developing coping mechanisms to manage stress and anxiety due to changes in condition or symptoms.

Learning objective 5: Discuss the nurse's role in working with people who have a chronic bowel condition.

The nurse's role is multifactorial, and involves educating, encouraging and supporting the individual and their family. Nurses also assist people with chronic bowel conditions with nutritional advice, encouraging exercise, smoking cessation, monitoring and sometimes during surgical interventions.

REVIEW QUESTIONS

1. What are the predominant symptoms that differentiate between ulcerative colitis and Crohn's disease?
2. What are the pharmacological treatments of IBD?

3. Identify four aspects you would include when educating a person and their family about IBD.
4. How would you differentiate between IBD and IBS in relation to symptoms and treatments?
5. Which multidisciplinary team members would you suggest in assisting a person in their IBS or IBD treatment journey?

RESEARCH TOPIC

Consider the lifestyle changes a 35-year-old male could face when he is advised the best treatment option for the ulcerative colitis he suffers is a subtotal colectomy and formation of an ileostomy. Explore how this change in body image could impact on both his physical and psychological wellbeing.

FURTHER READING

Abegunde, A. T., Muhammad, B. H. & Ali, T. (2016). Preventative health measures in inflammatory bowel disease. *World of Gastroenterology*, 22(34), 7625–44. doi: http://10.3748/wig.v22.i34.7625

Anastasi, J. K. & Capili, B. (2013). Managing irritable bowel syndrome: How to help patients control this life-altering condition. *American Journal of Nursing*, 113(7), 42–53. doi: http://10.1097/01.NAJ.0000431911.65473.35

Chey, W. D. Kurlander, J. & Eswaran, S. (2015) Irritable bowel syndrome. A clinical review. *Journal of the American Medical Association*, 313(9), 949–58.

Mulder, D. J., Noble, A. J., Justinich, J. & Duffin, J. M. (2014). A tale of two diseases: The history of inflammatory bowel disease. *Journal of Crohn's and Colitis*, 8, 341–8.

Schwartz, E. (2016). Perioperative parenteral nutrition in adults with inflammatory bowel disease: A review of literature. *Nutrition in Clinical Practice*, 31(2), 159–70.

REFERENCES

Abegunde, A. T., Muhammad, B. H. & Ali, T. (2016). Preventative health measures in inflammatory bowel disease. *World of Gastroenterology*, 22(34), 7625–44. doi: http://10.3748/wig.v22.i34.7625

Amiot, A. & Peyrin-Biroulet, L. (2015). Current, new and future biological agents on the horizon for the treatment of inflammatory bowel diseases. *Therapeutic Advances in Gastroenterology*, 8(2), 66–82.

Anastasi, J. K. & Capili, B. (2013). Managing irritable bowel syndrome: How to help patients control this life-altering condition. *American Journal of Nursing*, 113(7), 42–53. doi: http://10.1097/01.NAJ.0000431911.65473.35

Barboza, J. L., Talley, N. J. & Moshiree, B. (2014) Current and emerging pharmacotherapeutic options for irritable bowel syndrome. *Drugs*, 24, 1849–70.

Barrett, J. S. (2013). Extending our knowledge of fermentable, short-chain carbohydrates for managing gastrointestinal symptoms. *Nutrition in Clinical Practice*, 28(3), 300–6.

Canavan, C., West, J. & Card, T. (2014). The epidemiology of irritable bowel syndrome. *Clinical Epidemiology*, 6, 71–80.

Chey, W. D., Kurlander, J. & Eswaran, S. (2015) Irritable bowel syndrome. A clinical review. *Journal of the American Medical Association*, 313(9), 949–58.

Crocker, K., Chur-Hansen, A. & Andrews, J. (2013). Interpersonal relationships for patients with irritable bowel syndrome: A qualitative study of GPs' perceptions. *Australian Family Physician*, 42(11), 805–9.

Docherty, M. J., Jones, C. W. & Wallace, M. S. (2011). Managing pain in inflammatory bowel disease. *Gastroenterology & Hepatology*, 7(9), 592–600.

Duff, W., Haskey, N., Potter, G., Alcorn, J., Hunter, P. & Fowler, S. (2018). Non-pharmacological therapies for inflammatory bowel disease: Recommendations for self-care and physician guidance. *World Journal of Gastroenterology*, 24(28), 3055–70. doi: http://10.3748/wjg.v24.i28.3055

Farraye, F. A., Melmed, G. Y., Lichtenstein, G. R. & Kane, S. V. (2017). ACG clinical guidelines: Preventative care in inflammatory bowel disease. *The American Journal of Gastroenterology*, 112, 241–58.

French, J. (2017) Management of patients with intestinal and rectal disorders. In M. Farrell, *Smeltzer and Bare's Textbook of Medical-Surgical Nursing* (4th edn). Sydney: Wolters Kluwer Health.

Gastroenterological Society of Australia (GESA). (2006). *Irritable Bowel Syndrome: Clinical Update* (2nd edn). Melbourne: GESA.

——(2017). *Australian Guidelines for General Practitioners and Physicians. Inflammatory Bowel Disease* (4th edn). Melbourne: GESA.

Ghoshal, U., Shukla, R., Ghoshal, U., Gwee, K., Ng, S. C. & Quigley, E. M. M. (2012). The GUT microbiota and irritable bowel syndrome: Friend or foe? *International Journal of Inflammation*, 1, 46–50.

Goncalves, A., Roi, S., Nowicki, M, Dhaussy, A., Huertas, A., Amiot, M.-J. & Reboul, E. (2014). Fat soluble vitamin intestinal absorption: Absorption sites in the intestine and interactions for absorption. *Food Chemistry*, 172, 155–60.

Heizer, W. D., Southern, S. & McGovern, S. (2009). The role of diet in symptoms of irritable bowel syndrome in adults: A narrative review. *Journal of the American Dietetic Association*, 109(7), 1204–14. doi: http://10.1016/j.jada.2009.04.012

Hendrickson, B. A., Gokhale, R. & Cho, J. H. (2002) Clinical aspects and pathophysiology of inflammatory bowel disease. *Clinical Microbiology Reviews*, 15(1), 79–94.

Kaplan, G. G. (2015). The global burden of IBD: From 2015 to 2025. *Nature Reviews Gastroenterology & Hepatology*, 12, 720–7.

Lee, S. K., Yoon, D. W., Lee, S., Kim, J., Choi, K.-M., & Shin, C. (2017). The association between irritable bowel syndrome and the coexistence of depression and insomnia. *Journal of Psychosomatic Research*, 93, 1–5.

Lomer, M., Gourgey, R. & Whelan, K. (2014). Current practice in relation to nutritional assessment and dietary management of enteral nutrition in adults with Crohn's disease. *Journal of Human Nutrition and Dietetics*, 27(Suppl. 2), 28–35. doi: http://10.1111/jhn.12133

Lovell, R. M. & Ford, A. C. (2012). Global prevalence of and risk factors for irritable bowel syndrome: A meta-analysis. *Clinical Gastroenterology and Hepatology*, 10(7), 712–21.e4. doi: http://10.1016/j.cgh.2012.02.029

Mowat, C., Cole, A., Windsor, A., Ahmad, T., Arnott, I., Driscoll, R, ... & Bloom, S. (2011). Guidelines for the management of inflammatory bowel disease in adults. *Gut,* 60, 571–607.

New Zealand Ministry of Health (NZMOH). (2018). Inflammatory bowel disease. Wellington: Ministry of Health.

Nitzan, E. M., Elias, M., Peretz, A. & Saliba, W. (2016). Role of antibiotics for the treatment of inflammatory bowel disease. *World Journal of Gastroenterology,* 22(23), 1078–87.

Pedersen, N., Ankersen, D. V., Felding, M., Wachmann, H., Végh, Z., Molzen, L., ... & Munkholm, P. (2017). Low-FODMAP diet reduces irritable bowel symptoms in patients with inflammatory bowel disease. *World Journal of Gastroenterology,* 23(18), 3356–66.

Pullen, R. L. & Julian, M. K. (2012). Caring for a patient with inflammatory bowel disease. *Nursing Made Incredibly Easy,* 10(4), 36–45. doi: http://10.1097/01.NME.0000415009.50578.14

Purc-Stephenson, R., Bowlby, D. & Qaqish, S. T. (2015). "A gift wrapped in barbed wire". Positive and negative life changes after being diagnosed with inflammatory bowel disease. *Quality of Life Research,* 24, 1197–205.

Schwartz, E. (2016). Perioperative parenteral nutrition in adults with inflammatory bowel disease: A review of literature. *Nutrition in Clinical Practice,* 31(2), 159–70.

Singh, P., Staller, K., Barshop, K., Dai, E., Newman, J., Yoon, S., ... & Kuo, B. (2015). Patients with irritable bowel syndrome-diarrhea have lower disease-specific quality of life than irritable bowel syndrome-constipation. *World Journal of Gastroenterology,* 21(26), 8103–9. doi: http://10.3748/wjg.v21.i26.8103

Smith, G. D. (2017). Gut-directed hypnotherapy for irritable bowel syndrome. *Gastrointestinal Nursing,* 15(7), 2. Retrieved from www.magonlinelibrary.com/doi/10.12968/gasn.2017.15.7.20

Thompson, J. & Read, N. (2015). Managing the symptoms of irritable bowel syndrome. *Nurse Prescribing,* 13(5), 230–4.

Trindale, I. A., Ferreria, C. & Pinto-Gouveria, J. (2017). Chronic illness-related shame: Development of a new scale and novel approach for IBD patients' depressive symptomatology. *Clinical Psychology and Psychotherapy,* 24, 255–63.

Veilleux, S., Noiseux, I., Lachapelle, N., Kohen, R., Vachon, L., White Guay, G., ... & iGenoMed Consortium. (2018). Patient's perception of their involvement in shared treatment decision making: Key factors in the treatment of inflammatory bowel disease. *Patient Education and Counseling,* 101(2), 331–9.

Wilhelm, S. M., & Love, B. L. (2017). Management of patients with inflammatory bowel disease: Current and future treatments. *The Pharmaceutical Journal,* 9(3). doi: http:10.1211/CP.2017.20202316

Zhan, Y., Zhan, Y. & Dai, S. (2018). Is a low FODMAP diet beneficial for patients with inflammatory bowel disease? A meta-analysis and systematic review. *Clinical Nutrition,* 37, 123–9.

19

Eye, ear and dental health

Linda Deravin, Jennifer Manning
and Judith Anderson

LEARNING OBJECTIVES

After reading this chapter, you should be able to:

1. identify the main causes of chronic vision impairment
2. outline some of the causes of chronic hearing loss and its impact on individuals
3. explain the importance of good dental hygiene practices, and its impact on the health and wellbeing of individuals
4. explain the nurse's role in promoting health and reducing the risk of chronic conditions in relation to oral, eye and ear health.

Introduction

Even though eye, ear and dental health have not been identified among the national health priorities in Australia, they are still areas that require resources and funding so that nations like Australia and New Zealand can address the overall health and wellbeing of all their residents, regardless of location or socioeconomic status. Many of the chronic conditions that affect eye, ear and dental health are preventable. With this in mind, this chapter is included to highlight the importance of these chronic conditions in addressing the overall health and wellbeing of specific vulnerable population groups.

Eye health

The World Health Organization (WHO) estimated that 285 million people lived with a vision impairment and that 80 per cent were preventable or curable (WHO, 2013). As a result of this estimate, WHO established a universal eye health plan that outlined strategies to improve eye health and vision. In Australia, it has been estimated that by 2020, there may be over 800 000 people that will have a partial or complete loss of vision, and 90 per cent of these are preventable or treatable (Australian Government Department of Health, 2014; Foreman et al., 2016). Statistically, Indigenous Australians are three times more likely to have blindness or a vision impairment than non-Indigenous Australians (Foreman et al., 2016). Putting these figures into context, vision and hearing disorders only accounted for 2.2 per cent of the burden of disease in Australia in 2011 (Australian Institute Health and Welfare (AIHW), 2016). However, this calculation does not consider the personal cost and impact that vision impairment and blindness have on an individual.

Pathophysiology of the eye

The eye is a complex apparatus (see Figure 19.1). There are three main processes that are needed to have healthy vision. These are:

1. refraction – where the image is formed on the retina
2. stimulation of the photoreceptive cells in the retina, which are called **cones and rods**
3. conduction of the impulse along the optic nerve to the brain.

If there is anything that disrupts these processes, there is the possibility of vision impairment, ranging from temporary, partial or permanent loss of vision in one or both eyes.

There are many conditions and diseases that affect eye health and **visual acuity**. Individuals across the lifespan are diagnosed with conditions and diseases that affect eye health (Foreman et al., 2016; Vision Australia, 2018). *The National Eye Health Survey 2016* is the most recent report to reveal the main causes of blindness and vision impairment in Australia (Foreman et al., 2016). The overall cause of vision impairment or loss for both Indigenous and non-Indigenous Australians is an uncorrected **refractive error** (Australian Government Department of Health, 2014; AIHW, 2018a; Foreman et al., 2016). This condition can be corrected by having regular eye and vision

Cones and rods – the photoreceptor cells that are in the neural layer of the retina. The rods allow us to see in dim light and do not provide colour vision. Cones are stimulated by bright light and there are three types: blue, green and red. This is what gives us our colour vision.

Visual acuity – a testing process that is performed to assess the clarity of what is seen at either long or short distances.

Refractive error – occurs when light does not bend correctly causing blurred images.

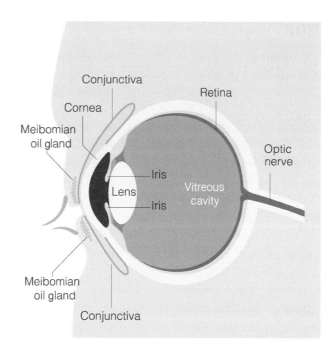

Figure 19.1   Anatomy of the eye

assessments, and having spectacles provided to correct the refractive error. Spectacles and/or contact lenses can correct this condition, but they are expensive and regular testing may indicate that vision aids need to be changed or modified. At a macro level, funding for eye health services is supported through the federal government. There are government-supported spectacle schemes in place to provide for those that meet the eligibility criteria, which may differ from state to state. Indigenous Australians have a three times higher burden of vision impairment or blindness from both refractive error conditions and preventable diseases (AIHW, 2018a).

Common conditions of the eye that affect vision

The main conditions that are common in affecting eye health or vision identified in *The National Eye Health Survey 2016* (Foreman et al., 2016) are:

- age-related macular degeneration (AMD) – where the macular region of the retina deteriorates and affects the person's central vision. Early detection is important to slow the progression by implementing treatment options and preventing further vision loss
- diabetic retinopathy – when the retinal capillaries in the back of the eye become damaged due to diabetes (either type 1 or 2) not being controlled or as a result of the chronic nature of the disease
- glaucoma – considered an umbrella term for a group of eye diseases that damage the optic nerve; it is usually associated with high intra-ocular pressure. Early detection allows interventions which can help prevent or slow the rate of vision loss

- cataracts — where the lens in the eye becomes opaque. Measures can be taken to prevent this, such as wearing sunglasses to reduce the exposure to ultraviolet light. Regular examinations can detect early changes and, if needed, cataract surgery is successful in restoring vision.

It is interesting to note that cataracts are the leading condition to affect vision (40 per cent) among Indigenous Australians, and AMD is the leading condition (71 per cent) causing non-Indigenous Australians to have vision impairment (Foreman et al., 2016).

Promoting health and reducing risk for chronic eye conditions

Prevention or correction

Eye health is important to maintain and there are strategies that help protect our eyes and vision. The leading cause for eye injuries that required admission to hospital in the last five years was falls, which were responsible for 35 per cent of reported cases. Assaults accounted for 23 per cent of eye injuries, mostly to males, and injury caused by an inanimate mechanical force was 20 per cent of hospital admissions. Other causes of injury were foreign bodies going into the eye, contusions to the orbital area, and sporting and work-related injuries. Traumatic eye injuries are the main cause of vision impairment or blindness in people under 46 years (Australian Institute Health and Welfare, Tovell & McKenna, 2018).

The areas identified for prevention in the 2014 National Framework recognised the World Health Assembly targets of risk reduction, improved early detection, and avoidance of vision loss and disease (Australian Government Department of Health, 2014). It is recommended that Indigenous Australians with diabetes undergo yearly eye health checks, and non-Indigenous Australians have biennial eye health checks to screen for preventable eye disease related to diabetes. *The National Eye Health Survey 2016* identified areas within Australia where prevention programs can still be improved. Data indicates that only 52.87 per cent of Indigenous Australians and 77.72 per cent of non-Indigenous Australians have the recommended number of eye checks (Foreman et al., 2016). Addressing inequities that exist within identified population groups, such as the elderly and Indigenous peoples, will help to reduce the personal impact felt and the burden on health care (Australian Government Department of Health, 2014).

There is also a similar disparity between the Indigenous Australians and non-Indigenous Australians in relation to cataract surgery. Only 61 per cent of Indigenous Australians who have cataracts have had them removed, compared to 88 per cent of non-Indigenous Australians (Foreman et al., 2016). It is recognised that there needs to be further measures taken to improve the eye health of the Australian Indigenous population (Australian Government Department of Health, 2014). In relation to cataract treatment, it has been identified that geographical location from a metropolitan centre increases the wait-time for surgery. Address-ing this issue and providing surgery for those with vision impairment resulting from cataracts could improve the person's overall health and wellbeing (Foreman et al., 2016).

Indigenous Australians with a refractive error condition have a lower incidence of having this corrected than non-Indigenous Australians. This is also consistent with other global Indigenous communities (Australian Government Department of Health, 2014; Foreman et al., 2016). Refractive errors can be corrected with spectacles. The Australian government is aware that the incidence of vision impairment and blindness is 10 times more common in Indigenous populations compared to non-Indigenous populations, and so the government is implementing programs to address the inequities (Australian Government Department of Health, 2014). In the aged population, estimates are difficult to ascertain as the expected increase in this population group is not known (Bourne et al., 2017).

REFLECTION

Consider what role nurses have in addressing the inequities in eye health. What assessment practices could be put into place to identify those who are at risk of developing eye or vision disorders? Are there any practices that can be implemented into your assessment of individuals to improve the eye health of all Australians, particularly Indigenous Australians?

Impact of having blindness or a vision impairment

Any vision impairment impacts an individual's quality of life and so preventative measures and eye health care should be integrated into primary health care strategies and programs to inform public health policy (Bourne et al., 2017). Vision impairment is not isolated to the aged — eye conditions are also commonly found as chronic issues in children (AIHW, 2009). There is a considerable cost — socially, financially and personally — for those with any form of vision impairment or eye disorder. The person may be restricted socially and experience a loss of independence, which could have a negative impact on their physical and mental health. These factors can lead to the person having greater risks of developing other health conditions or an increased mortality (AIHW, 2009).

SKILLS IN PRACTICE

Headaches and eye strain

Louise is a 51-year-old nurse who works on a medical ward. Lately she has noticed that her eyes are continually sore and that she suffers from headaches more frequently. You are a nurse working with Louise and you have noticed that she is struggling with the medication round; she often asks you to do the medication round for her and she will do some of your work. Louise has told you that she hates these new computer-based programs that are being implemented to provide and document patient care as it makes her eyes very sore by the end of the shift. She has always prided herself on her great eyesight and has had regular eye tests — the last one being two years ago. The thought of having to possibly wear glasses is something that she is concerned about.

QUESTIONS

1. What symptoms is Louise displaying that might make you think there is an issue with her eyesight?
2. What might be the underlying cause for her deteriorating eyesight?
3. How might you address this with your co-worker?

Ear health

There are a range of reasons for why an individual may experience hearing loss. Hearing loss can be caused by chronic ear infections, exposure to loud noises, ageing, birth complications or genetic disorders (AIHW, 2018b; New Zealand Ministry of Health (NZMOH), 2018a). The WHO estimates that approximately 466 million people worldwide (approximately 5 per cent of the world population) have a disabling hearing loss, and the expectation is that this number will double by the year 2050 (WHO, 2018). Specific vulnerable groups, such as the elderly and Indigenous populations, are more likely to suffer from a hearing impairment.

In Australia, the focus has centred on Indigenous children and the effects of otitis media, which is treatable and preventable. It is recognised that there is an increasing burden of hearing loss in this vulnerable population group. Statistics indicate that Indigenous children are 8.6 times more likely to have suffered from otitis media than non-Indigenous children (AIHW, 2018b). In New Zealand, middle ear disease is also known to be a common problem for Māori and Pacific Islander children, but available data on the prevalence within this demographic is limited (Deloitte Access Economics, 2017). For New Zealand, it is estimated that approximately 18.9 per cent of the total population (mainly the elderly over the age of 65) have a hearing impairment. In Australia, it is estimated that 74 per cent of people aged 71 years and over have some form of hearing loss (Punch & Horstmanshof, 2018). With the projected rates of hearing loss expected to increase in the next few generations, the need for preventative and restorative measures that can contribute to individual's wellbeing need to be considered.

Pathophysiology of the ear

There are three physiological components to an ear, and these are referred to as the external, middle and inner ear (see Figure 19.2). The external ear is the visible part of the ear which collects sound waves and directs them towards the middle ear. These sound waves then travel through the auditory canal towards the eardrum (tympanic membrane). The pressure of the sound waves causes the eardrum to vibrate. From this point, the sound wave is transmitted to the oval window via the middle ear bones, causing amplification of these waves in the inner ear (Martini et al., 2015)

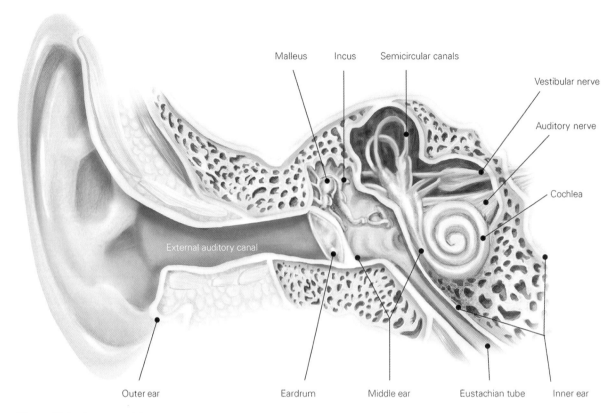

Figure 19.2   Anatomy of the ear

The middle ear bones are called the malleus (hammer), the incus (anvil) and the stapes (stirrups). The malleus is attached to the tympanic membrane, the incus connects the malleus to the stapes and the stapes is connected to the outer edges of the oval window. The Eustachian tube is also located in the middle ear and its function is to equalise pressure on the eardrum, ensuring that pressure within the ear does not build up. The inner ear contains the cochlear, the auditory nerve and the vestibular (balance mechanism). The cochlear converts sound waves into electrical impulses. The auditory nerve contains multiple nerve fibres that transmit the electrical impulses to the brain so that audible sounds are decoded. Also contained within the inner ear is the vestibular which has fluid filled passages that move in accordance with the position of the body. This helps the body keep its balance (Martini et al., 2015). When the messages are interrupted or the function of any part of the ear is not working as it should, then hearing loss may occur.

Common ear disorders

Table 19.1 is a list of common ear disorders that affect hearing function of individuals.

Table 19.1   Common ear disorders that affect hearing function

Ear condition	Description
Otitis media (also known as glue ear)	Presence of inflammation and/or infection of the middle ear. A build-up of fluid may occur reducing hearing function. Treatment may be antibiotics or the surgical insertion of grommets to assist with fluid drainage
Tinnitus	Constant ringing or noise in the ear. It is not a disease but is a symptom of a malfunction within the auditory system. It may be caused by a build-up of ear wax, a tumour on the auditory nerve, or it may indicate the presence of Ménière's disease or otosclerosis
External ear infections (also known as 'swimmer's ear')	Where water may be trapped in the ear canal trapping bacteria and causing inflammation and/or infection
Ear wax obstruction	Ear wax or cerumen normally builds up and self-dislodges from the ear either falling out or being wiped away. When this does not occur, ear wax may build up in the ear canal obstructing the tympanic membrane from functioning correctly. If the ear wax does not dislodge naturally then removal by a doctor may be required
Autoimmune inner ear disorder	An inflammatory condition where the person's own immune system attacks the inner ear, incorrectly perceiving the presence of a virus or bacteria
Cholesteatoma	A growth of skin in the middle ear behind the tympanic membrane. This may result from otitis media where the Eustachian tube does not function properly or can be present at birth
Perforated eardrum	When a hole occurs in the tympanic membrane; this can be spontaneous or through injury. Often this will heal on its own. In some cases, surgical intervention is required
Otosclerosis	The presence of abnormal bone growth in the middle ear (malleus, stapes and incus)
Ménière's disease	Affects the inner ear causing a person to experience difficulty with balance or vertigo, dizziness and tinnitus. It often occurs in one ear only and may lead to progressive hearing loss. There is no cure however symptoms can be managed

Source: Adapted from Deafness Foundation (2016); Martini et al. (2015)

Promoting health and reducing risk for chronic ear conditions

The impact of hearing loss on individuals

Living with a hearing impairment can have a significant effect on an individual's social and emotional wellbeing. For children, the experience of hearing loss may impede their ability to develop speech and language, which may also result in poor concentration, attention and listening skills vital to being able to learn. The social implications for living with hearing loss may lead to behavioural problems such as irritability and perceived disobedience, often resulting in poor school attendance, academic under-achievement, early attrition from secondary schooling and increased risk of injuries and social isolation (Choi, Kei & Wilson, 2017). This, in turn, may influence employment options, where a role may be dependent on adequate hearing. As a social determinant of health, lack of employment has been directly linked to an increase in antisocial behaviours and, in some instances, increased negative involvement with the criminal justice system (AIHW, 2018b). For the elderly, living with hearing loss may affect their ability to socialise and communicate, leading to feelings of social isolation and loneliness, contributing to their long-term mental health issues such as depression (Deloitte Access Economics, 2017).

At a meso level, early detection of hearing loss through health screening, to identify conductive hearing loss, is a recommended strategy to prevent long-term or chronic deafness (Choi et al., 2017). Through early identification and management of hearing loss, social and emotional impacts may be mitigated. In areas where populations have limited access to health and specialist medical services, the potential for hearing loss to go undetected and untreated is far greater (AIHW, 2018b).

Living with chronic hearing loss

Treatment for hearing loss will be influenced by the underlying cause. Where hearing loss may result from a build-up of fluid in the ears, surgery may be indicated with the insertion of a tympanostomy tube (grommet). Repeated bacterial infections, such as otitis media, can be treated with antibiotics or corticosteroids. Where hearing loss cannot be cured or reversed, the next step would be to consider hearing aids or other modifications and mechanisms that could improve hearing and communication; for example, cochlear implants, brain stem implants (where hearing is affected by nerve damage), or assistive devices like specialised sound systems, visual signals such as flashing lights and the use of subtitles on visual media. People with chronic and long-term hearing loss may also choose to learn sign language as a way to communicate when hearing; in some instances, the ability to speak may also be affected (Deloitte Access Economics, 2017). Nurses can participate in the early identification of hearing loss through health promotion programs and referral to other members of the multi-disciplinary team; this can lead to early treatment, and ongoing prevention and management of hearing loss.

SKILLS IN PRACTICE

My child cannot hear

Leona is a single mother, who lives in a small rural town. She comes in to visit the child and family health nurse (you) for a routine check-up for her six-month-old daughter, Morganna. You only visit this town once a week. Leona is accompanied by her other child, Michael, who will turn five in a few weeks time and start school next year. Michael is content to play with some blocks in the corner of the room and has his back facing you and Leona. While you are doing your routine milestone checks on Morganna, Leona accidently knocks a piece of equipment over which makes a very loud sound. You notice that Michael does not react to this loud sound and continues to play. You ask Leona if she has noticed whether Michael hears her normally in his own surroundings. Leona starts to tell you that Michael is a very 'naughty' boy as he never comes when she calls him. He tends to play on his own and does not take much notice of his baby sister, even when she cries. You ask more questions about Michael's general health, including if he has had any colds recently. Leona becomes defensive and replies that it would be no more than any other child. Later in the conversation, Leona admits that she is just too tired with the new baby anyway, and she does not really remember. You write a referral to the local general practitioner recommending an audiologist follow up for a hearing screening. Two weeks later, Leona returns to see you to tell you that Michael has been diagnosed with moderate to severe deafness in both ears. They are going to see an ear, nose and throat specialist in the city next month, which is three hours away, as that was the earliest appointment that she could get. She looks distressed and starts to cry saying that she is not coping and questions how she will manage with a child who cannot hear, as she does not know any sign language.

QUESTIONS

1. What would be the most likely clinical reason for Michael's apparent hearing loss?
2. What is the most likely treatment that would be recommended for Michael?
3. What resources or services might be available to help Leona when she attends the appointment in the city and possibly to follow up if it should be required?
4. As the nurse, what other social factors should you consider to help with this family situation?

Dental health

The impact of dental health problems for people with or without chronic conditions is an important area for consideration. Even though nurses do not provide dental care and treatment, they do have a role in providing education about dental care and nutrition to support improved dental health. People who have dental health issues may experience effects on their day-to-day living where there is a change to their self-image. This may result in an individual isolating themselves from social networks and supports. The loss of teeth or the effects of pain caused by dental health problems may also result in a person's reduced ability to participate in certain activities, such as eating, affecting their nutritional wellbeing. Nutrition and the socioeconomic level of individuals and communities have been shown to have a significant influence on dental health (Australian Institute Health and Welfare et al., 2016; Binns et al., 2017; Thornley et al., 2017). This section of the chapter will focus on some of the significant areas of dental health that affect how people can live well within their communities.

Dental caries

Dental caries are areas of decay that exist within teeth. In an Australian national survey, the latest data available showed that 42.8 per cent of children aged five years

Deciduous – teeth that are commonly known as either milk or baby teeth which are usually smaller than permanent teeth and generally fall out as permanent teeth grow.

had experienced dental caries and at aged nine this percentage rose to 68.7 per cent (AIHW, 2018c). Many of these dental caries existed in teeth which were **deciduous**. Once permanent teeth appeared, the rates varied from 7 per cent for children aged six years to 64.1 per cent for children aged 14 years (AIHW, 2018c). In New Zealand, similar rates of dental caries exist. One in three adults had evidence of tooth decay, and approximately 50 per cent of children aged 2–17 years showed evidence of dental decay (NZMOH , 2010; Thornley et al., 2017). In both Australia and New Zealand, Indigenous and Pacific Islander peoples, or those who lived in poorer socioeconomic circumstances, showed a higher prevalence of dental caries. This was attributed to exposure to high sugar foods, poor oral hygiene practices and the lack of access to dental care due to limited resources or the availability of services (Binns et al., 2017). Chronic conditions such as obesity and cardiovascular health are also compounded by poor nutrition and dental health.

Periodontal disease

Periodontal disease or gum disease refers to inflammation and swelling of the tissues surrounding the tooth. The most common cause of periodontal disease is a bacterial infection which may affect the gums, the ligaments and bone within the mouth cavity (AIHW, 2018c). Symptoms of periodontal disease may include toothache, swollen and bleeding gums (commonly known as gingivitis), **halitosis**, or the presence of an abscess in the tooth socket. If left untreated, loss of teeth or bone within the mouth area can occur, affecting an individual's ability to eat a nutritional diet (AIHW, 2018c; Australian Institute Health and Welfare et al., 2016). Regular dental hygiene practices, such as brushing teeth regularly after meals and flossing gums, may help in the prevention of periodontal disease.

Halitosis – presence of an unpleasant odour in a person's breath.

Promoting health and reducing risk for dental conditions: the fluoride debate

A topical area of debate in both Australia and New Zealand is the value of water fluoridation as a preventative measure for dental caries. The debate centres around the cost to fluoridate water supplies as a preventative measure, as opposed to the cost to individuals in managing dental health and the prevention of dental caries and disease (Cobiac & Vos, 2012). Fluoride is a naturally occurring substance that can strengthen and protect teeth from decay, limit the growth of bacteria which cause dental caries, and help to repair early stages of tooth decay. Fluoride is present in fresh water, sea water, plants and many foods that are consumed within a nutritious diet. Increased consumption of high-sugar foods and drinks can increase the acidity within the mouth, which removes essential minerals from teeth and can contribute to tooth decay (Thornley et al., 2017). Brushing teeth with fluoride toothpaste and drinking fluoridated water neutralises these damaging acids (NZMOH, 2018b).

Fluoridation of public water supplies is a key strategy under the Australian National Oral Health Plan (Oral Health Monitoring Group, 2015) and the New Zealand Oral Health Survey (Whyman, Mahoney & Borsting, 2016). The Australian strategy has been identified as a relatively low-cost approach that could potentially benefit many people by reducing the incidence of dental disease within the Australian population (Cobiac & Vos, 2012). In 2016, proposed legislative changes were introduced into New Zealand, which allowed district health boards to enforce local authorities to fluoridate the public water supply (NZMOH, 2018b). The counterargument to fluoridating water is that this may increase the risk of **fluorosis**, hypothyroidism and bone fractures (Awofeso, 2012). Current thinking supports fluoridation of water supplies as the benefits to dental health in the prevention of dental caries outweigh the potential risks of other health conditions (Awofeso, 2012), but the debate continues.

> **Fluorosis** – white or brown discolouration to the enamel on the surface of a tooth.

REFLECTION

Good dental hygiene and care of teeth and gums can help to prevent a range of dental conditions. Diet also plays an important part in the health of teeth and gums. Identify two or three chronic conditions where diet and dental health can have a significant impact on a person's wellbeing.

The nurse's role in the management of eye, ear and dental health

Providing education to reduce risk factors associated with each of these chronic conditions is a nursing responsibility and can be integrated into the nursing role in any setting. When a window of opportunity arises, an individual may be more open to this education rather than waiting for them to seek it out. Providing information, when a person can best understand the value of its impact, can support their decision making and, thereby, their autonomy. Dental caries, for example, can lead to pain, loss of teeth, systemic infection and nutritional deficiencies, but is frequently linked to low dental health literacy. Providing information about the use of **topical fluorides** (such as toothpaste and mouth rinses), consumption of **systemic fluoride** (like fluoridated water), good dental hygiene, and limiting the consumption of refined carbohydrates can mitigate these issues (Koo et al., 2016), particularly in the school setting prior to issues becoming overwhelming (Dudovitz et al., 2018). Screening for dental caries involves an oral examination; it can make parents more aware of the issues their children may be having and prevent further deterioration of the teeth (Arora et al., 2017). Screening in school-aged children can be a very effective role for nurses, not only in the prevention of dental caries, but also in the detection of hearing loss, which is commonly related to otitis media (especially when it occurs intermittently), and can be effectively treated with antibiotics, preventing long-term issues related to educational difficulties, speech and language impairments and compromising social development (Avnstorp et al., 2016; Kaspar et al., 2018). Supporting parents, who identify hearing loss in their children, to ensure that they are accurately assessed and appropriately treated, is part of the nurse's role. Due to poor services being available in remote areas of Australia and New Zealand, mobile screening and intervention units staffed with specialists can be cost-effective solutions in preventing chronic issues (Nguyen et al., 2015).

> **Topical fluoride** – applied directly to the teeth; it is absorbed by the surface of the teeth to strengthen them.
>
> **Systemic fluoride** – ingested into the body, it circulates through the blood and is incorporated into the growing tooth. It is also present in saliva where it can become a topical fluoride.

Advanced nursing practice

The role of nurse practitioners is extensive in the prevention of chronic conditions relating to oral, eye and ear health.

Keratoconus – a condition where the cornea thins and starts to bulge changing to be more conical in shape which causes distorted vision.

In terms of eye health, nurses can have particular success in the support of people with **kerataconus** to prevent eye rubbing, relieving irritation through antihistamine use and encouraging use of full ultraviolet protection through sunglasses and spectacles (Bonner & Winokur, 2017). Age-related macular degeneration is common but recent advances in the treatment of 'wet' neovascular AMD have led to an increased demand for intravitreal injections of ranibizumab, which not only prevents the loss of vision but also improves it for people with this condition. This increased demand has led to an expansion of the role of specialist ophthalmic nurses to administer the injections (Gregg, 2017; Samalia, Garland & Squirrell, 2016).

In terms of oral health, nurse practitioners in the United States have also developed their practice to include dental health by providing counselling, screening and fluoride varnish to develop healthy dental practices prior to children attending school (Koo et al., 2016).

REFLECTION

As a nurse providing care in any health setting, which population groups are more likely to have issues with chronic conditions related to eyes, ears and dental health?

SUMMARY

Learning objective 1: Identify the main causes of chronic vision impairment.
There are many conditions and diseases that affect eye health and visual acuity. Vision impairment is not isolated to the aged, and eye conditions and diseases are also commonly found as chronic issues in children. Common eye disorders are age-related macular degeneration, diabetic retinopathy, glaucoma and cataracts. Preventative and corrective measures are available to reduce the impact of vision impairment within society.

Learning objective 2: Outline some of the causes of chronic hearing loss and its impact on individuals.
Living with a hearing impairment can have a significant effect on an individual's social and emotional wellbeing. Early identification and treatment can reduce the impact of hearing loss. Hearing loss may be caused by chronic ear infections, exposure to loud noises, ageing, birth complications or genetic disorders. Specific vulnerable groups such as the elderly and Indigenous populations are more likely to suffer from a hearing impairment.

Learning objective 3: Explain the importance of good dental hygiene practices, and its impact on the health and wellbeing of individuals.
People who have dental health issues may experience effects on their day-to-day living where there is a change to their self-image. This may result in an individual isolating themselves from social networks and supports. The loss of teeth or the effects of pain caused by dental health problems may also result in a person's reduced ability to participate in certain activities, such as eating, which affects their nutritional wellbeing. Nutrition and the socioeconomic level of individuals and communities have a significant influence on dental health.

Learning objective 4: Explain the nurse's role in promoting health and reducing the risk of chronic conditions in relation to oral, eye and ear health.
Providing education in order to reduce risk factors associated with each of these chronic conditions is a nursing responsibility and can be integrated into the nursing role in any setting. Screening is usually beneficial, particularly in younger age groups prior to conditions becoming a significant issue.

REVIEW QUESTIONS

1. What are four main causes of vision impairment identified within Australia?
2. Which population groups are most susceptible to hearing loss?
3. What are some of the options to treat or manage hearing loss?
4. Does the benefit of fluoridation in the water outweigh the risks associated with artificially enhancing our public water supplies?
5. What information could you provide to a parent to promote dental health?

RESEARCH TOPIC

Hearing and vision loss have significant impacts on the daily lives of individuals. How does your local community support people with a hearing or vision impairment? Think about how easy or difficult it might be to undertake activities of daily living such as shopping, ordering a meal at a restaurant, or gaining employment. Find out what resources or aids are available to assist people to manage their lives while living with a hearing or vision impairment.

FURTHER READING

Australian Institute Health and Welfare (AIHW). (2018). *Australia's Health 2018-Australia's Health Series No. 16*. Canberra: AIHW.

Awofeso, N. (2012). Ethics of artificial water fluoridation in Australia. *Public Health Ethics*, 5(2), 161–72.

Eye Health Working Group of the Community Care and Population Health Principal Committee. (2015). *National Framework for Action to Promote Eye Health and Prevent Avoidable Blindness and Vision Loss. Third Progress Report to Australian Health Ministers Covering the Period 2011–2014*. Canberra: Department of Health.

Fred Hollows Foundation. (2015). *The National Trachoma Program*. Retrieved from www.hollows.org/au/what-we-do/indigenous-australia/trachoma-program

Nguyen, K. H., Smith, A. C., Armfield, N. R., Bensink, M. & Scuffham, P. A. (2015). Cost-effectiveness analysis of a mobile ear screening and surveillance service versus an outreach screening, surveillance and surgical service for indigenous children in Australia. *PLOS ONE*, 10(9), e0138369. doi: http://10.1371/journal.pone.0138369

REFERENCES

Arora, A., Khattri, S., Ismail, N., Sumanth, K. & Prashanti, E. (2017). School dental screening programmes for improving oral health of children. *Cochrane Database of Systematic Reviews*, 2017(12). doi: http://10.1002/14651858.CD012595

Australian Government Department of Health. (2014). *Implementation Plan under the National Framework for Action to Promote Eye Health and Prevent Avoidable Blindness and Vision Loss*. Canberra: Department of Health Retrieved from www.health.gov.au/internet/main/publishing.nsf/content/eyehealth-pubs-impl

Australian Institute Health and Welfare (AIHW). (2009). *A Guide to Australian Eye Health Data. Cat. no. PHE 119*. Canberra: AIHW Retrieved from www.aihw.gov.au/getmedia/aaaa9c6e-ff38-4ea3-9793-4a9d19834a17/phe-119-10786.pdf.aspx?inline=true

——(2016). *Australian Burden of Disease Study: Impact and Causes of Illness and Death in Australia 2011. Australian Burden of Disease Study Series No. 3. BOD 4*. Canberra: AIHW.

——(2018a). *Indigenous Eye Health Measures 2017*. Canberra: AIHW Retrieved from www.aihw.gov.au/reports/indigenous-australians/indigenous-eye-health-measures-2017/contents/summary

——(2018b). *Australia's Health 2018-Australia's Health Series No. 16*. Canberra: AIHW.

——(2018c). *Oral Health and Dental Care in Australia 2015*. Canberra: AIHW.

Australian Institute Health and Welfare, Chrisopoulos, S., Harford, J. E., & Ellershaw, A. (2016). *Oral Health and Dental Care in Australia- Key Facts and Figures 2015*. Cat. no. DEN 229. Canberra: AIHW.

Australian Institute Health and Welfare, Tovell, A. & McKenna, K. (2018). *Eye Injuries in Australia, 2010–11 to 2014–15. Injury Research and Statistics Series No. 194*. Canberra: AIHW and Flinders University.

Avnstorp, M. B., Homoe, P., Bjerregaard, P. & Jensen, R. G. (2016). Chronic suppurative otitis media, middle ear pathology and corresponding hearing loss in a cohort of Greenlandic children. *International Journal of Pediatric Otorhinolaryngology*, 83, 148–53. doi: http://10.1016/j.ijporl.2016.01.017

Awofeso, N. (2012). Ethics of artificial water Fluoridation in Australia. *Public Health Ethics*, 5(2), 161–72. doi: http://10.1093/phe/phs016

Binns, C., Howat, P., Smith, J. A. & Jancey, J. (2017). Children, poverty and health promotion in Australia. *Health Promotion Journal of Australia*, 27(3), 181–3.

Bonner, D. R. & Winokur, E. J. (2017). The "eyes" have it: Reviewing keratoconus, the nurse practitioner perspective. *The Journal for Nurse Practitioners*, 13(8), 532–7.

Bourne, R. R. A., Flaxman, S. R., Braithwaite, T., Cicinelli, M. V., Das, A., Jonas, J. B., ... & Taylor, H. R. MD on behalf of the Vision Loss Expert Group. (2017). Magnitude, temporal trends, and projections of the global prevalence of blindness and distance and near vision impairment: A systematic review and meta-analysis. *The Lancet Global Health*, 5(9), e888–97. doi: http://10.1016/S2214-109X(17)30293-0

Choi, S. M. R., Kei, J. & Wilson, W. J. (2017). Rates of hearing loss in primary school children in Australia: A systematic review. *Speech, Language and Hearing*, 20(3), 154–62. doi: http://10.1080/2050571X.2016.1259199

Cobiac, L. J. & Vos, T. (2012). Cost-effectiveness of extending the coverage of water supply fluoridation for the prevention of dental caries in Australia. *Community Dentistry & Oral Epidemiology*, 40(4), 369–76. doi: http://10.1111/j.1600-0528 .2012.00684.x

Deafness Foundation. (2016). Chronic diseases of the ear. Retrieved from www.deafness.org.au/hearing-loss/chronic-diseases-of-the-ear-2

Deloitte Access Economics. (2017). *Social and Economic Costs of Hearing Loss in New Zealand- The National Foundation for the Deaf*. Retrieved from www2.deloitte.com/ content/dam/Deloitte/au/Documents/Economics/deloitte-au-economics-social- economic-cost-hearing-loss-new-zealand-021216.pdf

Dudovitz, R. N., Valiente, J. E., Espinosa, G., Yepes, C., Padilla, C., Puffer, M., ... & Chung, P. J. (2018). A school-based public health model to reduce oral health disparities. *Journal of Public Health Dentistry*, 78(1), 9–16. doi: http://10.1111/jphd.12216

Foreman, J., Keel, S., Xie, J., van Wijngaarden, P., Crowston, J., Taylor, H. R. & Dirani, M. (2016). *The National Eye Health Survey 2016*. Melbourne: Vision 2020 Australia.

Gregg, E. (2017). Nurse-led ranibizumab intravitreal injections in wet age-related macular degeneration: A literature review. *Nursing Standard*, 31(33).

Kaspar, A., Newton, O., Kei, J., Driscoll, C. & Goulios, H. (2018). Prevalence of ear disease and associated hearing loss among primary school students in the Solomon Islands: Otitis media still a major public health issue. *International Journal of Pediatric Otorhinolaryngology*, 113, 223–8.

Koo, L. W., Horowitz, A. M., Radice, S. D., Wang, M. Q. & Kleinman, D. V. (2016). Nurse practitioners' use of communication techniques: Results of a Maryland Oral Health Literacy Survey. *PLOS ONE*, 11(1), e0146545. doi: http://10.1371/ journal.pone.0146545

Martini, F., Ober, W. C., Nath, J. L., Bartholomew, E. F. & Petti, K. (2015). *Visual Anatomy & Physiology:* New York: Pearson.

New Zealand Ministry of Health (NZMOH). (2010). Our oral health: Key findings of the 2009 New Zealand Oral Health Survey. Retrieved from www.health.govt.nz/publication/our-oral-health-key-findings-2009-new-zealand-oral-health-survey

—— (2018a). Hearing loss. Retrieved from www.health.govt.nz/your-health/conditions-and-treatments/disabilities/hearing-loss

—— (2018b). Fluoride. Retrieved from www.health.govt.nz/your-health/healthy-living/teeth-and-gums/fluoride

Nguyen, K. H., Smith, A. C., Armfield, N. R., Bensink, M. & Scuffham, P. A. (2015). Cost-effectiveness analysis of a mobile ear screening and surveillance service versus an outreach screening, surveillance and surgical service for indigenous children in Australia. *PLOS ONE*, 10(9), e0138369. doi: http://10.1371/journal.pone.0138369

Oral Health Monitoring Group. (2015). *Healthy Mouths Healthy Lives – Australia's National Oral Health Plan 2015–2024*. Adelaide: COAG Health Council.

Punch, R. & Horstmanshof, L. (2018). Hearing loss and its impact on residents in long term care facilities: A systematic review of literature. *Geriatric Nursing*. doi: http://10.1016/j.gerinurse.2018.07.006

Samalia, P., Garland, D. & Squirrell, D. (2016). Nurse specialists for the administration of anti-vascular endothelial growth factor intravitreal injections. *New Zealand Medical Journal*, 129(1438), 32–8.

Thornley, S., Marshall, R., Reynolds, G., Koopu, P., Sundborn, G. & Schofield, G. (2017). Low sugar nutrition policies and dental caries: A study of primary schools in South Auckland. *Journal of Paediatrics and Child Health*, 53(5), 494–9. doi: http://10.1111/jpc.13449

Vision Australia. (2018). Eye health. Retrieved from www.visionaustralia.org/information/eye-health

Whyman, R. A., Mahoney, E. K. & Borsting, T. (2016). Community water fluoridation: Attitudes and opinions from the New Zealand Oral Health Survey. *Australian & New Zealand Journal of Public Health*, 40(2), 186–92. doi: http://10.1111/1753-6405.12408

World Health Organization (WHO). (2013). *Universal Eye Health: A Global Action Plan 2014–2019*. Geneva: WHO. Retrieved from www.who.int/blindness/actionplan/en/

—— (2018). Deafness and hearing loss. Retrieved from www.who.int/news-room/fact-sheets/detail/deafness-and-hearing-loss

20

Disability

Sally Bristow
and Alison Devitt

With acknowledgement to Catherine Hungerford and Donna Hodgson

LEARNING OBJECTIVES

After studying this chapter, you should be able to:

1. describe the social model of disability and its link to the standards for disability services, including upholding the human rights of, and enabling self-determination for, people with disabilities
2. define the terms rehabilitation and habilitation in relation to supporting people with disabilities to live independent lives
3. outline how to involve families and/or carers in the rehabilitation or habilitation of people with disabilities
4. consider how best to communicate therapeutically with people who have disabilities and are seeking health and social services.

Introduction

The terms impairment and disability are closely connected. An impairment is any kind of health condition that impedes the way in which a person chooses to live; a disability is the result of the interaction between the person living with an impairment and the hurdles or barriers encountered (Government of Western Australia, 2014). These hurdles or barriers are contained in the physical, attitudinal, communication and social environments.

A disability can be temporary or permanent, visible or invisible, or acquired before or after birth. Disabilities arise from a range of impairments, including:

- physical
- sensory
- cognitive
- intellectual
- psychological
- those related to mobility.

For this reason, disabilities are often described as multidimensional, with a person's level of disability determined by their capacity to function in any given setting.

Over 4 million people in Australia (that is, one in five) have some form of disability (Australian Bureau of Statistics (ABS), 2015), with most people experiencing disability as a result of physical impairment. In New Zealand, the proportion of the population with a disability is even higher (24 per cent). Within this cohort, 64 per cent of adults with a disability report at least one physical impairment, with 42 per cent identifying the cause of the physical impairment as disease or illness. For children up to 14 years, a condition that existed at birth is the most common cause of disability. The most common impairment for children was reported as a learning difficulty, affecting 52 per cent of children aged under 15 years with a disability (Statistics New Zealand, 2014).

In both Australia and New Zealand, around 18 per cent of males and 19 per cent of females have a disability. Age is a significant contributor to disability. In New Zealand, the following age groups reporting at least one disability: 11 per cent of children aged 0–14 years; 21 per cent of people aged 15–24 years; 43 per cent of people aged over 55 years; and 59 per cent of people aged over 65 years (Statistics New Zealand, 2014). In both Australia and New Zealand, gender statistics and severity rates indicate that boys have higher rates of impairment than girls (ABS, 2015; Statistics New Zealand, 2014).

However, perhaps the most concerning statistic for both countries is that people with disabilities are twice as likely to be in the bottom 20 per cent of gross household incomes. With low income as one of the social determinants of poorer health outcomes, this statistic suggests that people with disabilities are more likely to have poorer health outcomes than people with no disability.

In this chapter, we consider the main principles to adhere to when delivering health services to people with disabilities. This includes consideration of the practice standards that frame the way in which nurses provide health care to people with disabilities, and ways of supporting people with disabilities to make the same kind of choices as people without disabilities. We also examine the difference between rehabilitation and habilitation for people with disabilities. For example, while some disabilities may be temporary or episodic, other disabilities will be long term and permanent, with varying degrees of impairment. It is the role of the nurse to support all people to reduce the impact of impairment – first, by overcoming the barriers they may encounter in the community; and second, by going on to live meaningful and contributing lives.

Another important focus of the chapter is the need for nurses to consider the way in which physical or mental impairments may affect individuals in quite different ways. These differences suggest the need for all health professionals to engage therapeutically with the person with a disability. In particular, we discuss the need to avoid making presumptions about a person's capacity to engage in a range of activities; such beliefs are often based on unhelpful stereotypes or ignorance, which inadvertently contribute to stigmatisation. We conclude the chapter with a section on therapeutic communication, including the strategies that can be used by nurses to connect with people with disabilities, together with their carers.

The social model of disability

According to the social model of disability, notions of disability are socially constructed; that is, the ways in which people understand what it means to have a disability are determined by the community and sociocultural context in which they live (Beckett & Campbell, 2015). The social model of disability is well aligned with the Innovative Care for Chronic Conditions Framework (ICCCF), developed by the World Health Organization (WHO), as a guide for health professionals and health service organisations to provide health care to people with complex and/or chronic conditions. For example, two of the principles that are promoted by the ICCCF – integration and adaptability – are also advocated by the social model of disability. It is only when communities adapt to the needs of people with disabilities that these people will be accepted and integrated into the communities. As noted earlier, disabilities result from the interaction between a person living with an impairment and the hurdles or barriers encountered by that person in society. Proponents of the social model of disability argue that impairment is an expected part of human diversity. For this reason, society must change to accommodate people living with impairment, rather than expecting people living with impairment to change to accommodate society (Goering, 2015). If the hurdles or barriers in society are reduced, then, conversely, the capacity of a person living with an impairment to participate in society on an equal basis with others improves.

SKILLS IN PRACTICE

Access and equity

Rahman injured his back in a car accident seven years ago. He has been unable to work since the accident and ambulates with the assistance of a walking stick. This means that Rahman finds it difficult to walk outside in areas such as grasslands, paving and gravel surfaces. He is much more stable on concrete or flat pathways. Inside buildings, Rahman is unable to navigate stairs without the risk of falling backwards.

Rahman has been attending physiotherapy, Pilates and massage therapy regularly to assist with pain management, core strengthening and skeletal mobilisation. He has an upcoming physiotherapy appointment; however, the (public) physiotherapist has recently relocated due to storm damage in the health centre. The new venue is nearer to where Rahman lives, but the building is older and there is no lift facility to the treatment room.

QUESTIONS

In this scenario, the absence of a functioning lift in the substitute building impacts on Rahman's ability to function autonomously in the community, and contributes to creating an access-to-service obstacle.

1. Without the provision of a lift, in what ways does this environmental obstruction impact on Rahman's independence, autonomy and overall sense of wellbeing?

2. How would you plan appropriate care given this scenario?

To enable the process of adaptation at the macro level of the ICCCF, and to assist with the process of reducing hurdles or barriers, governments in both Australia and New Zealand have legislated a range of laws, and developed a number of standards, to ensure that people with disabilities are protected from discrimination and other abuses of human rights. Australian and New Zealand legislation protects the rights of people with disability to ensure that they have the right to freedom, respect, equality and dignity. The United Nations' *Convention on the Rights of Persons with Disabilities* underpins the Australian government's commitment to coordinate, at all levels, in improving the lives of people with disability, and the lives of their families and carers (WHO, 2008). They are also in step with the principles of the ICCCF, and aim to ensure that people with disabilities receive the best and most appropriate health care possible. For example, in Australia, the *National Standards for Disability Services* comprise six standards, with each to be applied in the diverse situations or circumstances in which people with disabilities interact. Such situations or circumstances include health care settings. The National Standards aim to protect the human rights of people with disabilities, encour-

Equity – fairness in the distribution of services or resources, particularly for those in need.

age participation and inclusion, ensure **equity** by enabling access to well-managed services, and focus on individual outcomes (Department of Social Services, 2013).

A similar approach has been developed in New Zealand, where there are four standards that frame health and disability services. These four standards ensure that people with disabilities receive: safe services that comply with consumer rights and associated legislation; timely services that are planned, coordinated and appropriate; well-managed services that are efficient and effective; and services that are provided in a clean, safe environment (New Zealand Ministry of Health (NZMOH), 2008). Organisations and individual health professionals, including nurses located across Australia and New Zealand, must ensure the health care they provide to people with disabilities complies with these principles.

Adherence to the standards in both countries can be achieved by following the principles of normalisation and self-determination. These two principles are discussed in the next sections.

Normalisation

In the past, people with disabilities were often hidden away in institutions, stigmatised and treated poorly (Chowdhury & Benson, 2011). Today, the human rights of people with disabilities are protected, including the right to:

- respect and dignity
- choice and control
- confidentiality and privacy
- self-determination (Collins, 2015).

An important part of upholding the human rights of people with disabilities is to ensure that each person is encouraged and supported to live a full and contributing life, as an equal member of society (Department for Communities and Social Inclusion, 2012; Taua, Hepworth & Neville, 2012). This process is called **normalisation**.

The principle of normalisation means that people with disabilities are helped to lead a 'normal' life; that is, a life that provides the same choices and opportunities that are experienced by people who do not have disabilities (Jingree, 2015). To accomplish this, all health professionals, including nurses, must support the person with a disability to **access** the same range of health and social services that is available to the general population. Indeed, access is an important factor that supports the protection of the human rights of people with disabilities (Moodley & Ross, 2015). This is because people with disabilities encounter barriers to obtaining health and other services, and thereby experience inequity.

One challenge to the philosophy of normalisation is the assumption that mainstream health services are appropriate or suitable for people with disabilities who, in reality, may require specialist health or social services. For example, some people with one or more significant, long-term or permanent disabilities may present with chronic or complex issues that are beyond the experience or expertise of the general practitioner (GP) or generalist nurse (Madden et al., 2012). There is a need, then, for nurses who work for generalist health services, together with disability workers, who are employed by specialist disability services, to understand the many different services available in the community that support people with disabilities. Likewise, it is important for nurses to develop links that enable people with disabilities to bridge any disconnections between these services. A collaborative and consultative approach is required between all those involved, including nurses, disability workers, carers, families and other agencies (Madden et al., 2012).

Normalisation – the process of making available to all people with disabilities the same choices and conditions of life as those regularly experienced by the community as a whole.

Access – the means by which people with disabilities can obtain and use services or resources, or have the same opportunities as other people in society.

REFLECTION

What public services or non-government organisations are available in your local area to support people with disabilities? What information do you need to obtain to appropriately refer a person to these services? If there are inadequate suitable services, how will you solve this problem?

Self-determination

The term self-determination has long-standing political connotations, and first emerged in the disability literature in the early 1970s (Wehmeyer, 1998). The term was used to describe the principle of a person exercising control over their life and destiny by ensuring that their choices, wishes, desires and aspirations were taken into account during all decision-making processes, even if an optimal outcome was not achieved (Nirje, 1972).

The principle of **self-determination** is important in Western health contexts when providing health care to people with disabilities. In contemporary health settings, self-determination is closely connected to the notions of empowerment, choice and a person's freedom to make the life choices they see as being the best for them personally (Martinis, 2015). Empowerment and choice are the means by which self-determination is achieved.

The biomedical model of health care stands in contrast to the social model of disability, including the notions of empowerment, choice and self-determination. Most nurses will be familiar with the biomedical model because it has dominated the way in which health services have been provided in Western contexts for well over 100 years. The biomedical model promotes notions of **paternalism** with health professionals, including nurses, positioning themselves as 'knowing best' and handing out advice to passive 'patients' (Lantz & Marston, 2012). Biomedical approaches are very narrow in scope because they focus on the biological aspects of a person's illness, disease or condition, rather than the external barriers that can restrict a person's capacity to function at a higher level. In addition, the biomedical model is driven by medical practitioners who traditionally have held unquestioned authority in relation to the health and wellbeing of people, preventing them from making informed decisions. For this reason, biomedical approaches are not consistent with the disability standards, which advocate for independent decision making by people with disabilities, and their families or carers.

Self-determination – having the freedom, authority and support to exercise control over your life, including the right to choose your own health and social services.

Paternalism – policy or practice used by those in positions of power or authority to restrict the freedom or choices of, and make decisions for, other people.

SKILLS IN PRACTICE

Living with disability

Janelle, a 19-year-old female, experienced a car accident when she was 10 years old. This car accident left her with a complete fracture of spinal cord at the T6 level, resulting in paraplegia and being reliant on a wheelchair for mobility. Even so, in all personal aspects of daily living, Janelle is fully self-caring.

Janelle was seeing her GP to review an ongoing urinary tract infection. The GP required a urine sample and asked the practice nurse, Elizabeth, to assist. Elizabeth immediately took charge of the wheelchair and pushed Janelle into the treatment room; spoke slowly and loudly to her, repeating everything at least twice to ensure that she had understood what she was saying, and insisted on helping Janelle obtain the specimen. Because she felt sorry for Janelle, Elizabeth also made a point of patting her on the shoulder and addressed her as 'luvvy', even asking her if she would like a 'special cuppa' to help her 'obvious anxiety'.

Elizabeth felt quite offended when Janelle told her, in no uncertain terms, that she was neither a moron nor Elizabeth's 'luvvy'. Elizabeth said that if she wanted help, she would ask for it, and she did not want to be treated any differently to anyone else. Elizabeth felt that she had only been trying to help Janelle. She promptly asked the practice manager if another nurse could assist with the procedure.

QUESTION

Many people with disabilities consider their impairments in the same way that people think about, for example, their height – occasionally they might dream about being taller or shorter, but on the whole, their height is beyond their control and so they don't spend much time considering an alternative. In this scenario, what could Elizabeth have done to ensure that she respected Janelle's right to self-determine and support her independence?

The National Disability Insurance Scheme

The National Disability Insurance Scheme (NDIS) has been described as the most significant reform to disability services in Australia in a generation (Warr et al., 2017). The scheme is underpinned by the *National Disability Insurance Scheme Act 2013* and seeks to provide long-term, high-quality support for people under the age of 65 who have a permanent disability that significantly affects their capacity to communicate, move around, self-care or self-manage (Thill, 2015). The National Disability Insurance Agency (NDIA) is charged with implementing the NDIS across the country, which began rollout on 1 July 2016. Approximately 460 000 Australians are expected to participate in the scheme by 2019 (NDIS, 2018).

The NDIS operates in line with the social model of disability; that is, rather than focusing on the person's immediate illness, disease, condition or health needs, the NDIS will consider what is required across a person's lifetime, and how best to give the person a greater level of choice, control and self-determination by encouraging their social and economic participation. To maximise a person's choice and control, a strengths-based approach should be adopted by those involved in the planning process, which includes identifying a person's individualised goals and aspirations (NDIS, 2014). Strengths-based approaches tap into the person's strengths, such as positive attributes, existing knowledge, underdeveloped capabilities, ideas and motivations, to increase their involvement, decision making and ownership of issues (NDIS, 2014). It is 'a move away from a deficit "needs based" service model, were experts fix deficits and solve problems' to a partnership approach that amplifies a person's capabilities (Independent Advisory Council of the NDIS, 2015, p.7). The following strengths-based planning principles have been taken from the *National Disability Insurance Scheme Act 2013*:

(a) be individualised; and

(b) be directed by the participant; and

(c) where relevant, consider and respect the role of family, carers and other persons who are significant in the life of the participant; and

(d) where possible, strengthen and build capacity of families and carers to support participants who are children; and (da) if the participant and the participant's carers agree — strengthen and build the capacity of families and carers to support the participant in adult life; and

(e) consider the availability to the participant of informal support and other support services generally available to any person in the community; and

(f) support communities to respond to the individual goals and needs of participants; and

(g) be underpinned by the right of the participant to exercise control over his or her own life; and

(h) advance the inclusion and participation in the community of the participant with the aim of achieving his or her individual aspirations; and

(i) maximise the choice and independence of the participant: and

(j) facilitate tailored and flexible responses to the individual goals and needs of the participant; and

(k) provide the context for the provision of disability services to the participant and, where appropriate, coordinate the delivery of disability services where there is more than one disability service provider. (Australian Government, 2013, p. 34)

These planning principles also emphasise the establishment of the NDIS as an important step in supporting the ongoing needs of family members and carers. As will be discussed later in the chapter, family members or carers of people with disabilities tend to be either young carers aged under 24 years, or older carers aged over 65 years. For older carers of people with severe impairment, a significant concern is the future of their family member when the carer becomes frail or dies (Bibby, 2013). The NDIS provides a safety net for people in such circumstances, as well as supporting the person with a disability, and their family members or carers, to live life to their fullest potential.

Ongoing independent reviews of the NDIS will play an important role in continuing to improve and reinvigorate the scheme and its services. One recent study involved interviewing people using the NDIS to learn about their experiences of having more choice and control. The feedback was mixed, from positive changes to deep frustration with ongoing struggles to gain access to crucial resources (Warr et al., 2017). The identified challenges related to navigating a complex system and inflexible service providers. In regional areas, people had specific needs that could not be met by local service providers and a significant portion of their funding was being consumed by travelling to access services (Warr et al., 2017). Considering the complexity of the design of the NDIS and the diversity of its objectives and participants, ongoing evaluation will be vital for continuous improvement.

REFLECTION

The principles that frame the disability standards – including respect and dignity, choice and control, confidentiality and privacy, and the right to self-determine – are no different to the principles that frame the day-to-day lives of all people who live in Australia and New Zealand. Consider why there is a need for these principles to be made overt in national standards that frame the services provided to people with disabilities.

Rehabilitation and habilitation

Gauging the extent of a disability is complex, and may involve the assessment of a person's physical, sensory, mobile, cognitive, intellectual, learning and/or psychological status. For health professionals, including nurses, understanding these many different factors is important in enabling them to more effectively support the person, together with family members or carers, and identify the best interventions and ways of managing the disability (Department for Communities and Social Inclusion, 2012;Taua et al., 2012).

Rehabilitation is a term that describes the interventions that are employed to help a person to restore or improve functions for daily living that have been lost or impaired due to injury, illness or disease (Buys, Matthews & Randall, 2015). Rehabilitation services can be accessed in hospitals, through community-located services or in clinics. Habilitation, a related term, refers to the process of supporting a person to maximise their capacity to live independently (Crites & Howard, 2011). According to the WHO (2015), rehabilitation and habilitation are crucial in supporting people who have impaired functioning to live independently in their homes with their families, and contribute meaningfully to their communities.

Examples of rehabilitation and habilitation services include:

- physical therapy
- occupational therapy
- speech and language therapy
- audiology services
- psychiatric rehabilitation services.

Habilitation services, then, are very similar to rehabilitation services. The difference between rehabilitation and habilitation is the focus of these services – rehabilitation services aim to help the person regain what was lost; habilitation services aim to help the person manage their loss of function, and sustain and maintain function to live life to the fullest potential.

It is important that nurses understand the difference between habilitation and rehabilitation services. Even more importantly, all nurses must ensure that people with disabilities are aware of how to access rehabilitation and habilitation services. Utilising these services will help the person with a disability to minimise the consequences of impairment, improve their health, wellbeing and quality of life, and reduce the need for health services (WHO, 2015).

The nurse's role in supporting families or carers

People with disabilities, like other people, have families, friends, carers and, at times, advocates involved in their daily lives. In Australia, there are 2.7 million unpaid family and friend carers providing care and support to another person (Carers Australia, 2012). In a single calendar year, it is anticipated that these 2.7 million carers will provide 1.9 billion hours of unpaid care and support (Carers Australia, 2015). In New Zealand over 400 000 people are carers, which is approximately one in ten New Zealanders (Ministry of Social Development, 2014).

For some family members or carers, the caring role is a demanding one, with carers stating that they experience high levels of stress that impact detrimentally on their physical and mental wellbeing (Hungerford & Richardson, 2013). Family carers often have to rearrange their lives to accommodate their family member with a disability; they can become socially isolated, stigmatised and experience high levels of guilt, particularly if there are other family members that they no longer have time for (Dehghan et al. 2016). For this reason, carers are in need of ongoing emotional support, and also recognition from nurses of the important role they play in the lives of people with disabilities (Mental Health Council of Australia, 2012).

In addition, carers have expressed a desire to engage with health professionals and health services; and are keen to obtain the information they need for their caring role, particularly in relation to coordinating the health services that are required by the person for whom they are caring (Bass et al., 2013). Nurses can assist carers in navigating complex health systems and social services, enabling them to gain the additional skills and knowledge they must have to provide adequate care and resources for their family member. For example, the physical, psychological, emotional, social, financial, vocational and other stressors experienced by carers – that is, the carer burden – are amplified in the face of the barriers they experience when negotiating health services (Reid, Lloyd & de Groot, 2005).

Such barriers to negotiating health services include a lack of inclusion in the decision making that will affect the person with a disability (Wilkinson & McAndrew, 2008). When family members or carers are not involved in the process of health or discharge planning, and when they are not informed about the services that are available for them to access, they cannot fully support the person with a disability to make informed choices.

Who is the carer?

It is important that all health professionals, including nurses, avoid making assumptions about the identity of the primary or secondary carer. Carers are not always adults. For example, while 520 000 Australian carers are aged over 65 years, 300 000 carers are aged 24 years and younger, with 150 000 carers being aged less than 18 years (ABS, 2012).

For this reason, nurses must include all those who say that they are caring for the person with a disability in their care or discharge planning. Of course, such involvement must first include obtaining the permission of the person with a disability; however, generally speaking, it can be safely assumed that family members and/or carers will play a key role in supporting the person with a disability in the day-to-day activities of life. People with disabilities frequently attend outpatient clinics, accident and emergency departments, day-patient treatments and are admitted to hospital as in-patients (NSW Health, 2017). Often another person – a relative, a paid staff carer or a centre worker – accompanies them to these appointments, visits and admissions. It is important, therefore, to consider who the carer is and how they will support the person with disabilities while in hospital (Gibbs, Brown & Muir, 2008). During any interaction with the carer, it is important to also consider the impact of caring on their quality of life and facilitate any assistance, resources or services to improve their situation.

Overlooking family members or carers when giving out information about the person with a disability will have a detrimental effect on the health and wellbeing of all concerned. The best health care is collaborative, incorporating strong interpersonal skills that support close and rigorous working partnerships between nurses, the person with a disability, and family members or carers, because this will allow for continuity of care between health services, hospital and home (Gibbs, Brown & Muir, 2008).

REFLECTION

On the one hand, nurses are asked to support the rights of people with disabilities to self-determine. On the other hand, they are asked to support families, friends and carers to participate and/or be involved in decisions. How can nurses balance these two principles?

Therapeutic communication

To uphold the disability standards, including self-determination for people with disabilities, and to support achievement of the best possible outcomes of rehabilitation and habilitation, nurses must develop advanced skills in communication, including therapeutic communication. Therapeutic communication is the process of interacting with a person in a way that advances or promotes the physical and emotional wellbeing of that person (Kleier, 2013). Therapeutic communication is used to connect with a person and their family or carers, provide support and information to the person and their family or carers, and help the person and their family member or carers to grow or develop as people (Hungerford & Richardson, 2013).

Developing the skills for therapeutic communication takes time. An important aspect of therapeutic communication is listening to and validating the person's concerns. This will include overlooking the concerns that cannot always be immediately resolved. Therapeutic communication is about acknowledging the reality of an impairment, including the way in which it impacts on a person, and listening without giving advice or leaping in to 'fix' the problem. Therapeutic communication provides the person with a disability and/or their carer with an important means of talking through the issues involved. This, in turn, can lead to reductions in anxiety and feelings of helplessness in the person, and provides an important means by which the person can be empowered to consider how they can address the issues themselves (Duperouzel & Fish, 2010).

At the same time, therapeutic communication encourages a person to share information. If a nurse does not take the time to listen or does not stop talking long enough to allow others to express themselves, then the person with a disability and family member will presume the nurse is not interested in person-centred care. Instead, they will gain the impression that the nurse is only interested in handing out information and moving on to the next task.

Therapeutic communication is particularly important when helping people with disabilities. As already noted, there are many different types of disability. Some disabilities are not visible and so are not always quickly identified by health care providers. An example of this is visible hearing aids versus expressive aphasia, which may be present in a person as a result of a stroke or brain injury. A nurse who does not take the time to ask the person about their disability, including what the person *can* do, as well as their impairments, will not have the information needed to understand or assist the person (Crossley, 2015). Instead, the nurse will be basing their practice on unhelpful stereotypes and presumptions.

Some people with disabilities may have a limited capacity to communicate verbally. If this is the case, it is important that the nurse ask the person, their family member or carer, the following questions.

- How does the person communicate?
- What can the nurse do to support this mode of communication?
- Does the health setting have adequate resources to support the person to use their equipment, aids and/or devices?
- Does the person need additional aids, especially in health settings?

It may be that the way in which the person communicates is slow and takes time. Again, this can present challenges in busy or acute environments. For nurses working on in-patient wards in hospital, communication is essential as it is fundamental for delivering optimal care. People with disabilities can have complex health needs necessitating outpatient visits and frequent admission to hospital. Hence, effective communication with the person, their family member or carer is essential to ensure that they have been consulted and collaborated with in decisions related to their care (Sharkey et al., 2016).

As people with disabilities can have complex communication needs, identifying the communication impairment and communication supports that they use to convey their message is essential for therapeutic communication (Sharpe & Hemsley, 2016). Some of the methods used to communicate may include speech, signs or gestures, using pictures, facial expressions, the alphabet or communication devices (Department of Communities, Child Safety and Disability Services, 2018). For this reason, the question must also be asked: How can the systems that are in place be adapted so that the person with a disability is not disadvantaged?

There will often be times when the nurse will need to refer the person with a disability to those who can assist them to communicate in health settings. Such referrals must be made as soon as possible to avoid further disadvantage.

SKILLS IN PRACTICE

Hospitalised patient with complex communication requirements

Max is 23 years old and has an intellectual disability. He lives with his family and his mother, Libby, is his primary caregiver.

Max was admitted to hospital after experiencing severe abdominal pain. On further investigation, it was discovered that he had appendicitis and was going to the operating theatre for an appendectomy that evening. Libby decided to stay with Max while he was in hospital to assist with his physical care needs and facilitate his communication.

Libby felt that it was important to stay, as she feared that the hospital staff would neglect Max's needs due to his difficulties with expressing himself, despite her providing them with information regarding his care needs. She had already noted that staff spoke directly with her and not Max in relation to his operation. While Libby was staying in hospital, she observed that the nursing staff rarely came over to talk to them unless she called for them.

After the operation, Libby decided to discharge Max early as she felt isolated and unsupported by hospital staff. During her stay in hospital, she did not get a break; she slept in a chair next to Max's bed and found it difficult to get food and drinks. In addition, while in hospital, expensive items that she had brought in from home were misplaced, including Max's communication device, several drugs and incontinence pads (Gibbs et al., 2008).

QUESTIONS

1. What kind of provision could be considered necessary to respond to Max and Libby's needs while they are in hospital? Consider how nursing staff can improve communication needs for them both to improve their stay.

2. What type of support would the nursing staff need to put in place for Max's admission? Consider his communication needs as well as any environmental issues in relation to the in-patient setting.

Engaging in therapeutic communication with people with disabilities can sometimes have particular challenges; even so, these challenges provide nurses with opportunities to develop skills and enable people with disabilities, together with their family and carers, to self-determine and make their own choices. This work allows the person with a disability to live a full and productive life, and achieve the best possible health outcomes.

SUMMARY

Learning objective 1: Describe the social model of disability and its link to the standards for disability services, including upholding the human rights of, and enabling self-determination for, people with disabilities.

The social model of disability defines a disability as the result of the interaction between living with an impairment and the barriers a person encounters in the environment. The model highlights that when environmental barriers are reduced, the likely outcome is an improvement in the person's ability to independently function and participate in society on an equal basis with others. To help bring about the social changes required to reduce the levels of disability for people with impairments, governments in Australia and New Zealand have developed standards for health and disability services. These standards encourage participation and inclusion, enable access to well-managed services, and focus on individual outcomes.

Learning objective 2: Define the terms rehabilitation and habilitation in relation to supporting people with disabilities to live independent lives.

Rehabilitation includes the interventions or treatments that are employed to help a person restore or improve their functions for daily living, which were lost due to injury, illness or disease. Habilitation refers to the process of supporting a person to maximise their capacity to live independently. Both rehabilitation and habilitation are crucial in supporting people who have impaired functioning to live meaningful lives. However, to further differentiate between the two, rehabilitation services aim to help the person regain what was lost, whereas habilitation services aim to help the person to manage their loss of function, and to sustain and maintain function to live life to the fullest potential.

Learning objective 3: Outline how to involve families and/or carers in the rehabilitation or habilitation of people with disabilities.

Families and carers of people with disabilities often experience high levels of stress that impact detrimentally on their physical and mental wellbeing. Carers are in need of ongoing emotional support. Carers have also expressed a desire to engage with health profession-als and health services, and to obtain the information they need for their caring role, particularly in relation to care coordination. It is essential for nurses to include families and carers when planning health care for people with disabilities. The best health care involves strong partnerships between nurses, the person with a disability, and family members or carers.

Learning objective 4: Consider how best to communicate therapeutically with people who have disabilities and are seeking health and social services.

An important aspect of therapeutic communication is listening to and validating the person's concerns. Therapeutic communication does not deny the reality of impairment or its impact on the person, but instead means listening without giving advice or leaping in to 'fix' the problem, and providing the person with an important means of talking through the issues involved. This, in turn, leads to reductions in anxiety and feelings of helpless-ness, and provides an important means by which the person with a disability can be empowered.

REVIEW QUESTIONS

1. Why have governments in Australia and New Zealand legislated a range of laws and developed a number of standards related specifically to people with disabilities? Consider the standards for services provided to people with disabilities in both countries. What are the similarities and differences?
2. What are the main rights of people with disabilities? How are these different to those of the community as a whole?
3. Generally, health systems take a paternalistic approach to treating people, with medical practitioners prescribing treatment, and people being expected to follow it. How can nurses who work in these health systems help to safeguard the rights of people with disabilities?
4. What is the difference between rehabilitation and habilitation? Why are these differences important?
5. How can nurses apply the principles of therapeutic communication to people with disabilities who are unable to communicate through talking?

RESEARCH TOPIC

According to the ABS (2012), there are 300 000 carers aged 24 years and younger, with 150 000 carers being aged less than 18 years. Explore the main issues experienced by young people who are in a caring role. What services are provided and how do these services support them?

FURTHER READING

Carers Australia. (2015). *Young Carers*. Canberra: Carers Australia. Available at www.youngcarers.net.au

Krahn, G., Reyes, M. & Fox, M. (2014). Chronic conditions and disability: Toward a conceptual model for national policy and practice considerations. *Journal of Disability Health*, 7(1), 13–18.

Lollar, D. (2009). People with disabilities. In R. Detels, R. Beaglehole, M. Lansang & M. Gulliford (eds), *Oxford Textbook of Public Health* (5th edn). Oxford: Oxford University Press.

Playford, D. (2015). The international classification of functioning, disability and health. In V. Dietz & N. Ward (eds), *Oxford Textbook of Neuro-rehabilitation*. Oxford: Oxford University Press.

World Health Organization (WHO). (2015). *Rehabilitation*. Geneva: WHO. Retrieved from https://www.who.int/rehabilitation/en/

REFERENCES

Australian Bureau of Statistics (ABS). (2012). *Survey of Disability, Ageing and Carers*. Cat. no. 4430.0. Retrieved from www.abs.gov.au/ausstats/abs@.nsf/mf/4430.0.

—— (2015). *Disability, Ageing and Carers, Australia: Summary of Findings, 2015*. Cat. no. 4430.0. Retrieved from www.abs.gov.au/AUSSTATS/abs@.nsf/Lookup/4430 .0Main+Features982015?OpenDocument

Australian Government. (2013). *National Disability Insurance Scheme Act 2013*. Retrieved from https://www.legislation.gov.au/Details/C2013A00020

Bass, D., Judge, K., Lynn Snow, A., Wilson, N., Morgan, R., Looman, W., . . . & Kunik, M. E. (2013). Caregiver outcomes of partners in dementia care: Effect of a care coordination program for veterans with dementia and their family members and friends. *Journal of the American Geriatrics Society*, 61(8), 1377–86.

Beckett, A. & Campbell, T. (2015). The social model of disability as an opposition device. *Disability & Society*, 30(2), 270–83.

Bibby, R. (2013). 'I hope he goes first': Exploring determinants of engagement in future planning for adults with a learning disability living with ageing parents. What are the issues? *British Journal of Learning Disabilities*, 41(2), 94–105. doi: http://10.1111/j .1468-3156.2012.00727.x

Buys, N., Matthews, L. & Randall, C. (2015). Contemporary vocational rehabilitation in Australia. *Disability & Rehabilitation*, 37(9), 820–4.

Carers Australia. (2012). *About Carers*. Canberra: Carers Australia. Retrieved from www .carersaustralia.com.au/about-carers

—— (2015). *The Economic Value of Informal Care in Australia in 2015*. Retrieved from www.carersaustralia.com.au/storage/Access%20Economics%20Report.pdf

Chowdhury, M. & Benson, B. (2011). Deinstitutionalization and quality of life of individuals with intellectual disability: A review of the international literature. *Journal of Policy & Practice in Intellectual Disabilities*, 8(4), 256–65.

Collins, J. (2015). From hospital to home: The drive to support people with intellectual disabilities in the community. *International Journal of Developmental Disabilities*, 61(2), 76–82.

Crites, S. & Howard, B. (2011). Implementation of systematic instruction to increase client engagement in a day habilitation program. *Journal of Intellectual & Developmental Disability*, 36(1), 2–10.

Crossley, M. (2015). Normalizing disability in families. *Journal of Law, Medicine & Ethics*, 43(2), 224–7.

Dehghan, L., Dalvand, H., Feizi, A., Samadi, S. A. & Hosseini, S. A. (2016). Quality of life in mothers of children with cerebral palsy: The role of children's gross motor function. *Journal of Child Health Care*, 20(1), 17–26.

Department of Communities, Child Safety and Disability Services. (2018). Better communication. Retrieved from www.qld.gov.au/disability/community/communicating

Department for Communities and Social Inclusion. (2012). Disability Services: information sheet: Intellectual disability: The facts. Adelaide: South Australian Government.

Department of Social Services. (2013). *National Standards for Disability Services*. Canberra: Australian Government.

Duperouzel, H. & Fish, R. (2010). Hurting no-one else's body but your own: People with intellectual disability who self injure in a forensic service. *Journal of Applied Research in Intellectual Disabilities*, 23(6), 606–15.

Gibbs, S. M., Brown, M. J. & Muir, W. J. (2008). The experiences of adults with intellectual disabilities and their carers in general hospitals: A focus group study. *Journal of Intellectual Disability Research*, 52, 1061–77. doi: http://10.1111/j.1365-2788.2008 .01057.x

Goering, S. (2015). Rethinking disability: The social model of disability and chronic disease. *Current Reviews in Musculoskeletal Medicine*, 8(2), 134–8.

Government of Western Australia. (2014). *Disability Health Network Commitment to Inclusive Engagement*. Perth: Department of Health.

Hungerford, C. & Richardson, F. (2013). Operationalising recovery-oriented services: The challenges for carers. *Advances in Mental Health*, 12(1), 11–21.

Independent Advisory Council of the NDIS. (2015). Capacity building for people with disability, their families and carers. Canberra: Australian Department of Human Services.

Jingree, T. (2015). Duty of care, safety, normalisation and the Mental Capacity Act: A discourse analysis of staff arguments about facilitating choices for people with learning disabilities in UK services. *Journal of Community & Applied Social Psychology*, 25(2), 138–52.

Kleier, J. (2013). Disarming the patient through therapeutic communication. *Urologic Nursing*, 33(3), 110–33.

Lantz, S. & Marston, G. (2012). Policy, citizenship and governance: The case of disability and employment policy in Australia. *Disability & Society*, 27(6), 853–67.

Madden, R., Ferreira, M., Einfeld, S., Emerson, E., Manga, R., Refshauge, K. & Llewellyn, G. (2012). New direction in health care and disability: The need for a shared understanding of human functioning. *Australian and New Zealand Journal of Public Health*, 36(5), 458–61.

Martinis, J. (2015). 'The right to make choices': How vocational rehabilitation can help young adults with disabilities increase self-determination and avoid guardianship. *Journal of Vocational Rehabilitation*, 42(3), 221–7.

Mental Health Council of Australia. (2012). *Recognition and Respect. Mental Health Carers Report 2012*. Canberra: Mental Health Council Australia.

Moodley, J. & Ross, E. (2015). Inequities in health outcomes and access to health care in South Africa: A comparison between persons with and without disabilities. *Disability & Society*, 30(4), 630–44.

Ministry of Social Development. (2014). *The New Zealand Carers' Strategy Action Plan for 2014–2018*. Wellington: Ministry of Social Development. Retrieved from www .msd.govt.nz/about-msd-and-our-work/work-programmes/policy-development/ carers-strategy/index.html

National Disability Insurance Scheme (NDIS). (2014). *Operational Guideline – Planning and Assessment – Facilitating the Participant's Statements of Goals and Aspirations*. Retrieved from www.ndis.gov.au/html/sites/default/files/documents/ og_planning_assessment_facilitating_participants_statement_goals_ aspirations.DOCX

—— (2018). *About the NDIS*. Retrieved from www.ndis.gov.au/about-us/what-ndis.html

New Zealand Ministry of Health (NZMOH). (2008). *Health and Disability Services Standards. Standards New Zealand*. Wellington: Ministry of Health.

Nirje, B. (1972). The right to self-determination. In W. Wolfensberger (ed.), *Normalization: The Principle of Normalization* (pp. 176–200). Toronto: National Institute on Mental Retardation.

NSW Health. (2017). *Responding to needs of people with disability during hospitalisation*. Retrieved from www1.health.nsw.gov.au/pds/ActivePDSDocuments/PD2017_001.pdf

Reid, J., Lloyd, C. & de Groot, L. (2005). The psychoeducation needs of parents who have an adult son or daughter with a mental illness. *Australian e-Journal for the Advancement of Mental Health*, 4(2), 1–13.

Sharkey, S., Lloyd, C., Tomlinson, R., Thomas, E., Martin, A., Logan, S. & Morris, C. (2016). Communicating with disabled children when inpatients: Barriers and facilitators identified by parents and professionals in a qualitative study. *Health Expectations*, 19(3), 738–50.

Sharpe, B. & Hemsley, B. (2016). Improving nurse–patient communication with patients with communication impairments: Hospital nurses' views on the feasibility of using mobile communication technologies. *Applied Nursing Research*, 30, 228–36.

Statistics New Zealand. (2014). *Disability Survey: 2013*. Retrieved from www.stats.govt.nz/browse_for_stats/health/disabilities/DisabilitySurvey_HOTP2013.aspx

Taua, C., Hepworth, J. & Neville, C. (2012). Nurses' role in caring for people with a comorbidity of mental illness and intellectual disability: A literature review. *International Journal of Mental Health Nursing*, 21(2), 163–74.

Thill, C. (2015). Listening for policy change: How the voices of disabled people shaped Australia's National Disability Insurance Scheme. *Disability & Society*, 30(1), 15–28.

Warr, D., Dickinson, H., Olney, S., Hargrave, J., Karanikolas, A., Katsikis, V., . . .& Wilcox, M. (2017). *Choice, Control and the NDIS*. Melbourne: University of Melbourne.

Wehmeyer, M. L. (1998). Self-determination and individuals with significant disabilities: Examining meanings and misinterpretations. *Research and Practice for Persons with Severe Disabilities*, 23(1), 5–16.

Wilkinson, C. & McAndrew, S. (2008). 'I'm not an outsider, I'm his mother!' A phenomenological enquiry into carer experiences of exclusion from acute psychiatric settings. *International Journal of Mental Health Nursing*, 17(6), 392–401.

World Health Organization (WHO). (2008). *Convention on the Rights of Persons with Disabilities*. Geneva: WHO. Retrieved from www.un.org/development/desa/disabilities/convention-on-the-rights-of-persons-with-disabilities/convention-on-the-rights-of-persons-with-disabilities-2.html

——(2015). *Disabilities and Rehabilitation*. Geneva: WHO. Retrieved from www.who.int/disabilities/care/en

21

End of life care

Linda Deravin, Lyn Croxon,
Mooreen Macleay and Judith Anderson

LEARNING OBJECTIVES

After studying this chapter, you should be able to:

1. understand the relationship between chronic conditions and fatal burden in Australia and New Zealand
2. identify pain management and symptom-control techniques for the person at the end of life
3. consider the issues in providing emergency care for the palliative patient
4. describe the importance of the psychosocial aspects of end of life care
5. outline the importance of advanced care planning
6. understand the nurse's role in end of life care.

Introduction

End of life care or palliative care is defined by Palliative Care Australia (2018) as 'person and family-centred care provided for a person with an active, progressive, advanced disease, who has little or no prospect of cure and who is expected to die, and for whom the primary treatment goal is to optimise the quality of life'. On a global scale, chronic conditions such as non-communicable diseases, accounted for 71 per cent of all deaths in 2016 (World Health Organization (WHO), 2018).

Fatal burden – the prevalence of disease or injury in a population at a given time that leads to death.

Chronic conditions are attributed to be the cause of early death, significantly contributing to **fatal burden** worldwide. In Australia, chronic conditions accounted for the following mortality rates: cancer (29 per cent), cardiovascular disease (28 per cent), respiratory diseases (7 per cent), injuries (6 per cent) and diabetes (3 per cent) of the total burden. Non-communicable diseases were estimated to account for 89 per cent of all deaths in 2016 (WHO, 2018). Similarly, in New Zealand, non-communicable diseases accounted for 89 per cent of fatal burden comprising of: cardiovascular diseases (31 per cent), cancers (31 per cent), chronic respiratory diseases (7 per cent), injury (6 per cent) and diabetes (3 per cent) in 2016 (WHO, 2018).

Several national bodies exist which provide guidance and support to nurses working in the area of palliative care. In Australia, Palliative Care Australia (2018) provides a range of resources, as does Hospice New Zealand (2015) in New Zealand. These bodies provide useful guidelines for best practice that are current and contextualised to country of origin, which can be especially useful for legal issues. The exact model of palliative care used differs due to services and resources available, local legislation, demographics, and demand for services. Although health reforms are taking place worldwide, there is increasing evidence to demonstrate that patient- and family-focused palliative care improves quality outcomes related to pain control, symptom management, communication, emotional and spiritual support, quality of life, satisfaction, and cost (Palliative Care Australia, 2018).

End of life care is an essential consideration for the nursing care and management of people with chronic conditions. The prospect of impending death is an individual experience that people with chronic conditions may either be more prepared or less prepared to think about. Some of the issues they may consider are: who will be caring for the person in the palliative stage? Where will the person be cared for? And who will provide this care? Nurses need to be aware of a multitude of compounding factors that will influence how and where the person is cared for (Anderson, Croxon & Deravin, 2017; Anderson & Deravin, 2017). This chapter considers some of the important aspects of end of life care in nursing the person with a chronic condition.

Pain management and symptom control

Existential – pertaining to existence; for example, the value and meaning of a person's life, their worth in relationships, previous achievements, concerns about death and existence of an afterlife.

Pain is one of the most important issues and the most feared aspect concerning the dying person and family (Palliative Care Australia, 2015). Pain is an unpleasant sensory and emotional experience associated with actual or potential tissue damage. Pain is always subjective. It needs to be managed in a timely and effective manner to provide comfort and relieve suffering. Pain is a complex experience. It is multifactorial and is influenced by psychosocial and **existential** issues, and the disease process. To manage pain well, the type of pain needs to be identified and assessed so that effective pain medication can be given to the person for optimum pain relief and comfort. There are four types of pain.

1. *Nociceptive* pain relates to soft tissue pain. This is described as aching, sharp, throbbing and/or pressure-like.
2. *Visceral* pain is from organs. It is usually described as pain covering a large area and deep aching or throbbing pain.
3. *Neuropathic* pain relates to pain originating from nerve compression or dysfunction. It is described as sharp, cutting, burning, stinging or stabbing.
4. *Psychogenic* pain relates to pain that has no physical reason. It is increased or prolonged by mental, emotional, behavioural or physiological factors (Moore, 2012).

Assessment

There are six steps to effective pain assessment. These are outlined below.

1. Ask about pain and accept the person's description.
2. Ask where the pain is, what helps to ease the pain and whether it is exacerbated by activities or occurs at specific times of the day.
3. If the person has more than one pain, assess each pain individually.
4. Consider the extent of the person's condition, what stage it is at and if the pain is related to any current treatment.
5. Assess psychosocial and spiritual factors that may be contributing to or inhibiting an evaluation of the pain.
6. Reassess and consider if the pain is responding to treatment and review the person for new factors contributing to pain (Palliative Care Australia, 2015; Woodruff, 2013).

There are a range of pain scales that can be used to gauge the level of pain a person says they are experiencing. For example, for people who can communicate what they are experiencing a scale such as the Numeric Rating Scale (see Figure 21.1) or the Wong-Baker FACES Pain Rating Scale (see Figure 21.2) may be used. For those who are cognitively impaired or are unable to express how they are feeling, alternative pain assessment tools are available such as the Abbey Pain Scale.

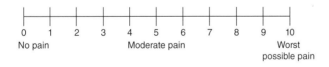

Figure 21.1   Numeric Rating Scale

Wong-Baker FACES® Pain Rating Scale

0	2	4	6	8	10
No Hurt	Hurts Little Bit	Hurts Little More	Hurts Even More	Hurts Whole Lot	Hurts Worst

Figure 21.2   Wong-Baker FACES Pain Rating Scale
Source: Wong-Baker FACES Foundation, 2016

Management

Medication is the mainstay of pain control. Analgesics range from non-opioids, such as paracetamol and non-steroidal anti-inflammatory drugs (NSAIDs), through to weak **opioids**, such as codeine-based medications, and then to stronger opioids, such as morphine, oxycodone and fentanyl. The choice of medication depends on the type and severity of pain. Different types of pain respond to different analgesics (Woodruff, 2013). It is common to use more than one type of analgesic; for example, a non-opioid such as paracetamol with an opioid such as oxycodone. Other medications used are antidepressants and anticonvulsants for neuropathic pain, and steroids.

The WHO has developed an 'analgesic ladder' to guide the use of pain relief; it is a useful basis for commencing and escalating pain management, as illustrated in Figure 21.3. Best practice is to commence with regular pain relief (that is, four hourly) and **titrate** to the requirements of the individual. Pain may occur between the scheduled doses, and this is referred to as breakthrough pain and may require additional medication or treatment (Palliative Care Expert Group, 2010).

> **Opioids** – substances that relieve pain by acting on the nervous system and reducing the intensity of pain signals that are sent to the brain. Opioids can affect areas that control emotion, further diminishing the effect of the painful stimulus.
>
> **Titrate** – the continual adjustment of a dose based on patient response. Dosages are adjusted until the desired clinical effect is achieved.

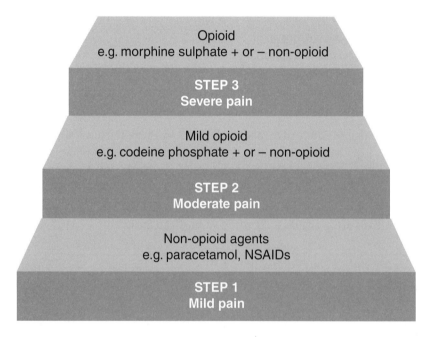

Figure 21.3 The WHO analgesic ladder
Source: Adapted from WHO (n.d.)

When pain levels have been stabilised with immediate-release opioids, sustained-release or long-acting opioids can be introduced. These forms of opioids provide a more even serum level over a longer period of time and help with patient compliance. Oral sustained-release and long-acting opioids' duration of action varies from 12–24 hours. Transdermal patches duration is from 72 hours to 7 days (Palliative Care Australia, 2015).

Analgesics come in many forms. In the palliative setting the preferred route of pain relief is the least invasive. Oral analgesics are given when the person is able to swallow safely. Transdermal patches can be used when safe swallowing is a concern or for the convenience of not having to take oral medications. The subcutaneous route can be used in the community setting after patient education and with support from palliative care services. Subcutaneous administration is preferred as it is less painful than intramuscular injections. Intravenous infusions are avoided as they are painful and create fluctuations in absorption in comparison with the subcutaneous route. Another form of pain management is **radiation therapy**. This is often given in the palliative setting for management of bone pain related to bone metastases (Palliative Care Expert Group, 2010).

Side effects of pain management

Pain management may have side effects that can create discomfort and reduce the quality of life. The most common side effects are constipation, nausea, vomiting, fatigue and sedation (Woodruff, 2013).

Up to 81 per cent of people taking opioids experience constipation (Bell et al., 2009). Opioids cause constipation by binding to specific **mu receptors** in the gastro-intestinal tract and nervous system (Peppin, 2012). This causes reduced motility through the bowel. The factors required for normal defecation are adequate fibre and fluid in the diet, normal peristalsis, normal abdominal and pelvic musculature, and normal rectal anal sensation. Palliative patients may not meet all of these requirements. Adding the effects of opioids on the bowel's motility may result in constipation.

Nausea with or without vomiting occurs in approximately 33 per cent of people started on an opioid (Smith, Smith & Seidner, 2012). Low dose opioids activate the mu receptors in the chemoreceptor trigger zone in the medulla. This is also compounded by morphine-related gastric stasis (Woodruff, 2013). Patients should be advised that nausea and vomiting may occur in the first couple of days once commencing an opioid, and nurses should have an anti-emetic available for them. If nausea and vomiting do not ease within a couple of days, titration of the opioid analgesic and opioid rotation should be considered (Smith et al., 2012). The use of cannabis to relieve nausea associated with chemotherapy treatment is currently an area of discussion, as the legal issues around use of this medication are contentious (Duran et al., 2010).

Opioid-induced fatigue and sedation is reported at the commencement of opioids and when the dose is increased. This usually subsides within the first two to five days (Levy & Swarm, 2015). It is important to educate the person (and family/carers) of this fatigue so they continue with the analgesia yet are aware of the possibility of falls. If the fatigue does not settle after the first week then further investigation as to the cause of the fatigue is warranted; possible reasons would be poor renal function and other causes of central nervous system depression, such as infection, metastases and the interaction with other medications.

Paediatric pain assessment and control

For children under the age of 11 there is a limited ability to self-report their feelings and needs (Goldman, Hain & Liben, 2012). For this reason, paediatric pain assessment and control requires a multidisciplinary approach (National Hospice and Palliative Care Organisation, 2016; Shaw, 2012; WHO, 2012).

For young or non-verbal children, we rely very heavily on the parents' or caregivers' report, which includes changes in behaviour, irritability, fatigue and decreased appetite. The changes in behaviour alert care givers to an underlying problem which the

Radiation therapy – a type of cancer treatment which is localised and affects cancer cells only in the treated area. The aim is to kill cancer cells in the treatment area. It is an energy beam likened to an X-ray beam but of extreme intensity.

Mu receptors – opioids produce effects on neurons by acting on receptors located on neuronal cell membranes. Mu receptors are mostly presynaptically located in the dorsal horn of the spinal cord, olfactory bulb, basal forebrain, cerebral cortex, nuclei of the temporal lobe and intestinal tract.

child may not be able to verbalise. Children and adult pain assessment are alike in the need to take a complete pain history, including what the child has and has not taken for pain management in the past and recently, and its efficacy.

For children three years and over, the use of the Wong-Baker FACES Pain Rating Scale is appropriate. Developmentally, the child should be able to point to the face which reflects their pain (see Figure 21.2).

The WHO three-step analgesic pain ladder used for adults is not recommended in the use of paediatric pain management. The WHO has revised its guidelines for treating paediatric persisting pain due to medical illness.

The two-step analgesic ladder for children is based on pain severity assessment, which is attained through the pain scale rating, observing the child and reports from the parents/caregivers. The steps are as follows:

- Step 1: mild pain, non-opioid analgesics, paracetamol, ibuprofen. Include comfort measures such as physical therapies (like massage), TENS machine and non-pharmacological methods such as music, play therapy and story reading
- Step 2: moderate and severe pain, strong opioids are used following the WHO guideline for dosing.

The WHO recommends this two-step analgesic ladder in conjunction with the following three key concepts to relieve persisting pain in children where the cause is due to medical illness:

1. *dosing at regular intervals* rather than on an as-needed basis (National Hospice and Palliative Care Organiztion, 2016; WHO, 2012). Schedule medication around the clock; that is, four-hourly, as well as additional breakthrough if required
2. *appropriate route of administration.* Avoid intramuscular injections for children due to the risk of fluctuations in absorption because of decreased muscle mass. Choosing a less invasive route will increase comfort and compliance, and will eliminate the association pain relief and analgesic administration. Examples of medication route considerations are oral, sublingual, transdermal and subcutaneous, via a portable pump
3. *adapting treatment to the individual child.* Tailor therapy to the individual child's circumstance, needs and response (Gregoire & Frager, 2006; WHO, 2012).

SKILLS IN PRACTICE

Paediatric pain assessment

Four-year-old Poppy presents to the emergency department. She has a history of acute lymphocytic leukaemia; diagnosis was at the age of two. All treatments have been unsuccessful and Poppy presents today after 12 hours of uncontrollable irritability.

QUESTION

What type of pain assessment would you consider using for a child?

End of life care emergencies

As a person approaches death, a change in their condition may result in a hospital admission. Often this will be as a result of a clinical emergency that is causing distress for the person and/or the family. Some of the reasons for unplanned admissions for palliative care patients can include uncontrolled symptoms, family or caregiver distress, not having sufficient medication or the medication regime needing review, and a lack of information about the disease trajectory and some of the possible complications that may occur. Sometimes the person or the family can change their mind about the place of death and present to the emergency department or be admitted to acute care facilities where the focus is on resuscitation rather than palliation (Swetenham, Grantham & Glaetzer, 2014).

The aim in end of life care is to provide the optimal quality of life, particularly in this end stage when death is near. Not all deaths go smoothly, and some patients will experience situations or conditions that could be considered life-threatening emergencies, where the quality of life for the person with the terminal illness is compromised. Common types of life-threatening emergencies that palliative patients may experience are spinal cord compression, dyspnoea, seizures, haemorrhage, acute anxiety and delirium, hypoglycaemia, medication toxicity or side effects, pneumothorax, pleural effusion, airway obstruction, gastrointestinal obstruction, and suicidal ideation and attempt (Mohammed Amrallah, 2014).

Fowell and Stuart (2011) affirm that the management of these palliative care emergencies and the decision to take action needs careful consideration, and that any action to treat the emergency must consider:

- the person's general condition
- the disease and the prognosis
- the person's wishes about care and treatment
- the distress caused by the symptoms.

Some emergencies can be managed with **conservative treatment** or non-invasive treatment, whereas others may require surgical intervention (Bosscher, van Leeuwen & Hoekstra, 2014). This can lead to additional anguish for the person, as well as the family members, who may feel distressed at seeing their loved one suffering or experiencing pain and discomfort as a result of the emergency condition.

Conservative treatment – care provided to a person with minimal intervention or active measures, and designed to provide comfort and avoid harm. Cure is often not an aim in conservative care.

Psychosocial aspects of caring

In end of life care, psychosocial aspects of care play a significant role in making a patient comfortable. A multidisciplinary team approach to this aspect of care can help, but it is also important for the nurse to have a basic understanding of their role, rather than merely referring such issues on to others (Anderson et al., 2017; Fordham & Howell, 2012). It has been found that a person-centred approach to palliative care reduces isolation, increases social support and encourages communication. Important factors for patients at the end of life include:

- their perspective of a safe environment where staff are available should they be needed
- a change of scenery to distract them and give them relief from the tedium or difficulties they face
- person-centred care, where they feel valued and respected
- social support from people in similar situations who may understand what they are going through
- overcoming isolation to obtain a different outlook
- communication with people who show genuine interest in their experiences and activities, which allows them to relax and feel less anxious (Bradley, Frizelle & Johnson, 2011).

Depression and anxiety

The discussion of mental health issues such as depression and anxiety with patients has been shown to be useful in predicting their subsequent receipt of mental health services. However, nurses in palliative care settings have been found to respond to patients' emotional concerns with non-empathic responses or with medical explanations. These nurses indicate that discussing emotional difficulties will make patients feel worse, and so they respond to patients by distancing themselves or speaking in a medically oriented framework (Hallford et al., 2012). Anxiety is a well-recognised clinical issue in patients at the end of their lives that nurses need to be aware of, and nurses may need to refer patients for further assessment in this area (Mah et al., 2013).

Depression is also prevalent in palliative care settings. It can cause a significant reduction in quality of life, increasing the frequency and intensity of physical symptoms, including pain and a hastened desire for death. Patients suffering from depression also have significantly higher care-related costs associated with them than non-depressed patients; however, the rates of detection are reasonably low and so it is not well treated. Poor recognition of depression is related to somatic symptoms being attributed to the end of life condition or medication, difficulty in distinguishing from preparatory grief, and nurses viewing depression as a typical reaction to terminal illness. A quick screening tool involving two questions ('Are you depressed?' and 'Have you lost interest or pleasure?') has been shown to be useful in palliative care settings to detect depression (Hallford et al., 2012).

Cultural considerations

When caring for palliative patients and their family, it is of the utmost importance that nurses take into consideration cultural attitudes to illness and death, because pain perception and behaviours are influenced by the sociocultural contexts of the individual. A person's culture can influence the degree of suffering associated with a terminal illness and strongly influence their decisions at the end of life (Palliative Care Australia, 2018). It is best practice to ask questions regarding the person's cultural beliefs and formulate a palliative care plan which incorporates these beliefs. It is important to communicate and document this information.

To be culturally competent, the nurse needs to be aware of their own culture, personal biases and assumptions; be capable of understanding the dynamics of difference; and be able to adapt to this diversity. The nurse should assess the person holistically by listening with empathy and acknowledging if there are differences with their own perceptions. The nurse needs to discuss the recommended treatment with the person and/or family member, and negotiate if it is required to suit their cultural needs (Husaini, 2014).

Spiritual care is also an important feature of psychosocial care and is influenced by culture. It is often overlooked, with many nurses claiming they do not have the time to attend to it effectively. Nurses working in acute care also commonly add that they are unable to provide a sufficiently private environment for this aspect of care. A key recommendation from evidence-based literature is that a nurse's comfort with their own spirituality is most important to providing spiritual care. Further education in the area can assist in this (Anderson & Deravin, 2017). Additional information about spirituality is provided in Chapter 4.

Stigma of death

Most people are not comfortable with the thought of dying. This is described as death anxiety, which is seen as a universal phobia (Peters et al., 2013). There has long been a stigma associated with the social experience of dying. It is often found that friends, colleagues and even family can cause the person suffering from a life-limiting condition to perceive negative attitudes or behaviour, or experience a sense of rejection. While friends may hear of illness, and visit and phone more often to help, some people sever relationships and contacts with a terminally ill person. The physical limitations of the condition may decrease the social opportunities of the individual. Sometimes, the terminally ill person may end friendships as they cannot cope with not being treated normally.

Advances in medical care have led to the medicalisation of end of life care, with the majority of people dying in acute care settings rather than their preference to die in the familiar environment of home (Coombs et al., 2015). Around half of deaths in Australia occur in hospitals, the majority being people over 75 years of age. Around one-third of New Zealand deaths occur in hospitals, one-third in residential aged care facilities, and one-third in the home (Broad et al., 2013).

The focus of end of life care has changed from caring for people with terminal cancer to include people suffering from other life-limiting conditions such as chronic obstructive pulmonary disease and chronic cardiac conditions. It is argued that staff in acute care areas do not always think in these terms. An Australian study found nurses have limited knowledge of palliative care principles. The focus was often on investigations and interventions responding to physical symptoms more effectively, rather than on support, relief of symptoms, and communication with the dying person and their family to find out about the person's wishes after their death (Shearer et al., 2014). It is often easier for health professionals to avoid the dying person. This may be due to the health professionals feeling there is little they can do to change the situation or that they have failed in their role.

REFLECTION

What are some of your own preconceived ideas about death and dying that might influence your nursing practice?

SKILLS IN PRACTICE

Living with a terminal condition

Lesley is a 35-year-old woman who has stage 3 ovarian cancer and is in the terminal phase of her condition. She lives with her husband and two children, aged four and six, and has family living nearby. Lesley lives in a rural town where there are palliative care outreach service providers who visit irregularly on an as-needed basis. Nursing care is provided by the community nurse who works Monday to Friday. Lesley has expressed a wish to die at home and she is anxious about the care of her children after she dies.

QUESTIONS

Consider the following aspects of the care of Lesley.

1. Identify the issues in providing end of life care for Lesley.
2. Consider how pain management and symptom control will be provided on a daily basis.
3. How will Lesley be supported at home and what services will she require?
4. What are some of the psychosocial aspects of care for Lesley and her family?

Advanced care planning

Advanced care planning is a term encompassing preparation for planning ahead should the health of the person deteriorate. It incorporates formulating an advanced care directive or health plan. It is also wise for the individual to consider preparing a will, power of attorney and enduring guardianship for circumstances when they are not able to make decisions for themselves (Raphael, Waterworth & Gott, 2014). Having conversations about what treatment they wish to have is critical. This could include the desire for cardiopulmonary resuscitation, intravenous therapy, or conservative treatment. It is important that the nurse has these discussions with the person and their family, for those situations which potentially lie ahead in the course of their illness (DeSpelder & Strickland, 2015).

An advance care directive or health directive involves discussion between the individual and family, and may include health professionals. The advance care directive articulates the person's wishes for care if their health deteriorates and they can no longer make these decisions for themselves. While a person can express their wishes orally, a written plan is required for their wishes to be recognised legally. This reduces ambiguity and makes the wishes accessible. It can include reference to specific care or treatment that the individual does not wish to undergo, or wishes to be avoided or ceased if commenced. It focuses on planning for near end of life scenarios. It is enacted when the person becomes legally incompetent (unable to make decisions) (Tan et al., 2013).

In 2011, the Australian Health Ministers' Advisory Council released a national framework for advance care directives. Each Australian state and territory has legislation that recognises advance care directives apart from New South Wales and Tasmania where such plans are currently recognised under common law. General practitioners are playing a greater role in advanced care planning in Australia, as funding for palliative care services has increased. Advanced care planning is comparatively new to the health care system in New Zealand (Raphael et al., 2014).

Children also suffer from chronic end of life conditions. Parents usually make decisions for children in Australia and New Zealand. The parents and young person's consent are generally sought between the ages of 14 and 16. A medical practitioner can intervene to treat a child against the parent's wishes if this is in the best interest of the child. However, in the United Kingdom, a decision around consent of a minor (under 16 years of age) has led to a test of 'Gillick competency' being applied. This ruling has led to a shift of decision-making power from the parents to the child – the court decides the child has reached sufficient maturity to understand and make their own decisions regarding their treatment. In such situations, the courts will rule in favour of the child's best interests (Atkins, de Lacey & Britton, 2014). This is not common in Australia or New Zealand, but it is a legal precedent that the nurse should be aware of as it could impact on future care.

REFLECTION

Why is it important to have an advance care directive or plan in place?

Euthanasia

Globally, within the nursing profession, position statements on euthanasia and assisted suicide vary. While the majority of countries reject the role of the nurse in assisting in acts of euthanasia and assisted suicide, countries such as the Netherlands have offered support to the role of the nurse for some time. Euthanasia is illegal in Australia under federal law, but the states and territories have introduced bills and debated the issues. The Northern Territory legalised assisted euthanasia in 1995, only to be overturned by the federal government two years later. In 2017, Victoria was the first state to legislate for voluntary assisted dying, with restrictive guidelines, which is expected to come into effect in 2019 (Department of Health and Human Services, 2018). While bills have been introduced into the New Zealand parliament, they have to date been unsuccessful. Euthanasia proponents argue for the ability of a competent person to be able to decide to end their life and request assistance to do so in a dignified manner in order to reduce their suffering (Department of Health and Human Services, 2018; Johnstone, 2012). Passive euthanasia or allowing the person to die is accepted by many who oppose euthanasia as being the natural course of a life-limiting disease. There is some concern that those people who are asking for someone to help end their life are not receiving adequate care (Palliative Care Expert Group, 2016). The active administration of a lethal dose of a medication to cause death, or assisting a person to do so, is a contentious issue as active euthanasia is seen to be the ending of a life. Palliative-care advocates argue that a request by a person to die offers an opportunity to ask why this alternative is being sought, and what could be done to assist with problems and to discuss options for care (Palliative Care Expert Group, 2016).

The use of analgesia to relieve pain for those who have a life-limiting condition can be a contentious issue. Large doses of medication may be necessary to control protracted pain. The doses that are needed may hasten the death of an individual. This comes under the doctrine of double effect (Wholihan & Olson, 2017). Very simply, this implies that while ending a person's life due to a lethal dose of medication to relieve pain is a bad act, if it relieves persistent, intolerable pain for the individual, it has a good consequence. In the same sense, the decision to withhold nutrition and hydration is debated, particularly in the last stages of dying when a person is unconscious. While withholding nutrition and hydration means a risk of people dying with the symptoms of thirst and hunger, providing this sustenance can prolong life and the process of dying. It is imperative that nurses provide relief for the symptoms of end of life, including mouth care in the case of thirst.

The nurse's role in palliative care

The nurse's role in palliative care can be divided into two areas: direct patient care (Palliative Care Australia, 2015) and indirect patient care. Direct patient care includes assessment, direct hands-on physical care such as helping with activities of daily living, and providing psychosocial support. Indirect care pertains to the nurse being part of the multidisciplinary team who use their specialist and management skills to meet the patient's and family needs (Husaini, 2014). The combination of direct and indirect nursing care is required to provide good-quality holistic care for the dying person and their family.

It is important to recognise that the family and carers also need support during end of life care, and that this should be extended beyond the death of the patient. Carers are often also suffering physically, financially, socially and psychologically. Their desire to care for their dying family member may lead them to neglect their own health and welfare. It is important that they be included in decision making, and be provided with information and support. Not only is support important for the carers themselves, but it also improves their ability to support the person at the end of life. Carers can be supported by nurses: increasing their awareness of their role, openly discussing what their role will be, talking through the implications of advanced care directives with them, recognising them as an important source of information, explaining services to them, having a case conference where they are involved, assessing their needs, planning their care, preparing them for death and contacting them after the patient's death to ascertain whether any more assistance is required (three to six weeks, and again six months after death are recommended). Complicated or chronic grief is experienced for extended periods of time and has been noted in 10–20 per cent of carers. It has been associated with a lack of preparation for death (Hudson et al., 2012).

SUMMARY

Learning objective 1: Understand the relationship between chronic conditions and fatal burden in Australia and New Zealand.
Chronic conditions can be the cause of early death, significantly contributing to fatal burden worldwide and resulting in loss of life years.

Learning objective 2: Identify pain management and symptom-control techniques for the person at the end of life.
There are a variety of tools available for the assessment of pain. Many of these are very useful in end of life care. A range of treatment options covering the use of non-opioids and opioids have a valuable place in palliative care. Potential side effects such as nausea and vomiting, fatigue and constipation can be managed when identified to support the person's quality of life.

Learning objective 3: Consider the issues in providing emergency care for the palliative patient.
Not all deaths go smoothly and some patients will experience situations or conditions that could be considered life-threatening emergencies; for example, pneumothorax, haemorrhage, seizures and difficulty in breathing. The nurse needs to be aware that these can occur and set plans in place to escalate treatment as per the person's wishes.

Learning objective 4: Describe the importance of the psychosocial aspects of end of life care.
In end of life care, psychosocial aspects of care play a significant role in making a patient comfortable. It has been found that a person-centred approach to palliative care reduces isolation, increases social support and encourages communication.

Learning objective 5: Outline the importance of advanced care planning.
Advanced care planning is a term encompassing preparation for planning ahead should the health of the person deteriorate. An advance care directive is a written statement that details the person's wishes for health and care when death is near, and the person is no longer able to express their wishes regarding treatment and care.

Learning objective 6: Understand the nurse's role in end of life care.
The nurse provides both direct and indirect care. Direct patient care includes assessment, direct hands-on physical care such as helping with activities of daily living, and providing psychosocial support. Indirect care pertains to the nurse being part of the multidisciplinary team, who use their specialist and management skills to meet the patient's and family's needs.

REVIEW QUESTIONS

1. What is the importance of palliative care for people with chronic illnesses?
2. What are some of the underlying principles and values that underpin palliative or end of life care?
3. List various pain management options used regularly in end of life care.
4. What factors influence people's thoughts about death and dying?
5. When should advanced care planning take place?

RESEARCH TOPIC

Anh is a married, 45-year-old father of three children, who migrated to Australia three years ago. He has been diagnosed with lung cancer and he is having difficulty breathing. His pain is not controlled on admission to hospital. Prior to his illness he ran his own business with the help of his wife and brother. Consider some of the psychosocial aspects of palliative care for Anh. What services are available in your area to support care for Anh and his family?

FURTHER READING

DeSpelder, L. A. & Strickland, A. L. (2015). *The Last Dance: Encountering Death and Dying* (10th edn). New York: McGraw Hill Education.

Hospice New Zealand. (2015). What is hospice? Retrieved from www.hospice.org.nz.

Matzo, M. & Sherman, D. W. (2018). *Palliative Care Nursing: Quality Care to the End of Life* (5th edn). New York: Springer Publishing Company.

Palliative Care Australia. (2018). *National Palliative Care Standards*. Canberra: Palliative Care Australia.

Woodruff, R. (2013). *Cancer Pain* (6th edn). Melbourne: Asperula.

REFERENCES

Anderson, J., Croxon, L. & Deravin, L. (2017). *Newly graduated nurses working in isolation with palliative patients*. Paper presented at the 14th National Rural Health Conference, Cairns, QLD.

Anderson, J. & Deravin, L. (2017). The importance of palliative care education. *Australian Nursing and Midwifery Journal*, 25(1), 39.

Atkins, K., de Lacey, S. & Britton, B. (2014). *Ethics and Law for Australian Nurses* (2nd edn). Melbourne: Cambridge University Press.

Bell, T. J., Panchal, S. J., Miaskowski, C., Bolge, S. C., Milanova, T. & Williamson, R. (2009). The prevalence, severity, and impact of opioid-induced bowel dysfunction: Results of a US and European patient survey (PROBE 1). *Pain Medicine*, 10(1), 35–42. doi: http://10.1111/j.1526-4637.2008.00495.x

Bosscher, M. R., van Leeuwen, B. L. & Hoekstra, H. J. (2014). Surgical emergencies in oncology. *Cancer Treatment Reviews*, 40(8), 1028–36. doi: http://10.1016/j.ctrv.2014.05.005

Bradley, S. E., Frizelle, D. & Johnson, M. (2011). Patients' psychosocial experiences of attending specialist palliative day care: A systematic review. *Palliative Medicine*, 25(3), 210–28. doi: http://10.1177/0269216310389222

Broad, J. B., Gott, M., Kim, H., Boyd, M., Chen, H. & Connolly, M. J. (2013). Where do people die? An international comparison of deaths occurring in hospital and residential aged care settings in 45 populations, using published and available statistics. *International Journal of Public Health*, 58(2), 257–67. doi: http://10.1007/s00038-012-0394-5

Coombs, M., Long-Sutehall, T., Darlington, A.-S. & Richardson, A. (2015). Doctors' and nurses' views and experience of transferring patients from critical care home to die: A qualitative exploratory study. *Palliative Medicine*, 29(4), 354–62. doi: http://10.1177/0269216314560208

Department of Health and Human Services. (2018). Voluntary assisted dying. Retrieved from www2.health.vic.gov.au/hospitals-and-health-services/patient-care/end-of-life-care/voluntary-assisted-dying

DeSpelder, L. A. & Strickland, A. L. (2015). *The Last Dance: Encountering Death and Dying* (10th edn). New York: McGraw Hill Education.

Duran, M., Pérez, E., Abanades, S., Vidal, X., Saura, C., Majem, M., ... & Capellà, D. (2010). Preliminary efficacy and safety of an oromucosal standardized cannabis extract in chemotherapy-induced nausea and vomiting. *British Journal of Clinical Pharmacology*, 70(5), 656–63. doi: http://10.1111/j.1365-2125.2010.03743.x

Fordham, P. & Howell, S. (2012). Effects of a psychosocial assessment tool on interdisciplinary team utilization in a palliative care unit (784). *Journal of Pain and Symptom Management*, 43(2), 470–1. doi: http://10.1016/j.jpainsymman.2011.12.262

Fowell, A. & Stuart, N. S. A. (2011). Emergencies in palliative medicine. *Medicine*, 39(11), 660–3. doi: http://10.1016/j.mpmed.2011.08.003

Georgoire, M.-C. & Frager, G. (2006) Ensuring pain relief for children at the end of life. *Pain Research Management*, 11(3). Retrieved from www.ncbi.nlm.nih.gov/pmc/articles/PMC2539002/

Goldman, A., Hain, R. & Liben, S. (2012). *Oxford Textbook of Palliative Care for Children* (2nd edn). Oxford: Oxford University Press.

Hallford, D. J., McCabe, M. P., Mellor, D., Davison, T. E. & Goldhammer, D. L. (2012). Depression in palliative care settings: The need for training for nurses and other health professionals to improve patients' pathways to care. *Nurse Education Today*, 32(5), 556–60. doi: http://10.1016/j.nedt.2011.07.011

Hospice New Zealand. (2015). What is hospice? Retrieved from www.hospice.org.nz

Hudson, P., Remedios, C., Zordan, R., Thomas, K., Clifton, D., Crewdson, M., ... & Bauld, C. (2012). Guidelines for the psychosocial and bereavement support of family caregivers of palliative care patients. *Journal of Palliative Medicine*, 15(6), 696–702. doi: http://10.1089/jpm.2011.0466

Husaini, A. (2014). The role of nurses in providing palliative care for dying cancer patients: A meta-ethnographic synthesis. *British Medical Journal Supportive and Palliative Care*, 4(Suppl. 1), A1–2. doi: http://10.1136/bmjspcare-2014-000654.3

Johnstone, M.-J. (2012). *Bioethics, Cultural Differences and the Problem of Moral Disagreements in End-of-Life Care: A Terror Management Theory* (vol. 37, pp. 181–200). New York: Oxford University Press.

Levy, M. H. & Swarm, R. A. (2015). Management of opioid-induced side effects. National Comprehensive Cancer Network 13th Annual Conference: Clinical Practice Guidelines & Quality Cancer Care. Retrieved from www.medscape.org/viewarticle/573016

Mah, L., Grossman, D., Grief, C. & Rootenberg, M. (2013). Association between patient dignity and anxiety in geriatric palliative care. *Palliative Medicine*, 27(5), 478–9. doi: http://10.1177/0269216312463111

Mohammed Amrallah, A. (2014). Scope of management of emergencies in palliative care. *Forum of Clinical Oncology*, 5, 11.

Moore, R. J. (2012). *Handbook of Pain and Palliative Care: Biobehavioral Approaches for the Life Course*. New York: Springer Science and Business Media.

National Hospice and Palliative Care Organization. (2016). Pain management with children. *ChiPPS E-Journal* (45). Retrieved from www.nhpco.org/sites/default/files/public/ChiPPS/ChiPPS_e-journal_Issue-45.pdf

Palliative Care Australia. (2015). Learn more about pain management. Canberra: Palliative Care Australia. Retrieved from http://palliativecare.org.au/wp-content/uploads/2015/05/PCA002_Pain-Management_FA.pdf

—— (2018). *National Palliative Care Standards*. Canberra: Palliative Care Australia. Retrieved from http://palliativecare.org.au/wp-content/uploads/dlm_uploads/2018/02/PalliativeCare-National-Standards-2018_web-3.pdf

Palliative Care Expert Group. (2010). *Therapeutic Guidelines: Palliative Care. Version 3*. Retrieved from www.tg.org.au/?sectionid=47

—— (2016). *Therapeutic Guidelines: Palliative Care. Version 4*. Retrieved from www.trove.nka.gov.autg.org.au/?sectionid=47

Peppin, J. F. (2012). Opioid-induced constipation: Causes and treatments. Retrieved from www.practicalpainmanagement.com/opioid-induced-constipation-causes-treatments

Peters, L., Cant, R., Payne, S., O'Connor, M., McDermott, F., Hood, K., . . . & Shimoinaba, K. (2013). How death anxiety impacts nurses' caring for patients at the end of life: A review of literature. *The Open Nursing Journal*, 7, 14–21. doi: http://10.2174/1874434601307010014

Raphael, D., Waterworth, S. & Gott, M. (2014). The role of practice nurses in providing palliative and end-of-life care to older patients with long-term conditions. *International Journal of Palliative Nursing*, 20(8), 373–9. doi: http://10.12968/ijpn.2014.20.8.373

Shaw, T. M. (2012) Pediatric palliative pain and symptom management. *Pediatric Annals*, 41, 8 329–34.

Shearer, F. M., Rogers, I. R., Monterosso, L., Ross-Adjie, G. & Rogers, J. R. (2014). Understanding emergency department staff needs and perceptions in the provision of palliative care. *Emergency Medicine Australasia*, 26(3), 249–55. doi: http://10.1111/1742-6723.12215

Smith, H. S., Smith, J. M. & Seidner, P. (2012). Opioid-induced nausea and vomiting. *Annals of Palliative Medicine*, 1(2), 121–9. doi: http://10.3978/j.issn.2224-5820.2012.07.08

Swetenham, K., Grantham, H. & Glaetzer, K. (2014). Breaking down the silos: Collaboration delivering an efficient and effective response to palliative care emergencies. *Progress in Palliative Care*, 22(4), 212–18. doi: http://10.1179/1743291x13y.0000000076

Tan, H. M., Lee, S. F., O'Connor, M. M., Peters, L. & Komesaroff, P. A. (2013). A case study approach to investigating end-of-life decision making in an acute health service. *Australian Health Review*, 37(1), 93–7. doi: http://10.1071/AH11125

Wholihan, D. & Olson, E. (2017). The doctrine of double effect: A review for the bedside nurse providing end-of-life care. *Journal of Hospice & Palliative Nursing*, 19(3), 205–11.

Woodruff, R. (2013). *Cancer Pain* (6th edn). Melbourne: Asperula.

World Health Organization (WHO). (n.d.). 'WHO's cancer pain ladder for adults'. Retrieved from www.who.int/cancer/palliative/painladder/en

—— (2012). *WHO guidelines on the Pharmacological Treatment of Persisting Pain in Children with Medical Illnesses*. Retrieved from http://apps.who.int/iris/bitstream/handle/10665/44540/9789241548120_Guidelines.pdf;sequence=1

—— (2015). The top 10 causes of death. Retrieved from www.who.int/mediacentre/factsheets/fs310/en/index3.html

—— (2018). Noncommunicable diseases country profiles 2018. Geneva: WHO.

Index